RESOURCE UTILIZATION IN CARDIAC DISEASE

199. Michele Mercuri, David D. McPherson, Hisham Bassiouny, Seymour Glagov (eds.):*Non-Invasive Imaging of Atherosclerosis*   ISBN 0-7923-8036-3
200. Walmor C. DeMello, Michiel J. Janse(eds.): *Heart Cell Communication in Health and Disease*   ISBN 0-7923-8052-5
201. P.E. Vardas (ed.): *Cardiac Arrhythmias Pacing and Electrophysiology.* The Expert View. 1998   ISBN 0-7923-4908-3
202. E.E. van der Wall, P.K. Blanksma, M.G. Niemeyer, W. Vaalburg and H.J.G.M. Crijns (eds.) *Advanced Imaging in Coronary Artery Disease, PET, SPECT, MRI, I VUS, EBCT. 1998*   ISBN 0-7923-5083-9
203. R.L. Wilensky (ed.) *Unstable Coronary Artery Syndromes, Pathophysiology, Diagnosis and Treatment. 1998.*   ISBN 0-7923-8201-3
204. J.H.C. Reiber, E.E. van der Wall (eds.): *What's New in Cardiovascular Imaging?* 1998   ISBN 0-7923-5121-5
205. Juan Carlos Kaski, David W. Holt (eds.): *Myocardial Damage Early Detection by Novel Biochemical Markers. 1998.*   ISBN 0-7923-5140-1
207. Gary F. Baxter, Derek M. Yellon, *Delayed Preconditioning and Adaptive Cardioprotection. 1998.*   ISBN 0-7923-5259-9
208. Bernard Swynghedauw, *Molecular Cardiology for the Cardiologist, Second Edition*
1998.   ISBN 0-7923-8323-0
209. Geoffrey Burnstock, James G.Dobson, Jr., Bruce T. Liang, Joel Linden (eds): *Cardiovascular Biology of Purines. 1998.*   ISBN: 0-7923-8334-6
210. Brian D. Hoit, Richard A. Walsh (eds): *Cardiovascular Physiology in the Genetically Engineered Mouse.* 1998.   ISBN: 0-7923-8356-7
211. Peter Whittaker, George S. Abela (eds.): *Direct Myocardial Revascularization: History, Methodology, Technology* 1998.   ISBN: 0-7923-8398-2
212. C.A. Nienaber, R. Fattori (eds.): Diagnosis and Treatment of Aortic Diseases. 1999.   ISBN: 0-7923-5517-2
213. Juan Carlos Kaski (ed.): *Chest Pain with Normal Coronary Angiograms: Pathogenesis, Diagnosis and Management.* 1999.   ISBN: 0-7923-8421-0
214. P.A. Doevendans, R.S. Reneman and M. Van Bilsen (eds): *Cardiovascular Specific Gene Expression.* 1999   ISBN:0-7923-5633-0
215. G. Pons-Lladó, F. Carreras, X. Borrás, Subirana and L.J. Jiménez-Borreguero (eds.): *Atlas of Practical Cardiac Applications of MRI.* 1999   ISBN: 0-7923-5636-5
216. L.W. Klein, J.E. Calvin, *Resource Utilization in Cardiac Disease.* 1999.   ISBN:0-7923-8509-8
217. R. Gorlin, G. Dangas, P. K. Toutouzas, M.M Konstadoulakis, *Contemporary Concepts in Cardiology, Pathophysiology and Clinical Management.*1999   ISBN:0-7923-8514-4

previous volumes are still available

KLUWER ACADEMIC PUBLISHERS - DORDRECHT/BOSTON/LONDON

RESOURCE UTILIZATION IN CARDIAC DISEASE

edited by

Lloyd W. Klein, M.D.
James E. Calvin, M.D.
Rush-Presbyterian-St. Luke's Medical Center
Rush Medical School
Chicago, IL

KLUWER ACADEMIC PUBLISHERS
Boston / Dordrecht / London

Distributors for North, Central and South America:
Kluwer Academic Publishers
101 Philip Drive
Assinippi Park
Norwell, Massachusetts 02061 USA
Telephone (781) 871-6600
Fax (781) 871-6528
E-Mail <kluwer@wkap.com>

Distributors for all other countries:
Kluwer Academic Publishers Group
Distribution Centre
Post Office Box 322
3300 AH Dordrecht, THE NETHERLANDS
Telephone 31 78 6392 392
Fax 31 78 6546 474
E-Mail <orderdept@wkap.nl>

 Electronic Services <http://www.wkap.nl>

Library of Congress Cataloging-in-Publication Data

A C.I.P. Catalogue record for this book is available
from the Library of Congress.

Resource utilization in cardiac disease/edited by Lloyd W. Klein,James E. Calvin.
  P. Cm. -- (Developments in cardiovascular medicine : 216)
ISBN 0-7923-8509-8(alk. Paper)
1. Heart--Diseases--Treatment--cost effectiveness. 2. Critical path analysis. I.
Klein, Lloyd W. II. Calvin, James E. III. Series: Developments in cardiovascular
medicine : v. 216.
[DNLM: 1. Critical Pathways. 2. Heart Diseases. WG 210 R434 1999]
RC683.8.R47 1999
616.1'2--dc21
DNLM/DLC for Library of Congress   99-24723
                                                                          CIP

Printed on acid-free paper.

Printed in the United States of America

TABLE OF CONTENTS

vi

LIST OF CONTRIBUTORS

Lloyd W. Klein, M.D.
Section of Cardiology, Department of Medicine
Rush Presbyterian St. Luke's Medical Center
1653 West Congress Parkway
Chicago, IL   60612-3833

James E. Calvin, M.D.
Section of Cardiology, Department of Medicine
Rush Presbyterian St. Luke's Medical Center
1653 West Congress Parkway
Chicago, IL   60612-3833

William H. Frishman, M.D.
New York Medical College
Department of Medicine
Munger Pavillion
Valhalla, NY   10595

Stephen Peterson, M.D.
New York Medical College
Department of Medicine
Munger Pavillion
Valhalla, NY   10595

Daniel Kombert, M.D.
New York Medical College
Department of Medicine
Munger Pavillion
Valhalla, NY   10595

Conor O'Shea, M.D.
Duke Clinical Research Institute
Duke Medical Center
Box 3275,
Durham, NC   27710

James E. Tcheng, M.D.
Duke Clinical Research Institute
Duke Medical Center
Box 3275,
Durham, NC   27710

Robert S. Rosenson, M.D.
Preventative Cardiology Center
Section of Cardiology, Department of Medicine
Rush-Presbyterian St.-Luke's Hospital
1653 W. Congress Parkway
Chicago, IL 60612

Lynne T. Braun, Ph.D., R.N.
Preventative Cardiology Center
Section of Cardiology, Department of Medicine
Rush Presbyterian St. Luke's Medical Center
Rush University College of Nursing
1653 W. Congress Parkway
Chicago, IL 60612

Philip R. Liebson, M.D.
Section of Cardiology, Department of Medicine
Rush Presbyterian St. Luke's Medical Center
1653 W. Congress Parkway
Chicago IL 60612

Henry R. Black, M.D.
Section of Cardiology, Department of Medicine
Rush Presbyterian St. Luke's Medical Center
1653 W. Congress Parkway
Chicago IL 60612

Ted Feldman, M.D.
University of Chicago Hospital
Hans Hecht Hemodynamics Laboratory
Pritzker School of Medicine
5841 S. Maryland Ave., MC5076
Chicago, IL 60637-1463

Marc A. Silver, M.D.
Department of Cardiology
Christ Hospital and Medical Center
4440 West 95th St.
Oak Lawn, IL 60453-2699

Durand E. Burns, M.D.
Minneapolis Heart Institute
920 E. 28th St., Suite 300
Minneapolis, MN 55407

Maryl Johnson, M.D.
Northwestern Memorial Hospital
Division of Cardiology
250 E. Superior St.
Wesley Pavilion, Suite 512
Chicago, IL 60611

Sudhir Wahi M.D., F.C.C.P.
Department of Cardiology Medicine / F15
The Cleveland Clinic Foundation
9500 Euclid Avenue
Cleveland, OH 44195

Allan L. Klein, M.D., F.R.C.P. (C), F.A.C.C.
Department of Cardiology Medicine / F15
The Cleveland Clinic Foundation
9500 Euclid Avenue
Cleveland, OH 44195

Warren Laskey, M.D.
University of Maryland, School of Medicine
Division of Cardiology, Department of Medicine
22 South Greene Street, RM. S3B08
Baltimore, MD 21201-1595

Eric R. Bates, M.D.
Department of Internal Medicine, Division of Cardiology
The University of Michigan Medical Center
University Hospital, B1-F245
1500 E. Medical Center Drive
Ann Arbor, MI 48109-0999

Mauro Moscucci, M.D.
Department of Internal Medicine, Division of Cardiology
The University of Michigan Medical Center
University Hospital, B1-F245
1500 E. Medical Center Drive
Ann Arbor, MI 48109-0999

William Weintraub, M.D.
Emory Heart Center
Emory University School of Medicine
Robert W. Woodruff Health Sciences Center
1364 Clifton Road, N.E., Rm. C404
Atlanta, GA 30322

Sergio L. Pinski, M.D.
Section of Cardiology, Department of Medicine
Rush Presbyterian St. Luke's Medical Center
1653 West Congress Parkway
Chicago, IL   60612-3833

Richard G. Trohman, M.D.
Section of Cardiology, Department of Medicine
Rush Presbyterian St. Luke's Medical Center
1653 West Congress Parkway
Chicago, IL   60612-3833

Foreword

Resource Utilization in Cardiac Disease

EDITORS: Lloyd W. Klein, MD
James E. Calvin, MD
Rush-Presbyterian-St. Luke's Medical Center, Chicago, IL

Why Evidence Based Medicine? Are Critical Pathways Really Necessary?

When physicians develop guidelines to assist other physicians in cost-effective practice, the skeptical recipient will immediately want to know why one's colleagues think they are so much more knowledgeable and in-touch than anybody else. When the critical pathways are published under the name of a national society, the physician community usually chooses to follow those items matching local prejudice but ignoring those that are not already consistent with current practice, assuming that what some "blue-ribbon panel" of politician - doctors think is irrelevant to them. Don't they know how complicated cardiology is? Don't they comprehend the weaknesses of the studies they quote? Why do they think it is so simple?

Well, what we are trying to do in this book is to provide a means that ultimately may systematize medical practice. Our rationale is that if doctors, hospitals, and medical care organizations, especially health maintenance organizations, practiced medicine consistently and on the basis of the best evidence, our patients' *and* our country's economic health would be best served. Further, we advocate that systems be created to measure the quality of what we do - not the mortality figures without assessments of risk published in newspapers willy-nilly, but incorporating intellectual analysis and corrected for patient selection. Further, the rational delivery of clinical care requires doctors to closely examine what they do and why. We want cardiologists to analyze their outcomes, and distinguish between what really works and what only sounds logical but doesn't work - and then share their experience with colleagues, our consumers, and the public. Michael L. Millenson calls this "doing the right thing and doing the right thing right". In his book <u>Demanding Medical Excellence</u> (University of Chicago Press, 1997), Millenson reminds us that the huge variability in physician practice dates back over 30 years, and is ascribable in part to geography, continuing education and physician individualism. He illustrates this point by showing that even as recently as 1993, many doctors did not employ thrombolysis and aspirin for acute myocardial infarction, in part out of fear of complications that were overblown and in part out of ignorance of its efficacy.

Lest we pat ourselves on the back for coming through these Dark Ages, consider a recent teaching rotation experience in our Coronary Care Unit. Neither cardiology fellow nor housestaff could point to the reason we prescribe heparin and aspirin for acute coronary syndromes, how we choose the anticoagulation parameters we do, when to advise an angiogram or do a stress test; worse, they actually felt that these were primarily judgment calls, individualized not so much for the patient as to the cardiologist and the payor! And alas - they may have had a point. Conclusions from scientific studies are increasingly being interpreted to suit the situation. Physicians openly question whether a contradictory study is relevant to their patient. We've allowed the critical evaluation of published studies to become sessions of open critique without emphasis on the correct conclusions.

We undertook this project because we think this leads to bad education and bad practice. While prudent economic decision making can be twisted into "penny pinching", bureaucracy, restrictions on choice of physician, denials of referrals to specialists and insane demands on hospital length of stay, it doesn't have to. We physician - practitioners have only ourselves to blame for administrators who do this to us because we did not govern ourselves when we had the control.

The editors challenge individual physicians of conscience to try to do their best - and we hope this book is one tool they can use. Better medicine at lower cost is, after all, a commendable goal. The authors who participated in this project have given their best attempt to be helpful to their colleagues.

Preface

Despite recent advances in the diagnosis and treatment of various cardiac illnesses, including ischemic, valvular and cardiomyopathic disease, the most cost effective means to employ laboratory testing and treatment modalities remains an issue in most practice settings. With the advent of managed care and vigilant third party payer evaluation of the use of diagnostic tests and hospital length of stay, the most effective medical and economic method to manage everyday cardiac illness is a question that arises daily in practice.

To this end, we will select well known and widely published experts in cardiac diagnosis and therapy to develop practical and informative approaches outlining the most cost-effective methods of patient management. The topics will include the entire range of cardiac diseases and emphasize the economics impact on decision making. We anticipate the development of guidelines and the presentation of general strategies for the practicing cardiologist and general internist. Additionally, the editors, who have 10 years of experience in this area, will discuss the methods necessary to bring critical pathways and practice guidelines into clinical use. Both in-hospital and out-patient phases of illness will be considered. Special concerns of hospital, private practice, managed care and group practice settings will specifically be addressed.

Lloyd W. Klein, M.D.

James E. Calvin, M.D.

Chicago, Illinois

ACKNOWLEDGEMENT

To our teachers and students, without whom it would never been thought of; and to our wives, Barbara and Sadie, without whom it could never have been completed.

1

COST EFFECTIVE EVALUATION
OF CHEST PAIN

Lloyd W. Klein, MD
James E. Calvin, MD
Rush-Presbyterian-St. Luke's Medical Center, Chicago, IL

INTRODUCTION

The accurate and cost effective evaluation of patients presenting with chest pain can be vexatious because it is a common symptom with an extensive differential diagnosis. Some etiologies are life threatening, others treatable if diagnosed early, and a few are aggravating but not serious. Although thorough attention to the details of the history and a careful examination often provide clues that narrow the diagnostic possibilities, further testing is frequently required. Laboratory studies are appropriately employed to confirm clinical suspicions, eliminate unlikely but dangerous processes, and to delineate the extent and functional severity of disease. However, the cost of pursuing a comprehensive investigation in complex cases can be staggering, rendering a prudent selection of testing modalities mandatory, tailored to the individual case.[1-4]

Each year in the U.S., more than 6 million persons are evaluated for chest pain or other symptoms redolent of cardiac ischemia. A correct, cost-effective approach to the evaluation of chest pain syndromes is consequently required in modern practice.

Differential Diagnosis

The most common cardiac and non-cardiac conditions causing chest pain is summarized in **Table 1**. Each condition should be considered in every case of chest pain, and discarded only with unmistakable evidence. The following discussion emphasizes the findings in ischemic heart disease, which is the crucial diagnosis to be entertained, as patients with acute coronary syndromes are at risk for death and heart attack; further, outcomes are improved if appropriate medical therapy is delivered.

Table 1. Etiologies of Chest Pain Syndrome and Distinguishing Attributes

Cardiovascular

Ischemic Heart Disease	Exercise or stress induced. Occurs at rest in severe cases
Coronary Spasm	Pain at rest with transient ST elevation in young people, cocaine, 5-FU
Aortic Stenosis	Systolic murmur, delayed carotid upstole
Hypertrophic Cardiomyopathy	Murmurs change with maneuvers, brisk/bisferiens carotid upstroke
Cardiomyopathy	Cardiomegaly
Myocarditis	Sudden onset, CK elevation, fever, recent URI
Pericarditis	Pleuritic, positional, presence of rub
Dissecting aortic aneurysm	Sharp or tearing, prolonged, often in back
Mitral valve prolapse	Transient, non-exertional, click + murmur
Costochondritis	Chest wall tenderness, worse with inspiration
Neuromuscular Radicular syndromes (i.e. cervical spine disease)	Characteristic distribution: neck and arm; positional, rash of herpes zoster
Arthritis	Pain and swelling localized to joint, worse on palpation.

Gastrointestinal

Esophageal spasm	Worse with cold liquids, relief with NTG
Hiatal Hernia	Reflux, non-exertional, worse with eating, relieved with antacids, occ. relief with NTG.
Ulcer/Gastritis	Epigastric, worse 2-3 hrs. after eating or recumbency, non-exertional, relieved with antacids.
Cholecystitis	RUQ tenderness, abdominal pain, worse with fatty food ingestion.

Pulmonary

Pulmonary embolism	Tachypneia, dyspnea, cough, pleuritic , RV failure
Pulmonary hypertension	RV failure, hypoxia, chest x-ray.
Pneumothorax	Sudden onset pain and dyspnea, chest x-ray.
Pleuritis	Sharp pain, worse with inspiration.

Others

Musculoskeletal	Positional, worse with movement, local tenderness
Hyperventilation	Tachypnea, anxiety attack

Symptoms of Angina Pectoris

Any form of discomfort experienced between the umbilicus and the ear lobes should be initially regarded as potentially cardiac in origin. This view has been reinforced by personally witnessing documented angina with complaints of: toothache; tongue-tingling with exertion; neck stiffness; and/or elbow discomfort[5].

Table 2. Diagnosis of Myocardial Ischemia

Clinical Presentation (Symptoms)
Typical: Usually retrosternal with or without radiation to inner arms, jaw, neck, upper back, epigastrium; lasts 30 sec to 15 min.
Atypical: (1) only in areas of radiation; (2) sharp, fleeting pains, or other uncharacteristic presentations of chest discomfort but in appropriate location.
Anginal equivalent: diaphoresis, breathlessness, anxiety, nausea, vomiting, occurring in response to ischemia that may develop without pressure or pain.
Physical Findings During Angina Attack
Transient S_4 gallop, mitral regurgitation murmur, paradoxically split S_2, abnormal pericardial systolic impulse.
Electrocardiographic Findings (Rest or Exercise)
Transient ST depression or elevation 0.08 sec after J-joint, associated with J-joint depression or elevation of 1 mm or more from baseline (TP interval at rest, PR segment with exercise
Radionuclide Scan Findings (Exercise)
Filling defect with exercise that fills at rest (perfusion imbalance during exercise with viable myocardium at rest).
Echocardiographic Findings
Segmental decrease in systolic endocardial wall motion and thickening with exercise compared with rest.

From: Liebson and Klein, Ischemic Heart Disease In Current Diagnosis,Edition 9.[6]

In eliciting the history, questions should be carefully worded to obtain an accurate account of the symptomatology. This is especially true when interviewing individuals with differing cultures and/or languages. The history should determine whether the pain is recurrent or a single episode, the factors which precipitate and ameliorate it, the precise location of the pain and radiation, and its quality, severity, frequency and duration. Associated symptoms should be sought, including dyspnea, diaphoresis, nausea, vomiting, palpitations, dizziness, and syncope. The presence of cardiac risk factors should be ascertained, including both the classical ones of tobacco use, hypertension, diabetes, hyperlipidemia and family history, and non-traditional factors such as cocaine use (particularly as "crack"), use of oral contraceptives and occurrence of menopause.[7]

Angina is typically described as substernal chest discomfort, a pressure, heaviness or squeezing sensation; it is not "painful". A nearly pathognomic sign is when the patient clenches his fist in front of his chest when describing the discomfort (Levine's Sign). Occasionally the pain may radiate to, or be experienced solely, in the shoulders, arms, neck, jaw, wrist or epigasturim. It is exacerbated by physical exertion, emotional stress, or cold and windy weather.[8] **Table 3** suggests questions to be asked to establish functional class.

Table 3. Clinical Classifications of Angina Pectoris Severity

Diagnosis of Angina Pectoris Presence and Severity*	
Presence of pain or discomfort in chest	(Y/N)
Location of pain or discomfort in chest	(Indicate)
Characteristics of pain and discomfort:	
When walking uphill or hurrying	(Y/N).
When walking on level or ordinary pace	(Y/N).
Response in activity to pain or discomfort:	
Stopping, slowing down, continued activity.	
Does pain/discomfort go away when standing still?	(Y/N)
How soon?	(<10 min, >10 min)

Functional Classifications of Activity Leading to Angina Pectoris

Class	New York Heart Association	Canadian
I	Greater than ordinary activity	Strenuous or prolonged exertion
II	Ordinary activity	Walking or climbing stairs rapidly
		Walking uphill
		Regular or climbing after meals, in cold, wind, with emotional stress
		Walking more than 2 blocks on level
III	Less than ordinary activity	Walking 1 to 2 blocks on level
		Climbing 1 flight normally
IV	Any activity or at rest	

From Liebson and Klein, Ischemic Heart Disease In Current Diagnosis, Edition 9.[6]

Physical Examination

The physical examination rarely excludes ischemia, but evanescent signs during an anginal episode can be suggestive (Table 4). These signs include the development of a systolic pulsation over the precordium; a fourth heart sound; rarely a third heart sound; paradoxical splitting of the second heart sound; and an apical systolic murmur. Although increases in heart rate and blood pressure are typical of ischemia, they are nonspecific, and may be absent with inferior wall ischemia or patients on certain medications.

Other causes of chest pain may be evaluated by the physical examination. The pain of pericarditis is positional and relieved by sitting up. A two- or three-component friction rub may be heard over the precordium. Aortic dissection may be accompanied by the decrescendo diastolic murmur of aortic regurgitation and pulse deficits. Hypertrophic cardiomyopathy with obstruction often presents as a bifid carotid pulse and an early to midsystolic murmur over the base that increases with the Valsalva maneuver. Aortic stenosis or regurgitation must be evaluated as a possible cause of angina. The presence of significant coronary artery disease may correlate with tendinous or tuberous xanthomas or xanthelasmas over the eyelids, suggesting lipid abnormalities.

Diagnostic Studies

The chest radiograph is of little assistance in diagnosing ischemia, but it is useful in evaluating heart size, vascular redistribution typical of congestive heart failure, a dilated ascending aortic shadow that may suggest dissection or aneurysm, and calcification of the aortic valve and coronary arteries.

The resting ECG may be entirely normal, especially when angina is not being experienced. The ECG can provide evidence of previous infarction and other cardiac causes of angina or chest discomfort. Prior infarction may be diagnosed by the presence of Q waves. Voltage and ST-T criteria for left ventricular hypertrophy may support the diagnosis of hypertension or aortic valve disease. Ambulatory electrocardiographic monitoring can be used to evaluate ST-segment changes during usual daily activity.

Table 4. Evaluation of Non-Cardiac Chest Pain

Diagnosis	*Test Modality*
Esophageal reflux	Bernstein Test, CXR to detect hiatal hernia, consider trial of antacids
Esophageal mortality disease	Manometry
Peptic ulcer disease	GI endoscopy, upper GI series, consider trial of H$_2$ blockers
Pancreatitis	Serum anylase, lipase
Cholecystitis	Abdominal ultrasound, HIDA scan
Muscloskeletal	Anti-inflammatory agents
Pulmonary embolism	V/Q scan
Pulmonary hypertension	CXR, Cardiac echo
Pneumonia	CXR, fever, leukocytosis, sputum exam
Pleurisy	CXR
Pericarditis	Echo, ESR, Anti-inflammatory agents
Mitral valve prolapse	Cardiac echo, B blockers
Psychogenic	Anxiolytic, referral to specialist
Cervical radiculopathy	C-spine x-rays, neurologic exam

Initial Management Strategy

Following the history and physical examination, an assessment regarding additional evaluation and therapy must be made (Figure 1). The information gathered from the history and physical may allow the exclusion of angina pectoris with no further investigation (i.e., rib fracture). Another possible conclusion is that the chest pain may be due to angina pectoris; in this case, further diagnostic evaluation is necessary. A third possibility is that the chest pain is definitely angina pectoris; then, the next step is to classify the condition as either chronic stable (mild or severe) angina pectoris or unstable angina pectoris. Chronic stable angina pectorisis present in patients whose chest pain has remained unchanged in terms of severity, frequency, and duration over a period of weeks to months. Mild angina pectoris typically occurs only after marked exertion and does not require the patient to alter lifestyle to prevent the pain (Table 3). Severe chronic stable angina occurs frequently and results in modifying daily routine in order to exclude strenuous activities, while mild chronic stable angina usually does not require hospitalization, and evaluation and treatment can be performed on an outpatient basis. Patients with

Figure 1. Critical Pathway For Chest Pain Triage

CCCF: Canadian Cardiovascular Society Functional Class

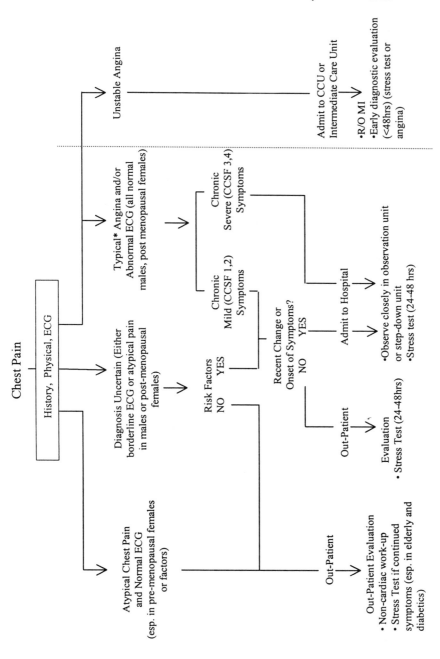

* Typical Angina = A+B; atypical chest pain = A or B where A = chest pain described as pressure or squeezing, 2 - 15 min. duration, substernal, jaw, neck, arm pain. B = Precipitated by exertion/emotional stress and relieved by rest.

severe chronic stable angina may not require hospitalization for evaluation and treatment; the decision to hospitalize depends on the severity of the symptoms and must be made on an individual basis. Patients categorized as having unstable angina pectoris (who by definitive are at medium to high risk of in-hospital complication) should be hospitalized. Features common to all definitions of unstable angina include new onset of angina; more severe, prolonged or frequent episodes of angina superimposed on chronic stable angina; and angina occurring at rest.

Differentiating chest pain due to acute ischemic syndromes from pain due to other causes can be difficult. Because the number of patients complaining of chest pain is large, it is impractical to admit all of them to coronary care units for further cardiac evaluation. However, to send home a patient actually suffering a myocardial infarction or unstable angina with a diagnosis of chest pain of noncardiac origin can be catastrophic. Thus, one should have a low threshold for admitting patients when there is any reasonable doubt about diagnosis and symptoms are progressive. An abnormal electrocardiogram, especially with new or transient changes during chest pain, should ordinarily be sufficient reasoning for further observation[9].

Many important decisions about the evaluation and treatment of patients with angina pectoris are made on the basis of the initial history and physical exam. For this reason, it is important to be aware of how accurately these tools can reflect the presence and degree of coronary artery disease. Numerous studies have demonstrated that even the most skillfully and carefully conducted clinical history has limitations. Most series report that patients classified clinically as having unstable angina pectoris have a 10% to 80% incidence of normal coronary arteries when coronary angiography was performed.

Non-Invasive Evaluation

The history, physical examination, resting ECG, and ambulatory ECG can detect more than 80 percent of the diagnoses of myocardial ischemia. When required, further noninvasive evaluation may include exercise stress testing using electrocardiography, thallium-201 (^{201}Tl) or technetium-99m sestamibi (^{99m}Tc-sestamibi) nuclear imaging and echocardiography or resting studies using dipyridamole or dobutamine. These studies can help diagnose ischemia and define coronary artery disease according to location and severity.

Stress testing is optimally performed 24-48 hrs. after admission for chest pain once myocardial infarction is ruled out. Recently, stress testing 6-12 hours after admission in those with possible, but not unstable, angina has been advocated. This additional testing is primarily used to assess vulnerability to myocardial infarction and risk for sudden cardiac death based on the severity of coronary artery disease and the extent of ischemia. However, because these non-invasive diagnostic studies are expensive, care and skill is required when choosing the modality to evaluate each patient.

Utility of Non-Invasive Testing

It is axiomatic that stress testing is imperfect; to understand its utility, it is necessary to know when it is most and least useful. The accurate interpretation of a diagnostic procedure requires the knowledge of 3 characteristics: its sensitivity, specificity, and the pre-test likelihood of disease in the population to be tested. Sensitivity is equivalent to the frequency of an abnormal test result in the presence of disease, and specificity is equivalent to the frequency of a normal test result in the absence of disease. These values, expressed as finite percentages, are relative and are highly dependent on the specific criteria used to define "abnormal test result" and "presence of disease". Thus, sensitivity and specificity are very sensitive to any modification in test and analysis criteria. Additionally, these values will be different when applied to different populations with varying disease prevalences.

The post-test likelihood of disease in a given individual can be calculated, if one has accurate knowledge of these 3 parameters, by the equation:

$$\text{Post-Test likelihood} = \frac{\text{Pre-test likelihood} \times \text{Sensitivity}}{(\text{Pre-test likelihood} \times \text{Sensitivity}) + (1\text{-pretest likelihood})(1\text{-specificity})}$$

Bayes' Theorem analyses for chest pain were popularized by Diamond and others in the 1970's, and continue to provide the theoretic foundation for their utility. However, it has become clear that accurately quantitating pre-test likelihood is very difficult and limits the value of this approach in clinical practice. Nevertheless, Bayes Theorem does emphasize several crucial points of great use in this era of cost awareness. First, ordering stress tests in *all* patients with chest pain is cost inefficient, since it will (or should) not enhance confidence in the diagnosis or alter management strategy in patients very unlikely (on the basis of the history, physical and ECG) or, alternatively, almost certainly, to have disease. It will have the most impact in the population of most diagnostic complexity - those with an intermediate pre-test probability of disease. Consequently, patients with atypical chest pain and no risk factors for CAD proceed with a non-cardiac work-up first(Table 4). We reserve non-invasive testing for those with chest pain syndrome of intermediate or indeterminate likelihoods (see Figure 1) in whom the test result would significantly impact subsequent management.

Use of Coronary Angiography

Patients with high probability of disease - those with typical angina and the presence of risk factors - constitute more of a dilemma because usefulness of a stress test depends on the exact question being posed. If one wants to know for certain if disease is present, we advise early coronary angiography.   Proceeding directly to angiography is appropriate when the presence of CAD is not in doubt but when knowing the specific anatomy is needed to determine therapeutic strategy. If a functional assessment is required to make a judgement about stenosis severity or physiologic significance, the length of exercise and the size and location of induced abnormalities can be helpful. Together with the number of vessels diseased, LV ejection fraction, and the location and severity of coronary stenoses, the best management plan can usually be arrived at.

The traditional concept of using stress testing as a "screening test" and angiography as a "definitive" examination fails to recognize both the limitations of angiographic demonstration of stenosis severity and the value of functional class assessment prognostically.[10]   Ideally, the utilization of stress testing and coronary angiography should be individualized to optimize diagnostic relevance but not be wasteful of resources. A rational approach to the patient with chest pain requires a general estimate of pre-test likelihood of disease, which then provides a framework for a selective approach to testing (Figure 1). However, when a patient or family member is uncomfortable with any degree of uncertainty, coronary angiography will usually be required.[11]

Coronary Calcium Screening

Although the American Heart Association has not endorsed Fast CT scanning for routine screening for coronary disease, preliminary studies suggest that it may have use in some low risk cases. (See Figure 2). A total calcium score >100 is the key threshold for further evaluation, although values between 100-300 are borderline and those >1000 usually correlate with advanced disease.

Figure 2. Critical Pathway Using Coronary Calcification as Initial Screening Test

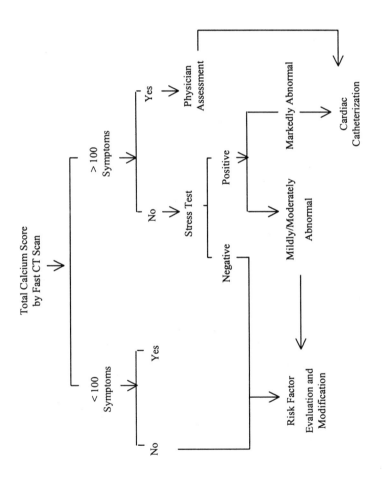

Purpose: Provide guidelines for the physician for the management of patients with coronary calcification.

Nuclear Stress Testing

Familiarity with indications, contraindications, predictive limitations, situations in which false positives and false negatives are increased, costs of the proposed test and alternative testing strategies are required to develop the most rational schemes for the individual patient. One way to safely save money without compromising patient care is to avoid ordering tests that are not optimally suited to settle the diagnostic problem, especially when the test result may lead to incorrect conclusions.

The estimated sensitivity and specificity of electrocardiographic treadmill testing is 60 per cent and 85 per cent, respectively. Nuclear imaging, which demonstrates exercise-induced perfusion defects that are reversible with rest, has a sensitivity of 80 per cent and a predictive value of 90 percent. Patients with symptomatic exercise-induced ischemia have a higher prevalence of severe coronary artery disease than do those without angina during exercise testing. However, in patients without prior myocardial infarction, ST-segment depression is a better predictor of significant coronary artery disease. The heart rate may affect the degree of ST depression in response to ischemia. Normalization is obtained by dividing ST-segment change by heart rate change.[13-16]

^{201}Tl myocardial imaging studies can demonstrate regional myocardial perfusion imbalance with exercise and thereby provide evidence of significant epicardial coronary artery disease. ^{201}Tl is a potassium analogue that functions as a marker for myocardial perfusion and viability, because only intact myocardial membranes retain the tracer. ^{201}Tl stress images reflect relative perfusion modified by myocardial extraction, which is, in turn, dependent on regional blood flow. In necrotic tissue, even with adequate flow, the tracer is not retained by the tissue and appears as a filling defect. Usually two scans are performed, one at the time of peak exercise just after intravenous injection of ^{201}Tl and another 3 to 4 hours later. Absence of ^{201}Tl uptake during the exercise phase, with filling in during the rest phase, indicates ischemia. A defect present in both phases suggests myocardial infarction of unknown age. If myocardial stunning or hibernation has occurred, redistribution takes from 18 to 72 hours. To visualize these areas, a second injection of ^{201}Tl can be performed after the delayed image scan. Images can be obtained using both planar and single-photon emission computed tomography (SPECT) techniques. The former approach obtains images in three views, and individual coronary artery beds are superimposed on one another. SPECT technology acquires images in a 180-degree arc around the patient, with reconstruction of the heart in three dimensions. The radioisotope uptake is then evaluated by tomographic slices in three orientations, separating individual coronary arteries. Abnormal regions are identified by decreased uptake relative to other regions; consequently, left main or multivessel disease is a not uncommon cause of false negative tests.

^{99m}Tc-sestamibi nuclear stress studies are considered slightly more specific than thallium tests, and have fewer false positives, especially in women and obese patients. This is likely due to the enchanced penetration of sestamibi, rendering breast alternative and other artifacts less problematic. However, there is the disadvantage of lengthening the testing procedure because the radiotracer does not redistribute as quickly after injection; consequently, the rest scan usually has to be performed 24 hours later. Also, for this reason, myocardial viability can not be assessed with this technique.

^{99m}Tc-sestamibi can also be used to evaluate patients at the time of spontaneous chest pain. The sensitivity for detecting significant coronary artery disease is more than 95 per cent, but the specificity is less than 80 per cent, indicating frequent false-positive results. The perfusion defect, when present, closely with the location of significant coronary artery disease. In unstable angina, perfusion defects are frequently found at rest with or without chest pain or electrocardiographic evidence of ischemia.

Stein et al[16] recently evaluated the hypothesis that a diagnostic evaluation of chest pain syndrome performed by a primary care physician is less expensive than performed by a cardiologist. In a 14 month experience in which 1,902 consecutive radionuclide stress tests were performed, non-cardiologists ordered more non-indicated tests than cardiologists, but both over-utilized nuclear stress tests. When the ECG is entirely normal there is very little additional incremental to diagnostic value to performing a nuclear imaging test, but the cost becomes far higher. Referral to a cardiologist before ordering tests could have saved $63,000 in costs and $170,000 in charges. Thus, the "gate keeper" hypothesis is unsubstantiated in evaluating chest pain syndrome.

Nuclear Imaging With Pharmacologic Stress Testing

For patients who cannot perform exercise, pharmacologic stress testing may be performed with dobutamine, dipyridamole, and adenosine. The diagnostic results obtained are nearly as good as with exercise, but functional capacity is not assessed. For example, ^{99m}Tc sestamibi SPECT imaging with dipyridamole has provided a sensitivity for detection of significant CAD as high as 95 percent, with close to 80 percent identification of the diseased coronary arteries.

Echocardiographic Stress Testing

The principle of echocardiographic stress testing is based on ischemia-induced regional degradation of left ventricular myocardial performance. The technique permits a choice between treadmill stress testing and pharmacologic studies at rest; dobutamine stress echocardiograms are most common. With exercise stress echocardiography, four tomographic views are obtained at rest and immediately after treadmill exercise. An absolute decrease in regional wall motion denotes an abnormal test result. The absence of increased contraction with higher dobutamine dosage constitutes an equivalent result with about 50% specificity. Exercise echocardiographic testing overall has sensitivities ranging from 63 to 100 per cent and specificities ranging from 64 to 100 per cent. The sensitivity and specificity for dobutamine stress echocardiography is comparable to that for nuclear imaging studies in two- and three-vessel coronary artery disease, when it especially effective. Also, it is a very elegant and accurate method to detect myocardial viability, correlating well with improvement in myocardial function after revascularization, although less sensitive in detecting PET scan abnormalities compared to 24 hour re-injection thallium tests.

SUMMARY

In comparing the utility of stress testing generally to angiography, the preferred test depends on the clinical context. When the diagnosis of coronary artery disease is very likely and symptoms are rapidly progressive, the most cost-effective strategy may be to perform angiography rapidly. However, when the diagnosis is in doubt or is unlikely, stress testing is the preferred means of screening. Which stress testing imaging technique is also dependent on the specific situation. When the ECG is normal and the patient can exercise, a regular ECG stress test is most cost effective. Pharmacologic stress is necessary only when the patient can not walk for (i.e. CHF, arthritis, amputations). Echo is a better imaging technique when multivessel disease is likely; cardiolyte when obesity on breast shadow alternation may occur, and double injection thallium when viability is at issue.

References

1. Lee TH, Cook EF, Weisberg M, Sargent RK, Wilson C, Goldman L. Acute chest pain in the emrgency room. Indentification and examination of low risk patients. Ann Intern Med 1985; 145:65-69.

2. Lee TH, Rowan GW, Weisberg MC, et al. Clinical characteristics and natural history of patients with acute myocardial infarction sent home from the emergency room. Am J Cardiol 1987; 10:219-224.

3. Kaul S. Evaluation of chest pain in the emergency department. Ann Int Med 1994; 121:976-978.

4. Jesse RL, Kontos MC. Evaluation of chest pain in the emergency department. Curr Probl in Card 1997; 22:149-236.

5. Mukerji B, Alpert MA, Mukerji V. Chest Pain. In Conn RB, (editor) Current Diagnosis, edition 9, page 5-8.

6. Liebson PR, Klein LW. Ischemic heart disease. In Conn RB, Current Diagnosis 9, pages 362-368.

7. Anton R, Pepine C. Angina Pectoris. Card Rev Rep 1996; 24-32.

8. Ryan TJ. A clinician's approach to chest pain. Proceedings from the First Maryland Chest Pain Center Research Conference 1997, page 14-17.

9. Hlatky MA. Evaluation of chest pain in the emergency department. N Engl J Med 1997; 337:1687-1689.

10. Bodenheimer M. Risk stratification of coronary disease: A contrary viewpoint. Ann of Int Med. 1992; 116:927-936

11. Van Miltenberg-Van Zijahn AJM et al. Variation in the use of coronary angiography in patients with unstable angina. Eur H J 1996; 17:1828-36.

12. TIMI IIIB Investigators - Effect of t-PA and a comparison of early invasive and conservative strategies in unstable angina and non Q wave myocardial infarction. Circulation 19976; 89:1545-1552.

13. Kontas MC, Jesse RL, Schmidt KL, Omato JP, Tatum JL. Value of acute rest sestamibi perfusion imaging for evaluation of patients admitted to the emergency department with chest pain. JAAC 1997; 30:976-982.

14. Christian TF, Miller TD, Bailey KR, Gibbons RJ. Exercise tomographic thallium -201 imaging in patients with severe coronary artery disease and normal electrocardiogram. Ann Inter Med 1994; 121:825-832.

15. Zabel KM, Califf RM. The value of exercise thallium imaging. Ann Int Med 1994; 121:891-883.

16. Ritchie JL, Trobaugh GB, Hamilton GW, et al. Myocardial imaging with thallium-201 at rest and during exercise. Circulation 1997; 56:66-71.

17. Iskandrian AS, Wasserman LA, Anderson GS, et al. Merits of stress thallium-201 myocardial perfusion imaging in patients with normal exercise electrocardiogram. Am J Cardial 1980; 46:553-558.

18. Stein JH, Uretz EF, Parrillo JE, Barron JT. Cost and appropriateness of radionuclide exercise stress testing by cardiologists and non-cardiologists. Am J Cardiol 1996; 77:139-142.

2

MANAGEMENT OF STABLE ANGINA PECTORIS

William H. Frishman MD
Stephen Peterson MD
Daniel Kombert MD
New York Medical College, Valhalla, NY

INTRODUCTION

Angina occurs when there is an imbalance between myocardial perfusion and the oxygen needs of the myocardium, and the chest discomfort may be associated with transient left ventricular dysfunction. The important features of angina chest discomfort are its location, relationship to exercise, character, and duration.

Regarding location, the discomfort is typically described as originating in the retrosternal area, but it frequently radiates across the precordium, up the neck, and down the ulnar surface of the left arm or down both arms. Frequently the pain can start in one of these other areas and later spread to the midsternal area. Angina pain occurring above the mandible or below the epigastrium is rare (1). The chest discomfort may be associated with or even overshadowed by dyspnea, fatigue, lightheadedness, fatigue and mild epigastric discomfort.

Regarding character, terms used to describe angina are heaviness, pressure, squeezing, crushing or a strangling sensation. The pain may vary in its intensity from a mild localized discomfort to severe pain. Other descriptions of chest pain that are not typical of angina pectoris include pinpricks, pins and needles, pain relieved by changes in position or constant pain that lasts for hours (1,2).

Regarding duration, typical angina begins gradually during exercise and usually is relieved within 3 minutes of rest. The discomfort may last up to 10 minutes or even longer after very strenuous exercise or emotional duress. Chest pain lasting for more than 30 minutes may suggest an acute myocardial infarction. Angina episodes related to Syndrome X are frequently longer in duration and less consistent in their relation to exercise than those in patients with atherosclerotic CAD (1,2).

Regarding the relation to exercise, angina pectoris is typically induced by exertion related to the increased myocardial oxygen demands seen with exercise or other stressors, and is relieved by rest. Emotional stress may be another provocative stimulus for angina. Angina occurring at rest would suggest coronary artery vasospasm, an arrhythmia, or unstable angina (1,2,3).

The differential diagnosis of chest pain includes both cardiac and non-cardiac causes. Cardiac causes of chest pain unrelated to CAD include Syndrome X, severe pulmonary hypertension, pulmonary embolus, pericarditis, aortic stenosis, hypertrophic cardiomyopathy, mitral valve prolapse, and arrhythmia. Non-cardiac causes include esophageal reflux, peptic ulcer disease, pneumonia, cholelithiasis, musculoskeletal disorder, and anxiety states. The pretest likelihood of having CAD in male and female patients having typical and atypical angina pain (2) is shown in Table 1.

Table 1: Pretest Likelihood of Coronary Artery Disease in Symptomatic Patients According to Age and Sex

Age (yrs)	Typical Angina		Atypical Angina		Non-anginal Anginal Chest Pain	
	Male	*Female*	*Male*	*Female*	*Male*	*Female*
30-39	69.7+3.2	25.8+6.6	21.8+2.4	4.2+1.3	5.2+0.8	0.8+0.3
40-49	87.3+1.0	55.2+6.5	46.1+1.8	13.3+2.9	14.1+1.3	2.8+0.7
50-59	92.0+0.6	79.4+2.4	58.9+1.5	32.4+3.0	21.5+1.7	8.4+1.2
60-69	94.3+0.4	90.1+1.0	67.1+1.3	54.4+2.4	28.1+1.9	18.6+1.9

From Ref. 2 with permission.

Epidemiology: Impact of Gender, Age and Race

Population-based studies using various data collection methodologies have revealed that among middle-aged individuals, angina pectoris is more than twice as common in men as it is in women (2,4). The prevalence of angina increases with age and occurs in 11-20% of men in the age group of 65-74 years, and occurs in 10-14% of women in this age group. After age 75, the prevalence of angina in men and women is about the same (2).

Data from the Framingham Study have revealed that the most common presentation of coronary artery disease in women is angina pectoris, which occurs, on average, 10 years later than in men (5). Men often present with a myocardial infarction as their first manifestation of CAD. However, after 75 year, both men and women experience the same myocardial infarction and sudden death rate (6).

In Framingham, the prevalence of obstructive CAD is less commonly seen in women with angina pectoris than in men (5). In the Asymptomatic Cardiac Ischemic Pilot (ACIP) trial, we compared the demography and clinical outcomes of men and women of comparable age with stable angina pectoris who participated in the study (7). Subjects needed to have a positive stress ECG exam, evidence of obstructive CAD on angiography, and evidence of silent myocardial ischemia on a 48 hour ambulatory ECG to be considered for this trial. Qualified subjects were then randomized into two medical treatment arms and a surgical treatment arm. One medical treatment arm utilized antianginal drug therapies titrated to relieve symptoms only; the second treatment arm utilized antianginal drug therapies to relieve both symptoms and silent ischemia on the ambulatory ECG. For the surgical treatment arm, subjects were treated either with coronary angioplasty or coronary bypass surgery, depending on the severity of the obstructive CAD on angiography (8).

In ACIP, there were many more men than women randomized into the study. Although the mean ages were the same, women had more risk factors for CAD than men (7), including a higher prevalence of diabetes and hypertension. In contrast, men had more obstructive CAD than women (7). In a large retrospective experience from Emory, comparing men and women with CAD, similar findings were noted (9). In ACIP, despite having more CAD, men could perform better on the treadmill than women, however both groups demonstrated similar amounts of ischemia on the ambulatory ECG exam. Women had higher left ventricular ejection fractions than men (7).

Of interest is the observation that Black women have a higher mortality rate from CAD than white women, and in Black women aged 35-39 years, CAD is the leading cause of death (10-12).

Prognosis

Chronic stable angina is associated with a relatively good prognosis in the majority of patients, with an annual mortality rate of 2-3% and a new non-fatal myocardial infarction rate that is similar (2,13,14). There are, of course, high risk subgroups with severe three vessel disease and left main CAD, with and without left ventricular dysfunction. In the evaluation of patients with chronic stable angina, it is important to identify these high risk subgroups that might benefit more from coronary revascularization procedures than from medical therapy. The medical prognosis of stable angina pectoris may become more favorable with the advent of aggressive lipid-lowering therapy and aspirin. Estrogen replacement, which is now being evaluated with the Women's Health Initiative trial (15) and the Hormone

Estrogen/Progestin Replacement Study, may also be shown to favorably influence the prognosis of women with angina pectoris.

Diagnostic Evaluation

After a careful history is taken and a complete physical exam is performed, a non-invasive diagnostic evaluation is performed to definitively establish CAD as the most likely cause for angina pectoris. This evaluation also helps to quantitate the severity of ischemic heart disease and rules out/in other causes of angina pectoris, such as aortic stenosis and hypertrophic cardiomyopathy.

Resting ECG

The first part of the non-invasive evaluation is the resting ECG. This ECG can be normal or show an infarct pattern or an ischemic repolarization pattern suggestive of underlying CAD (2). Women with suspected CAD show a higher prevalence of ECG repolarization abnormalities than men (7,16).

ECG Stress Testing

The diagnostic value of stress testing is lower in women than in men because of the lower prevalence of CAD, especially in younger women with chest pain (**Table 2**) (2). Women more commonly have a false positive stress ECG (38-67%) than men (7-44%) related to a lower pretest likelihood of disease in younger women (17). Some of these repolarization abnormalities with exercise may be caused by estrogen (18). In women older than 50, the likelihood increases that an abnormal stress ECG is predictive of CAD (2). A negative exercise test has a similar specificity for demonstrating the absence of coronary disease in both men and women.

Ambulatory 24 Hour ECG

In predicting the presence or absence of CAD, the specificity and sensitivity of the ST segment abnormalities obtained with ambulatory ECG monitoring are lower than that seen with the stress ECG (2). For the most part, those subjects with strongly positive ECG stress tests will show the most ambulatory ischemia and subjects with negative stress tests will show little ambulatory ischemia (19). Therefore, the ambulatory ECG for diagnosis provides little additional information beyond that obtained from the stress ECG, except for the detection of rest ischemia.

Table 2: CAD Post-Test Likelihood (%) Based on Age, Sex, Symptom Classification and Exercise-Induced ECG ST Segment Depression

Age (years)	ST depression (mV)	Typical Angina		Atypical Angina		Non-anginal Chest pain		Asymptomatic	
		Male	Female	Male	Female	Male	Female	Male	Female
30-39	0.00-0.04	25	7	6	1	1	<1	<1	<1
	0.05-0.09	68	24	21	4	5	1	2	4
	0.10-0.14	83	42	38	9	10	2	4	<1
	0.15-0.19	91	59	55	15	19	3	7	1
	0.20-0.24	96	79	76	33	39	8	18	3
	>0.25	99	93	92	63	68	24	43	11
40-49	0.00-0.04	61	22	16	3	4	1	1	<1
	0.05-0.09	86	53	44	12	13	3	5	1
	0.10-0.14	94	72	64	25	26	6	11	2
	0.15-0.19	97	84	78	39	41	11	20	4
	0.20-0.24	99	93	91	63	65	24	39	10
	>0.25	>99	98	97	86	87	53	69	28
50-59	0.00-0.04	73	47	25	10	6	2	2	1
	0.05-0.09	91	78	57	31	20	8	9	3
	0.10-0.14	96	89	75	50	37	16	19	7
	0.15-0.19	98	94	86	67	53	28	31	12
	0.20-0.24	99	98	94	84	75	50	54	27
	>0.25	>99	99	98	95	91	78	81	56
60-69	0.00-0.04	79	69	32	21	8	5	3	2
	0.05-0.09	94	90	65	52	26	17	11	7
	0.10-0.14	97	95	81	72	45	33	23	15
	0.15-0.19	99	98	89	83	62	49	37	25
	0.20-0.24	99	99	96	93	81	72	61	47
	>0.25	>99	99	99	98	94	90	85	76

From Ref. 2 with permission.

Myocardial Perfusion Scintigraphy

The advent of radionuclide perfusion imaging during stress testing or after inotropic stress has increased the sensitivity of the non-invasive evaluation of CAD in women (**Table 3**) (2,20). In addition, individuals who cannot exercise can receive vasodilators such as dipyridamole or adenosine to enhance perfusion in areas where the coronary supply is normal, in order to augment the difference from abnormal areas (21).

Table 3: Functional Tests of CAD

	Exer ECG	Thallium Scint with Exercise or Vasodilator Drugs	Stress Echo with Etiher Exercise or Inotropic Agents
Detection of CAD			
Sensitivity	50-80%	65-90%	65-90%
Specificity	80-95%	90-95%	90-95%
Greatest Sensitivity	Multivessel disease	Single vessel disease	Single & multivessel disease
Location of CAD		80% LAS 60% RCA	No influence
Use in patients with abnormal ST at rest	Difficult	Unhampered interpretation	Unhampered
Recommended use	First Choice in most patients	To provide additional data in some patients, particulary location of myocardial ischemia.	First choice in patients unable to exercise. Limited value in patients with poor echo quality.

Exer=exercise; Scint=scintigraphy; Echo=echocardiography; CAD=coronary artery disease; LAD=left anterior descending; RCA=right coronary artery.

From Ref. 2 with permission.

It has been shown that thallium (TL-201) perfusion scintigraphy with exercise is less sensitive in detecting CAD in women than in men (22). The increased false positive rate in women is attributed to breast soft tissue attenuation artifacts (22). These are caused by increased attenuation and low energy scatter. Higher energy radionuclides, such as technetium-99m (Tc-99m) sesta-mibi have also been studied. Amanullah et al (23) studied the accuracy of adenosine Tc-99m sesta-mibi in detecting CAD and found this radionuclide to be a highly reliable agent in perfusion scintigraphy with the overall sensitivity, specificity and predictive accuracy to be 93%, 78% and 88% respectively. Studies have also been done comparing the sensitivity and specificity of TL-201 to Tc-99m sesta-mibi SPECT imaging in detecting CAD in women (24,25). The overall sensitivity was similar for TL-201 and Tc-99m sesta-mibi (75% and 71.9% respectively) (24). Specificity was found to be higher with Tc-99m sesta-mibi (24,25).

The diagnostic accuracy of radionuclide myocardial perfusion scintigraphy is affected by the patient population, the heart rate response, the type of imaging acquisition and the degree of soft tissue attenuation artifact. Therefore, the type of stress test (e.g. exercise vs drug), the type of tracer and imaging protocol, are important.

Iskandrian (26) recommends that the ideal radionuclide tracer have a high extraction fraction at high flow rates. The highest extraction fraction is achieved by teboroxime → thallium → sesta-mibi and tetrofosmin. The greatest impact on myocardial flow is achieved by adenosine → dipyridamole → dobutamine → exercise.

Stress Echocardiography

Another non-invasive modality for the detection of CAD is stress echocardiography using exercise dobutamine or similar substances (2,21). Echocardiographic images are compared before and during the stress. A normal myocardial image shows an increase of wall motion and wall thickening during stress, while ischemia is recognized by reduced regional wall thickening of the ventricle and transient contractile abnormalities. It appears to be as accurate as perfusion scintigraphy for detecting or ruling out CAD (Table 3) (2). Stress echocardiography is becoming the test of first choice in patients unable to exercise. Its value is limited, however, in patients where good echocardiographic images cannot be obtained.

Coronary Angiography

It remains controversial whether or not a gender bias is the reason why women with a positive non-invasive evaluation for CAD undergo cardiac catheterization less often than men. In 1987, Tobin et al (27) reported that the referral pattern for cardiac catheterization after abnormal radionuclide scans was 4% for women vs 40% for men (p<0.001). After adjusting for age, myocardial infarction, chest pain characteristics, and test results, the gender difference remained.

In a recent study, Lauer et al (28) examined whether or not post-test gender bias influenced referrals for cardiac catheterization. They found that women were less likely than men to undergo coronary angiography, 6% vs 14% respectively. Also, women were less likely to have positive or abnormal thallium scans, 8% vs 29%. After adjusting for age and thallium test results, women were less likely than men to be referred for coronary angiography. Results from coronary angiography reinforced the fact that women have a lower prevalence of severe CAD disease and mortality.

In contrast, Shaw et al (29) reported that with a similar prevalence of abnormal stress tests in men and women, additional testing was only obtained in 38% of women vs 62.3% of men. The incidence of coronary events was 14.3% in women and 69% in men. All events occurred in patients who had not undergone revascularization.

Another study by Steingart et al (30) highlights these differences in the management of CAD in women vs men. The men and women in this study had similar risk factors and medical therapy. The women had chest pain as frequently as the men, and complained of more disabling symptoms. Yet, women underwent coronary angiography less often than men. The authors try to explain the difference as follows:

1. Many women with angina do not have coronary disease. If they do, it is usually non-obstructive. This is true of studies in younger age groups.

2. Women in older age groups have a higher incidence of CAD They may not be referred for coronary angiograhy because they are more likely to experience vascular

and renal complications secondary to age and smaller body size.   But the complications of myocardial infarction, stroke and death are similar in men and women.

Coronary angiography can be considered in women with abnormal results at the time of radionuclide imaging, or in those in whom there is a high index of suspicion of disease because of an increased number of risk factors for CAD (24) or where there are unsatisfactory or inconclusive results from non-invasive testing (Table 4) (24).

Table 4: Use of Diagnostic Tests in Women with Chest Pain

Likelihood of CHD	Initial Test	Subsequent Test

Low (<20%)
  No major and ≤1 intermediate
  or ≤2 minor determinants*
	None indicated	None indicated

Moderate (2-=80%) 1 major or multiple intermediate and minor determinants	Routine ETT Negative Inconclusive Positive	 None indicated Further testing indicated; selection must be individualized Imaging test or catheterization
	Imaging ETT Negative Inconclusive Positive	 None Indicated Catheterization Catheterization
High (>80%) ≥2 major or 1 major +>1 Intermediate or minor determinants.	Routine ETT Negative Inconclusive Positive	 None Indicated; observe patient Catheterization Catheterization
	Imaging #TT	None Indicated

CHD=coronary heart disease; ETT=exercise tolerance test; * Determinants of CHD in women with chest pain include **major** (typical angina pectoris, postmenopausal status without hormone replacement, diabetes mellitus, peripheral vascular disease); **intermediate** (hypertension, smoking, lipoprotein abnormalities, especially low HDL cholesterol levels); **minor** (age >65 yrs, obesity, especially central obesity, sedentary lifestyle, family history of CHD, other risk factors for CHD such as psychosocial or hemostatic).

From Douglas PS, Ginsburg GS: The evaluation of chest pain in women. N Engl J Med 1996; 334: 1311-15.

Clinical Recommendations

General Management

Patients with stable angina pectoris related to CAD and Syndrome X have good medical prognoses and specific non-pharmacologic approaches should be followed (Tables 5 & 6).

Smoking should be strongly discouraged and patients warned to avoid second-hand smoke. Nicotine replacement therapies (patches, gum) appear to be as effective in women as in men, as part of a smoke-ending program (31,32). There appears to be no contraindication to nicotine replacement therapy in patients with stable angina pectoris (33).

Anemia and infection should be treated since both conditions will increase myocardial oxygen demands, while a low hematocrit in anemia will also decrease oxygen supply. A diagnostic search should be made to rule out the presence of thyroid disorders which are more common in women than in men.

Hypertension and diabetes need to be vigorously treated with diet (see next section). A diet rich in vegetables, fruit, fish and poultry, and low in fat should be prescribed, and weight reduction encouraged in overweight individuals. Alcohol in moderation may be beneficial (34). The safety of antiobesity drugs has not been determined in patients with angina pectoris, and their use should be discouraged for now (35).

Regular isotonic exercise has been shown to be of benefit regarding the prevention of cardiovascular events, and patients with angina pectoris should be encouraged to be as active as possible within the limits of their symptoms (36).

Patients with angina are often anxious and/or depressed. Anxiolytic agents may be used, and the selective serotonin reuptake inhibitors may be used to treat depression, even though there is no good evidence as yet to demonstrate their safety in patients with angina pectoris (37).

Table 5: Medical Approach to Patients with CAD and Angina Pectoris

NON-PHARMACOLOGIC

1. Weight control (role of antiobesity drugs in patients with CAD unknown)
2. Low fat diet (20-22% of daily food calories as fat, 1/3 can be polyunsaturated fat)
3. Diet high in fiber and vegetables
4. Salt restriction if CHF present
5. Diabetic diet if hyperglycemia is present
6. Smoking cessation (treatments are safe in patients with angina pectoris)
7. Alcohol in moderation (less than 1 oz. alcohol daily)

PHARMACOLOGIC

Risk Factor Control

1. Lipid lowering therapy with diet to reduce LDL-cholesterol below 100mg%
2. Aspirin 75-160 mg daily if tolerated
3. Vitamin E, 400 IU/daily
4. Folate 5, mg/day
5. Pharmacologic control of systolic and diastolic hypertension
6. Pharmacologic control with diet of hyperglycemia
7. Estrogen, with and without progestin, unless contraindicated Antianxiety and antidepressant medication as needed (selective serotonin reuptake inhibitors in patients with angina, although they are probably the preferred drug for depression in patients with CAD

Antianginal Control

1. Beta-adrenergic blockers
2. Nitrates
3. Calcium-channel blockers
4. Combinations of above
5. Estrogens in postmenopausal women? (improved vasomotor function)
6. Lipid-lowering therapies? (improved vasomotor function)

Table 6: Medical Treatment of Syndrome X

1. Nitrates
2. Calcium-channel blockers
3. Estrogens?

Drug Therapy

Treatment of the Complications of Atherosclerosis

The pharmacologic approach to treating patients with chronic stable angina pectoris involves both the prevention of the complications of atherosclerotic heart disease and the relief of chest pain symptoms. Aspirin, lipid-lowering agents, antihypertensives, hypoglycemic agents, antioxidant vitamins, and hormone replacement therapies are utilized for the prevention of myocardial infarction and stroke. Nitrates, beta-adrenergic blockers and calcium-channel blockers are used for both prophylaxis and treatment of chest pain episodes.

Aspirin – In patients with angina pectoris, there is a 33% reduction in vascular events with aspirin (37,38). Aspirin is absorbed more rapidly in women than men, and, therefore, aspirin's bioavailability may be higher in women (40,41). Women may also have a decreased antiplatelet effect with aspirin (42,43), and early studies suggested that women benefited less than men (26,44,45) regarding the clinical endpoints of myocardial infarction and stroke. However, the Nurse's Health Study did demonstrate a reduction in myocardial infarctions with aspirin use (46) in women and other studies have revealed benefits of aspirin use in high-risk women who are older and who have a previous history of myocardial infarction (47,48).

Lipid-Lowering Therapy - Elevated cholesterol, LDL-cholesterol and triglycerides, and low levels of HDL-cholesterol are predictors of CAD. These abnormalities appear to be less important in pre-menopausal women where it is suggested that estrogen interferes with the uptake of LDL-cholesterol by the arterial wall. In post-menopausal women, levels of LDL-cholesterol and HDL-cholesterol are higher than in age-matched men, and our group did confirm an increased risk of LDL-cholesterol for CAD in older women (49). Other studies have shown an increased risk for CAD in post-menopausal women with low HDL-cholesterol, high triglycerides, high apolipoprotein-a levels, and high Lp(a) levels (50).

Studies using various HMG-CoA reductase inhibitors have demonstrated similar reductions in total cholesterol and LDL-cholesterol when comparing men and women with hypercholesterolemia (51-54). Studies have also shown a slowing of coronary artery plaque progression on repeat angiographic studies, and a reduction in cardiovascular events has been observed in a study of patients with angina pectoris and/or myocardial infarction who had hypercholesterolemia (52).

Studies with bile acid resins have shown no beneficial effects on the primary prevention of coronary artery events in women; fibric acid derivatives have been shown to be effective in secondary prevention; and probucol, although effective, has been shown to induce cardiac electrophysiologic abnormalities, specifically in women (55).

Based on the available information, it is recommended that all patients with angina pectoris have their LDL-cholesterol reduced below 100mg%. The National Cholesterol Education Program Guidelines recommend estrogens as first-line lipid-lowering therapy in women (56), however, their effects on cholesterol and LDL-cholesterol are much more modest than with the HMG-CoA reductase inhibitors, which should be considered now as the first-line lipid-lowering drug therapy for women.

Antihypertensive Treatment – Combined systolic and diastolic hypertension and isolated systolic hypertension are poserful predictors of CAD (57). Systolic hypertension also is an aggravator of angina pectoris because of its effect on raising myocardial oxygen demands by increasing ventricular wall stress. Left ventricular hypertrophy induced by hpertension many also cause angina pectoris without concomitant large-vessel CAD (58). Coronary vasodilator reserve has been shown to be impaired in patients with left ventricular hypertrophy, most likely due to medial thickening of the microvasculature of the myocardium (58). Also, the hypertrophy of individual myocytes without a parallel increase in the coronary microvasculature could result in a supply-demand imbalance and the development of anginal symptoms (58).

Treatment of hypertension, therefore, is imperative in patients having angina pectoris. Beta-adrenergic blockers as first-line therapy and calcium antagonists as alternative or additional treatment are ideal because of pharmacologic toerance. Additional blood pressure-lowering treatments without direct antianginal activity would include diuretics, angiotensin converting enzyme inhibitors, angiotensin II receptor blockers, and clonidine. The best treatment for left ventricular hypertrophy is not known, and the ALLHAT study is currently investigating how different blood pressure-lowering drugs might affect cardiovascular disease endpoints (60).

The amount of blood pressure lowering which is safe in patients with angina has not been determined and the question has been raised about the safety of reducing the diastolic blood pressure below 85 mmHg. The results of the HOTS Study (Hypertension Optimal Therapeutic Study), which looked at diastolic blood pressure lowering below 85 mmHg found that a diastolic blood pressure of 83 mmHg and a systolic blood pressure of 138 mmHg was associated with maximal cardioprotection. However, values of diastolic blood pressure were associated with no evidence of harm (61).

Treatment of Congestive Heart Failure – Angina pectoris can be aggravated in patients with systolic dysfunction because left ventricular dilation increases wall stress and myocardial oxygen demands. Attempts should be made to minimize ventricular dilation with diuretics and vasodilators. Beta blockers can be used in patients with stable stage II-III NYHA congestive heart failure, for treatment of both angina and congestive heart failure (62).

Treatment of Diabetes – Diabetes mellitus is a powerful determinant of CAD risk in women, and every attempt should be utilized to control hyperglycemia by both non-pharmacologic and pharmacologic means. No specific study has been done, however, analyzing the effects of glycemic control on cardiovascular outcomes in patients with angina pectoris.

Hormone replacement – The evidence that estrogen, with and without progestin, can protect against CAD and tis complications is getting stronger (63). The Women's Health Initiative (14) in the general post-menopausal population, and the Hormone Estrogen/Progestin Replacement Study in wowmen with known CAD will provide additional information about the safety and eficacy of hormone replacement for primary and secondary prevention.

Estrogen does favorably affect plasma lipids and lipoproteins, and its direct effcts on the vasculature may protect against coronary ischemic events. Estrogen therapy may also have a direct antianginal benefit on both symptoms and exercise tolerance (64,65).

With the evidence in hand, it is probably reasonable now to recommend estrogen replacement to post-menopausal women with angina pectoris who have a hysterectomy. Estrogen plus progestin should be used in women with an intact uterus. Hormone replacement may also be useful in patients having Syndrome X, where reduced coronary artery vasodilator reserve and endothelial cell dysfunction in blood vessels have been described (Table 6) (66). All women with angina pectoris being considered for hormone replacement should undergo both a mammography and pelvic exam prior to treatment.

Antioxidants and Folate - The theoretical benefits of supplementary antioxidant therapy have not been confirmed in definitive prospective clinical trials, however, the available evidence is suggestive of benefit against CAD and its complications (67). The Nurse's Health Study in 90,000 women showed the benefits of vitamin E supplementation (68), and in another study in 34,000 women without known CAD vitamin E in the diet was associated with fewer coronary events (69).

There are ongoing prospective, controlled studies examining the effects of vitamin E supplementation (400-600 IU/daily) in 40,000 post-menopausal women and in 8,000 women with known cardiovascular disease (67). However, until the results of these studies are available, it is probably reasonable to recommend the use of 400 IU/daily of vitamin E supplement in women with angina pectoris.

Homocysteinemia has also been shown to be a risk factor for CAD (70) in men and women. Until definitive studies are done, folate supplementation, which lowers homocysteine levels, may be recommended.

Antianginal Therapies

There is no justification for treating men and women differently with angina pectoris and CAD, and they appear to accrue the same benefits from medical therapy and coronary artery revascularization.

The three main classes of drugs are nitrates, beta-adrenergic blockers, and calcium-channel blockers. The aim of antianginal treatment is to reduce myocardial oxygen requirements and to increase myocardial perfusion.

Nitrates - Sublingual nitroglycerin is the only available treatment for rapid relief of angina episodes (71). Long-acting nitrates (isosorbide mononitrate and isosorbide dinitrate) are available in multiple formulations for antianginal prophylaxis, using nitrate-free intervals to avoid tolerance. There are no studies as yet demonstrating a mortality benefit with nitrates in patients with angina pectoris. Nitrates may also be metabolized differently in women than in men, which may require different dosing regimens related to gender (72,73).

Beta-Adrenergic Blockers - Beta blockers are the cornerstone therapy for long-term antianginal prophylaxis (74). All available beta blockers appear useful as antianginal treatments, and they can be used, albeit with caution, in patients with class II-III congestive heart failure (e.g. carvedilol) (75). Beta blockers should be dosed to achieve a reduction in heart rate, both at rest and during exercise.

Calcium-Channel Blockers - Calcium-channel blockers are coronary and peripheral vasodilators which can lower blood pressure, heart rate and myocardial contractility (76). They are divided into 2 major groups: dihydropyridines (e.g. nifedipine, amlodipine, nicardipine), which do not lower heart rate; and the rate-lowering agents (e.g. bepridil, diltiazem, verapamil).

The calcium antagonists should be used with caution in patients with angina pectoris and left ventricular dysfunction. Unlike the beta blockers, calcium-channel blockers have not been shown to reduce mortality after myocardial infarction, although there is some evidence that verapamil and diltiazem may reduce the risk of reinfarction (76).

Combination Therapy - Many studies have demonstrated additive antianginal effects when a beta blocker is combined with a calcium-channel blocker or nitrate. Special care needs to be taken when beta blockers are combined with diltiazem or verapamil in patients having myocardial conduction abnormalities or left ventricular dysfunction.

The additional benefit of combining different antianginal drugs is not always evident, and a recent study suggests that the improvement in anginal symptoms may be related to a clinical response to the new drug and not an additive action (77). There is also little evidence to suggest that triple therapy provides any additional benefit over one or two drugs. In severe, disabling stable angina, bepridil may be combined with beta blockers to achieve additional antianginal effects.

Choice of Agents

In patients with stable angina pectoris, sublingual nitroglycerin and a beta blocker should be used as first-line therapy. Calcium antagonists can be substituted for beta blockers if the latter drugs are not well tolerated or contraindicated. Long-acting nitrates and/or calcium blockers can be added to beta blockers to achieve angina control if higher doses of beta blockers cannot achieve maximal pain relief.

Other Antianginal Treatments

The HMG-CoA reductase inhibitors and estrogen, in addition to their lipid-lowering actions, may have effects on vascular endothelial function to improve coronary flow reserve in patients with angina (63,64). Studies are now being done looking at both treatments as potential antianginal treatments..

Invasive Procedures

Percutaneous Transluminal Coronary Angioplasty and Coronary Bypass Surgery

As with medical therapy, men and women should be offered angioplasty or bypass surgery if clinically indicated. The indications for performing an invasive intervention for CAD in patients depend on the previous response to medical therapy and whether the patient is at a high risk of death. If a patient's symptoms are not controlled satisfactorily with medical treatment, the decision for angioplasty with or without stenting or bypass surgery is made by the severity of coronary obstructive disease, the presence or absence of left main coronary disease, the underlying ventricular function, and concomitant diseases. Reperfusion not only relieves symptoms of angina, but will often improve ventricular function as a consequence of augmented blood flow to the myocardium (78).

CONCLUSION

Patients with angina pectoris benefit equally from aggressive lifestyle interventions and from pharmacologic therapies that target the atherosclerotic process and the clinical syndrome of angina pectoris. Surgical therapies should be reserved for those patients who do not respond to medical therapy or who are at high risk of myocardial infarction and death with continued medical treatment (14) (See **Algorithm**).

ALGORITHM

Diagnosis and Treatment of Stable Angina Pectoris

Stable Angina Pectoris (r/o aortic stenosis and hypertrophic cardiomyopathy)

Diagnostics

Conventional Stress ECG if unable to perform
Myocardial Perfusion Scintigraphy or
Dobutamine Stress Echocardiography

If strongly positive (drop in BP with
exercise, ischemia on ECG with low
heart rate and exercise level)

If positive (without BP drop
And ability to exercise to or above 90)

Coronary Arteriography

Medical Therapy

? revascularization depending
on anatomy

(nitrates, ß blockers, calcium
blockers, aspirin), reducing
elevations in BP, plasma lipids
and blood sugar, folic acid, ?
antioxidants, ? estrogen ±
progestin in postmenopausal women

References

1. Braunwald E: The History. In, Braunwald E, Heart Disease: A Textbook of Cardiovascular Medicine, 5th ed. Philadelphia: Saunders ; 1997, 1-14.

2. Recommendations of the Task Force of the European Society of Cardiology: Management of stable angina pectoris. Eur Heart J 1997; 18: 394-413.

3. Mohri A, Koyanagi M, Egashira K, et al: Angina pectoris caused by coronary microvascular spasm. Lancet 1998; 351: 1165-1169.

4. Mittelmark MB, Psaty BM, Rautaharju PM, et al: Prevalence of cardiovascular diseases among older adults. The Cardiovascular Health Study. Am J Epidemiol 1993; 137: 311-317.

5. Lerner DS, Kannel W: Patterns of heart disease morbidity and mortality in the sexes: a 26 year follow up of the Framingham population. Am Heart J 1986; 111: 383-390.

6. Nadelmann J, Frishman WH, Ooi WL, et al: Prevalence, incidence and prognosis of recognized and unrecognized myocardial infarction in persons aged 75 years or older: The Bronx Aging Study. Am J Cardiol 1990; 66: 533-537.

7. Frishman WH, Gomberg-Maitland M, Hirsch H, et al: Differences between male and female patients with regard to baseline demographics and clinical outcomes in the Asymptomatic Cardiac Ischemia Pilot (ACIP) Trial. Clin Cardiol 1998; 121: 184-190.

8. ACIP Investigators: Asymptomatic Cardiac Ischemia Pilot (ACIP) Study. Am J Cardiol 1992; 70: 744-747.

9. Weintraub WS, Kosinski AS, Wenger NK: Is there a bias against performing coronary revascularization in women? Am J Cardiol 1996; 78: 1154-1160.

10. Feild SK, Savard MA, Epstein KR: The female patient. In, Douglas PS (ed) Cardiovascular Health and Disease in Women. Philadelphia: Saunders; 1993: 4-20.

11. Liao V, Copper RS, Ghali JK, Szocka A: Survival rates with coronary artery disease for black women compared with black men. JAMA 1992; 268: 1867-1871.

12. National Center for Health Statistics: Vital Statistics of the United States, 1986. Vol. II, Mortality, Part A. DIIIIS Pub. No. (PHS) 89-1101, Washington, D.C., U.S. Public Health Service, 1989.

13. Brunelli C, Cristofani R, L'Abbate A: Long term survival in medically treated patients with ischaemic heart disease and prognostic importance of clinical and echocardiographic data. Eur Heart J 1989; 10: 292-303.

14. Peduzzi P, Kamina A, Detre K: Twenty-two-year follow-up in the VA Cooperative Study of coronary artery bypass surgery for stable angina. Am J Cardiol 1998; 81: 1393-1399.

15. Womens Health Initiative Study Group: Design of the Womens Health Initiative Clinical Trial and observational study. Controlled Clin Trials 1998; 19: 61-109.

16. Weiner DA, Ryan TJ, McCabe CH, Kennedy JW, et al: Correlations among history of angina, ST segment response and prevalence of coronary artery disease in the Coronary Artery Surgery Study (CASS). N Engl J Med 1979; 301: 230-235.

17. Gibbons RF: Exercise ECG testing with and without radionuclide studies. In, Wenger NK,Speroff L, Packard B (eds): Cardiovascular Health and Disease in Women.   Greenwich: LeJacq Communications; 1993: 73-90.

18. Stress testing in women.   In, Ellestad MH (ed): Stress Testing: Principles and Practice, 4th ed. Philadelphia: F.A. Davis; 1996; 361-363.

19. Stone PH, Chaitman B, McMahon RP, et al: Relationship between exercise-induced and ambulatory ischemia in patients with stable coronary disease: The Asymptomatic Cardiac Ischemia Pilot (ACIP) Study. Circulation 1996; 94: 1537-1544.

20. Friedman TD, Greene AC, Iskandrian AS, Hakki AH, Kane Sa, Segal BL: Exercise thallium-201 myocardial scintigraphy in women: correlation with coronary arteriography. Am JCardiol 1982; 49: 1632-1637.

21. Meisner JS, Shirani J, Strom JA, Frishman WH: Use of pharmaceuticals in noninvasive cardiovascular diagnosis. In, Frishman WH, Sonnenblick EH: Cardiovascular Pharmacotherapeutics Companion Handbook. New York: McGraw Hill Inc., 1998: 427-442.

22. Hung J, Chaitman BR, Lam J, Lesperance J, Dupras G, Fine P, Bourassa MG: Noninvasive diagnostic test choices for the evaluation of coronary artery disease in women: a multivariate comparison of cardiac fluoroscopy, exercise electrocardiography, and exercise thallium myocardial perfusion scintigraphy. J Am Coll Cardiol 1984; 4: 8-16.

23. Amanullah AM, Kiat H, Friedman JD, Berman DS: Adenosine technetium-99m sestamibi myocardial perfusion SPECT in women: diagnostic efficacy in detection of coronary artery disease. J AmColl Cardiol 1996; 27: 803-809.

24. Taillefer R, DePuey EG, Udelson JE, Beller GA, Latour Y, Reeves F: Comparative diagnostic accuracy of thallium 201 and technetium-99m sestamibi SPECT imaging (perfusion and ECG-gated SPECT) in detecting coronary artery disease in women. J Am Coll Cardiol 1997; 29: 69-77.

25. Amanullah AM, Berman DS, Hachamovitch R, Kiat H, Kang X, Friedman JD: Identification of severe or extensive coronary artery disease in women by adenosine technetium 99-msestmibi SPECT. Am J Cardiol 1997; 80: 132-137.

26. Iskandrian AE: Gender differences in noninvasive testing: editorial. J NoninvasiveCardiol 1997; Jan/Feb, 14-16.

27. Tobin JN, Wassertheil-Smoller S, Wexler JP, et al: Sex bias in considering coronary bypass surgery. Ann Intern Med 1987; 107: 19-25.

28. Lauer MS, Pashkow FJ, Snader CE, Harvey SA, Thomas JD, Marwick TH: Gender and referral for coronary angiography after treadmill thallium testing. Am J Cardiol 1996; 78: 278-283.

29. Shaw LJ, Miller DD, Romeis JC, Kargl D, Younis LT, Chaitman BR: Gender differences in the noninvasive evaluation and management of patients with suspected coronary artery disease. Ann Intern Med 1994; 120: 559-566.

30. Steingart RM, Packer M, Hamm P: Sex differences in the management of coronary artery disease. N Engl J Med 1991; 325: 226-230.

31. Lando HA, Gritz ER: Smoking cessation techniques. JAMA 1996; 51: 31-34.

32. Sachs DP, Sawe U, Leischow SJ: Effectiveness of a 16 hour transdermal nicotine patch in a medical practice setting, without intensive group counseling. Arch Intern Med 1993; 153: 1881-1890.

33. Frishman WH, Ismail A: Tobacco smoking, nicotine, and nicotine replacement. In, Frishman WH, Sonnenblick EH: Cardiovascular Pharmacotherapeutics. New York: McGraw Hill Inc., 1997; 499-509.

34. DelVecchio A, Frishman WH, Fadel A, Ismail A: Cardiovascular manifestations of substance abuse. In, Frishman WH, Sonnenblick EH: Cardiovascular Pharmacotherapeutics. New York: McGraw Hill Inc., 1997; 1115-1149.

35. Frishman WH, Weiser M, Michaelson MD, Abdeen MA: The pharmacologic approach to the treatment of obesity. J Clin Pharmacol 1997; 37: 453-473.

36. Blair SN, Kampert JB, Kohl HW III, et al: Influence of cardiorespiratory fitness and other precursors on cardiovascular disease and all-cause mortality in men and women. JAMA 1996; 276: 205-210.

37. Frishman WH, Nurenberg JR, Frishman E: Cardiovascular considerations with use of psychoactive medications. In, Frishman WH, Sonnenblick EH: Cardiovascular Pharmacotherapeutics. New York: McGraw Hill Inc., 1997: 1039-1052.

38. Ridker PM, Manson JE, Gaziano JM, Buring JE, Hennekens CH: Low dose aspirin therapy for chronic stable angina. Ann Intern Med 1991; 114: 835-839.

39. Antiplatelet Trialists' Collaboration: Collaborative overview of randomised trials of anti-platelet therapy-1: Prevention of death, myocardial infarction and stroke by prolonged antiplatelet therapy in various categories of patients. Br Med J 1995; 308: 81-106.

40. Aarons L, Hopkins K, Rowland M, Brossel S, Thiercelin JF: Route of administration and sex differences in the pharmacokinetics of aspirin, administered as its lysine salt. Pharm Res. 1989; 6: 660-666.

41. Ho PC, Triggs EJ, Bourne DWA, Heazlewood VJ: The effects of age and sex on the disposition of acetylsalicylic acid and its metabolites. Br J Clin Pharm 1985; 19: 675-684.

42. Escolar G, Bastida E, Garrido M, Rodriguez-Gomez J, Castillo R, Ordinas A: Sex-related differences in the effects of aspirin on the interaction of platelets with subendothelium. Thromb Res 1986; 44: 837-847.

43. Spranger M, Aspey BS, Harrison MJC: Sex differences in antithrombotic effect of aspirin. Stroke 1989; 20: 34-37.

44. Paganini-Hill A, Chao A, Ross RK, Henderson BE: Aspirin use and chronic diseases: a cohort study of the elderly. Br Med J 1989; 299: 1247-1250.

45. The Aspirin Myocardial Infarction Study Research Group: The Aspirin Myocardial Infarction Study: final results. Circulation 1980; 62 (Suppl V): V79-84.

46. Manson JE, Stampfer MJ, Colditz GA, Willet WC, Rosner B, Speizer FE, Hennekens CH: A prospective study of aspirin use and primary prevention of cardiovascular disease in women. JAMA 1991; 266: 521-527.

47. Second International Study of Infarct Survivors (ISIS-2) Collaborative Group: Randomized trial of intravenous streptokinase, oral aspirin, both, or neither among 17,187 cases of suspected acute myocardial infarction: ISIS-2. Lancet 1988; 2: 349-360.

48. Harpaz D, Benderly M, Goldbourt U, Kishon Y, Behar S: Effect of aspirin on mortality in women with symptomatic or silent myocardial ischemia. Am J Cardiol 1996; 78: 1215-1219.

49. Zimetbaum P, Frishman WH, Ooi WL, et al: Plasma lipid and lipoproteins and the incidence of cardiovascular disease in the old old: The Bronx Longitudinal Aging Study. Arterio & Thrombo 1992; 12: 416-423.

50. Fetters JK, Peterson Ed, Shaw LS, Newby LK, Califf RM: Sex-specific difference in coronary artery disease risk factors, evaluation and treatment: have they been adequately evaluated? Am Heart J 1996; 131: 796-813.

51. LaRosa JC, Applegate W, Crouse JR III, et al: Cholesterol lowering in the elderly: Results of the Cholesterol Reduction in Seniors Program (CRISP) pilot study. Arch Intern Med 1994; 154: 529-539.

52. Scandinavian Simvastatin Survival Study Group: Randomized trial of cholesterol lowering in 4444 patients with coronary heart disease: the Scandinavian Simvastatin Survival Study (4S): Lancet 1994; 344: 1383-1389.

53. Frishman WH, Clark A, Johnson B: Effects of cardiovascular drugs on plasma lipids and lipoproteins. In, Frishman WH, Sonnenblick EH (eds): Cardiovascular Pharmacotherapeutics. New York: McGraw Hill Inc., 1997: 1515-1559.

54. D'Agostino RB, Kannel WB, Stepanians MN, D'Agostino LC: Efficacy and tolerability of lovastatin in women. Clin Ther 1992; 14: 390-395.

55. Walsh JM, Grady D: Treatment of hyperlipidemia in women. JAMA 1995; 274: 1152-1158.

56. Adult Treatment Panel II: Summary of the Second Report of the National Cholesterol Education Program (NCEP) Expert Panel on Detection, Evaluation and Treatment of High Blood Cholesterol in Adults. JAMA 1993; 269: 3015-3023.

57. Saltzberg S, Stroh JA, Frishman WH: Isolated systolic hypertension in the elderly: pathophysiology and treatment. Med Clinics N Amer 1988; 72(2): 523-547.

58. Kahn S, Frishman WH, Weissman S, Ooi WL, Aronson M: Left ventricular hypertrophy on electrocardiogram: prognostic implications from a 10 year cohort study of older subjects. A report from the Bronx Longitudinal Aging Study. J Am Geriat Soc 1996; 44: 524-529.

59. Frishman WH, Michaelson MD: Use of calcium antagonists in patients with ischemic heart disease and systemic hypertension. Symposium issue. Am J Cardiol 1997; 79(10A): 33-38.

60. Davis BR, Cutler JA, Gordon DJ, et al for the ALLHAT Research Group: Rationale and design for the Antihypertensive and Lipid Lowering Treatment to Prevent Heart Attack Trial (ALLHAT). Am J Hypertens 1996; 9: 342-360.

61. Hansson L, Zanchetti A, Carruthers SG, et al for the HOT Study Group: Effects of intensive blood-pressure lowering and acetylsalicylic acid in patients with hypertension: principal results of the Hypertension Optimal Treatment (HOT) randomised trial. Lancet 1998; 351: 1755-1762.

62. Task Force of the Working Group on Heart Failure of the European Society of Cardiology: The treatment of heart failure. Eur Heart J 1997; 18: 736-753.

63. Gomberg-Maitland M, Frishman WH, Karch S, Schwartz J, Freeman R, Shapiro J: Hormones as cardiovascular drugs: estrogens, progestins, thyroxine, growth hormone, corticosteroids and testosterone. In, Frishman WH, Sonnenblick EH: Cardiovascular Pharmacotherapeutics. New York: McGraw Hill Inc., 1997: 787-835.

64. Holdright GR, Sullivan AK, Wright JL, Sparrow JL, Cunningham D, Fox KM: Acute effect of oestrogen replacement therapy on treadmill performance in post-menopausal women with coronary artery disease.. Eur Heart J 1995; 16: 1566-1570.

65. Rosano GMC, Sarrel PM, Poole-Wilson PA, Collins P: Beneficial effect of oestrogen on exercise-induced myocardial ischaemia in women with coronary artery disease. Lancet 1993; 342: 133-136.

66. Egashira K, Inou T, Hirooka Y, Yamada A, Urabe Y, Takeshita A: Evidence of impaired endothelium-dependent coronary vasodilation in patients with angina pectoris and normal coronary angiograms. N Engl J Med 1993; 328: 1659-1664.

67. Vakili BA, Frishman WH, Lin TS, Boczko J, Gurell D, Hussain J: Antioxidant vitamins and enzymatic and synthetic scavengers of oxygen-derived free radical scavengers in the prevention and treatment of cardiovascular diseases. In, Frishman WH, Sonnenblick EH: Cardiovascular Pharmacotherapeutics. New York: McGraw Hill Inc., 1997: 535-556.

68. Stampfer MJ, Hennekens CH, Manson JE, Colditz GA, Rosner B, Willett WC: Vitamin E consumption and the risk of coronary disease in women. N Engl J Med 1993; 328: 1444-1449.

69. Kushi L,H Folsom AR, Prineas RJ, Mink PJ, Wu Y, Bostick RM: Dietary antioxidant vitamins and death from coronary heart disease in post menopausal women. N Engl J Med 1996; 334: 1156-1162.

70. Schwartz SM, Siscovick DS, Malinow MR, et al: Myocardial infarction in young women in relation to plasma total homocysteine, folate, and a common variant in the methylenetetrahydrofolate reductase gene. Circulation 1997; 96: 412-417.

71. Abrams J: The organic nitrates and nitroprusside. In, Frishman WH, Sonnenblick EH: Cardiovascular Pharmacotherapeutics. New York: McGraw Hill Inc., 1997: 253-265.

72. Bennett BM, Twiddy DAS, Moffat JA, Armstrong PW, Marks GS: Sex related difference in the metabolism of isosorbide dinitrate following incubation in human blood. Biochem Pharmacol 1983; 32: 3729-3734.

73. Tam GS, Marks GS, Brien JF, Nakatsu K: Sex and species related differences in the bio-transformation of isosorbide dinitrate by various tissues of the rabbit and rat. Can JPhysiol Pharmacol 1987; 65: 1478-1483.

74. Frishman WH; Alpha- and beta-adrenergic blocking drugs. In, Frishman WH, Sonnenblick EH: Cardiovascular Pharmacotherapeutics. New York: McGraw Hill Inc., 1997: 59-94.

75. Frishman WH: Carvediolol. N Engl J Med 1998 in press.

76. Frishman WH: Calcium channel blockers. In, Frishman WH, Sonnenblick EH: Cardiovascular Pharmacotherapeutics. New York: McGraw Hill Inc., 1997: 101-130.

77. Savonitto S, Ardissiono D, Egstrup K, et al: Combination therapy with metoprolol and nifedipine versus monotherapy in patients with stable angina pectoris. Results of the International Multicenter Angina Exercise (IMAGE) Study. J Am Coll Cardiol 1996; 27: 311-316.

78. LeJemtel TH, Sonnenblick EH, Frishman WH: The diagnosis and management of heart failure. In, Alexander RW, Schlant RC, Fuster V (eds): Hurst's The Heart, 9th ed. New York: McGraw Hill Inc., 1998: 745-781.

3

MANAGEMENT OF UNSTABLE ANGINA USING RISK STRATIFICATION METHODS

James E. Calvin, MD and Lloyd W. Klein, MD
Rush-Presbyterian-St. Luke's Medical Center, Chicago, Illinois

INTRODUCTION

In the current era of health care reform, the efficacies of various management strategies are being scrutinized using measures of patient outcomes, quality of life, and costs. Acute coronary ischemic syndromes such as acute myocardial infarction (AMI) and unstable angina (UA) have received a great deal of attention because of their frequency (approximately 1,500,000 myocardial infarctions and 570,000 admissions for unstable angina annually in the US), their potential morbidity and mortality, and the costliness of newer treatment modalities. Some studies evaluating cost-effectiveness of care have suggested that many patients with suspected myocardial infarction or unstable angina can be adequately treated in a coronary stepdown or intermediate care unit at lower cost than if they are admitted to a coronary care unit. The inference is that the highest level of care is neither necessary nor cost-effective for all patients with suspected myocardial infarction or unstable angina[1-4] and better patient triage might be a reasonable cost effective strategy.

RISK STRATIFICATION - RATIONALE

Risk stratification is the initial goal in evaluating all patients with chest pain, as the appropriate level of risk inherent in any strategy must match the anticipated degree of risk and the likelihood of preventing adverse events. Timing and therapeutic initiatives are guided by the risk and the capability to intervene effectively. The traditional approach has been to focus on the patient at high risk in whom rapid therapy can improve outcome.

The primary issue to be addressed in the patient with an acute ischemic syndrome is to identify those patients who are candidates for thrombolytic therapy or angioplasty: ST segment elevation myocardial infarction must be excluded immediately. Beyond this, ST depression and new T wave changes have been shown to be associated with adverse outcomes in both non-Q infarcts and unstable angina.

An alternative approach receiving high interest recently is to emphasize identification of the low risk patient. This strategy reduces CCU admissions, hence cost, of patients at low risk (the "soft R/O MI") by identifying those treatable in step down or observation units. This strategy recognizes the need to improve patient care through the effective allocation of resources and enhanced efficacy while reducing cost overall.   It is critical to recognize that using tests appropriately to identify those patients with ischemia at moderate or high risk allows both reduction of total resource consumption while ensuring that expenditures are rationally adjusted to risk, improving outcomes. Several reports have demonstrated cost reductions or improved resource utilization and outcome but no study addresses whether both are compatible. Gaspoz[5] showed that step-down, non-CCU admissions or early home discharge could be accomplished with cost saving, but the rate of complications was similar to those admitted to the CCU. Gomez[6] randomized patients to a rapid rule out protocol vs. standard care and showed significant cost savings but no difference in outcome. Calvin[4] showed that step-down unit admissions for moderate risk patients saved substantially compared to admission to the CCU with no difference in complications. Our group also recently showed that guideline reminders can improve outcomes subtly, with cost savings overall compared to standard care, but the guidelines used did not seek to influence physician decision regarding unit triage.

MODELS PREDICTIVE OF RISK

Incorporating the clinical elements predictive of adverse outcome in unstable angina and acute chest pain syndromes into mathematical models has been attempted by numerous investigators.[7-12] All are sensitive tools, comparable to physician judgment, for identifying patients at short-term increased risk. However, they perform better at identifying those at highest risk, compared to expert judgment, than those determined to be at lower risk, resulting in fewer patients being considered candidates for hospital admission and observation. This is likely because most of these models assign high values to clinical factors other than the quality, frequency or severity of the chest pain syndrome, as a treating physician would. This likely explains why these algorithms have not achieved widespread clinical use - the absence of a factor for "clinical judgment" - which the physician appears to value, even though this creates a tendency for physicians to overestimate the risk of patients at low risk, resulting in increased, possibly unnecessary, hospital admissions.

FACTORS ASSOCIATED WITH INCREASED RISK IN PATIENTS WITH UNSTABLE ANGINA

The standard clinical factors predictive of an increased risk of developing coronary artery disease, (such as hypertension, smoking, hypercholesterolemia, diabetes, obesity and family history), are not useful in assessing the likelihood of the occurrence of myocardial infarction or other adverse events (death, ventricular arrhythmia, need for revascularization) in the patient presenting with acute coronary syndrome. Lee et al[13] retrospectively analyzed factors predictive of outcome in 596 patients admitted with unstable angina and found that only older age and male gender were predictive. In a later study,[14] only a history of prior angina or MI and age >40 years were predictive of MI. Selker[15] and Goldman[16] showed that only age >60 and male gender were strongly predictive of cardiac ischemia.

Fuchs and Scheidt[17] analyzed a group of 414 consecutive admissions with known or suspected coronary artery disease, finding that one or more of 3 variables (ongoing chest pain, pulmonary rales, and one or more ventricular premature beats) identified 306 high risk patients, 41% of whom received lifesaving interventions. In a group of 108 patients without any of these criteria, only 6% received lifesaving interventions. Gheorghiade and co-workers[18] determined in 2162 consecutively admitted patients with a diagnosis of suspected myocardial infarction that 16 clinical criteria could identify a low-risk group that had a 0.9% risk of life-threatening complications and 10% likelihood of actually ruling in for myocardial infarction. This ability to predict not only myocardial infarction but also the risk of a life-threatening complication was underscored by Fineberg et al,[1] who demonstrated the cost effectiveness of treatment in an intermediate care unit for patients with a low probability (< 5%) of acute myocardial infarction.

RISK STRATIFICATION STRATEGIES

Other investigators[7, 10, 19-21] have developed algorithms or models for the management of all chest pain syndromes including, but not limited to, unstable angina. These studies usually use either multiple logistic regression or recursive partitioning to stratify subjects into risk groups. However, this earlier work is not specific enough to make it useful for stratifying unstable angina patients. The low risk categories in these models still have a 2-5% rate of myocardial infarction.

In a multiple center study of 5,773 emergency room patients, Selker and colleagues[15] developed, using multiple logistic regression analysis, a predictive model based on 3,453 of these patients and tested its prognostic ability on the subsequent 2,320 patients. The overall incidence of acute cardiac ischemia was 36% and of myocardial infarction was 19% . The model, developed to predict acute cardiac ischemia, was based on seven easily obtained clinical factors (age, sex, chest pain presence on admission, chest pain as chief complaint, Q waves, ST shift, and T wave changes). Quartiles based on the probability of cardiac ischemia estimated from the model identified low, medium, and high-risk populations where the incidence of myocardial infarction ranged from 0.17-1.8%, to 49.7-53.3%, respectively. However, patients with estimated probabilities of acute ischemia greater than 10% had observed rates of infarction that varied from 4.4-53.3%.

Goldman and colleagues[10] analyzed 482 patients admitted to a single center. Using recursive partitioning they developed a decision tree based on the identification of myocardial infarction.

Of these 482 patients, 60 (12.4%) had an acute myocardial infarction. In prospective testing on 468 other patients, 85 (18%) had acute myocardial infarction. Validation of the protocol in the prospective cohort showed that patients were at low risk of having sustained an acute myocardial infarction if the probability estimate of such an occurrence was < 1/15. This model correctly identified 80 of 85 patients with acute myocardial infarction. However, 10% of patients judged to be at low risk sustained an acute myocardial infarction. Of patients who were not expected to have an infarction, 5% did.

In a subsequent study, Goldman and colleagues[14] refined the decision tree on a group of 1,379 patients admitted with acute chest pain and tested the model prospectively in 4,770 patients. The overall incidence of acute myocardial infarction in the validation population was 8%. In patients who were judged to have < 7% chance of myocardial infarction and who largely had atypical chest pain the acute infarction rate was 2%. It is unclear whether patients with a high likelihood of unstable angina on clinical grounds would demonstrate the same low risk of acute myocardial infarction or death.

Tierney[19] considered a group of patients who ultimately had an incidence of myocardial infarction of 34%. In contrast to the previous three studies, Tierney demonstrated that the lowest risk category had an incidence of acute myocardial infarction of 8.1%. In none of these studies was early stress testing used to identify a very low risk group of patients with an incidence of serious cardiac complication <1%.

In 1995, the Agency for Health Care Policy and Research (AHCPR) published guidelines for the management of unstable angina, proposing an evidenced-based approach to acute chest pain syndromes.[22] Unstable angina was categorized into 3 tiers: high, intermediate and low risk. Low risk was defined in such a way as to encompass the spectrum of very atypical pain syndromes in which immediate hospitalization was not required. The relative merits of an early invasive versus conservative approach was addressed, and the various diagnostic and therapeutic modalities discussed. These AHCPR Guidelines stress two important components in the initial assessment of unstable angina patients: 1) an assessment of the likelihood of coronary artery disease (Tables 1 and 2) an assessment of the risk of adverse outcomes (Table 2). These two assessments allow a stratification of patients into high, intermediate, and low risk. Low risk patients were free of rest pain and had a normal ECG. This category only constitutes 5-6% of potential patients presenting to the emergency room[23] and recent data from our group suggests that the MI or death rate to be 4.8%.[24]

We recently published a predictive model that elaborates on a scheme proposed by Braunwald.[11, 12] Six predictors including recent MI, age, diabetes, ST depression, prior antianginal therapy and ongoing chest pain are used to calculate an actual probability of major complications. We have validated this model statistically and on a new population of patients[24] and have found that the likelihood of a complication predicts resource consumption.[25] This model is particularly good at predicting low and medium risk patient, making it a useful tool for triage in the emergency room. In our predictive model low risk patients may have rest pain but only one of the following risk factors, age > 65y, ST depression, ≥ 1 mm, diabetes, but does not allow the presence of prolonged chest pain. Using this model we can identify a low risk group who had an event rate of 2% (AHA abstract, 1997) and comprise more than 25% of patients presenting with chest pain. Another advantage of our model is that all predictors are readily attainable without the need of expensive testing and is a fairly straightforward way to estimate a patient's overall odds or probability of suffering a major cardiac complication. The primary limitation is that the low-risk group has an estimated probability of early cardiac complication of 4.2%, although the risk of myocardial infarction or death is 1.4%.

Table 1. Short-term risk of death or nonfatal myocardial infarction in patients with unstable angina

High Risk	Intermediate Risk	Low Risk
At least one of the following features must be present:	No high-risk feature but must have any of the following:	No high- or intermediate-risk feature but may have any of the following features:
Prolonged ongoing (>20 mins) rest pain	Prolonged (>20 mins) rest angina, now resolved, with moderate or high likelihood of CAD	Increased angina frequency, severity, or duration
Pulmonary edema, most likely related to ischemia	Rest angina (>20 mins or relieved with rest or sublingual nitroglycerin	Angina provoked at a lower threshold
Angina at rest with dynamic ST changes ≥1 mm	Nocturnal angina	New onset angina with onset 2 weeks to 2 months prior to presentation
Angina with new or worsening MR murmur	Angina with dynamic T-wave changes	Normal or unchanged ECG
Angina with S3 or new/worsening rales	New onset CCSC[1] III or IV angina in the past 2 weeks with moderate or high likelihood of CAD	Normal or unchanged ECG
Angina with hypotension	Pathologic Q waves or resting ST depression #1 mm in multiple lead groups (anterior, inferior, lateral	

[1]*CCSC = Canadian Cardiovascular Society classification*

Table 2 Calvin - Klein Predictive Model

Predictors of All Major Cardiac complications: Results of Multiple Logistic Regression Using Braunwald Criteria, Diabetes, and Age*

Variables	Odds Ratio	95% Confidence Intervals
Post MI (< 14 d)	5.72	1.92-16.97
Requiring IV NTG on admissions	2.33	1.31-4.17
No β-blocker or rate-lowering calcium channel blocker	3.83	1.55-9.42
Baseline ST depression	2.81	1.45-5.47
Diabetes Mellitus	2.19	1.25-3.83
Incremental decade of age	1.48	1.21-1.90
Constant	0.11	0.07-0.18

*MI indicates myocardial infarction; IV, intravenous; and NTG, nitroglycerin

PRACTICE GUIDELINES, CRITICAL PATHWAYS, AND CLINICAL PROTOCOLS IN CLINICAL PRACTICE

Since the mathematical models have failed to significantly influence triage decisions, primarily because of their complex numerical nature and their insensitivity to physician judgment, a different approach is currently in vogue. This strategy entails the development of a structured pre-defined formula or outline of management applied by the physician. These instruments have the additional advantage of being developed at the location of use to incorporate the usual practice pattern among participating physicians. The disadvantage, of course, is that they become a document produced by committee, affected as much by local opinion and political concerns as scientific evidence. Nevertheless, by narrowing the variations in clinical care, it is hoped that adherence would raise the quality of medical care and correct inappropriate resource utilization.

Actual experience in the field, however, shows that while the AHCPR guidelines were developed by expert opinion, and wide consensus supported by the latest research, local implementation can be met with resistance and lack of adherence. Weingarten[26] showed that guidelines can be affective in reducing hospital length of stay but were only adhered to when reminders were placed on charts. Calvin[27, 28] showed that guideline reminders can be effective, even after being maintained for 1 year.

THE ROLE OF STRESS TESTING IN UNSTABLE ANGINA

Although it may be possible to identify a low-risk group of patients based on clinical factors, some form of further testing will be necessary. Noninvasive testing for risk stratification in unstable angina has been proposed by several authors, especially for patients who have responded initially to medical therapy over the first few days of admission. Noninvasive or functional stress testing refers to tests that provoke myocardial ischemia by either exercise or pharmacological means. They are based on the premise that progressive physiological stresses increase myocardial workload and oxygen demand and can induce heterogeneity of regional blood flow, which can be detected by either electrocardiographic, nuclear or echocardiographic means. Markers of functional capacity under physiological stress, such as exercise duration and metabolic equivalents (METs), can be used to identify high-risk patients. These patients develop ischemia at low workloads (< 6 METs) or develop hypotension and marked or prolonged ST depression. Large areas of reversible ischemia detected by nuclear scanning or echocardiography also suggest higher risk. Low-risk patients, who have excellent exercise tolerance, have a good prognosis and may be considered for conservative strategy. Pharmacological stresses such as dipyridamole[29] and dobutamine,[30] infusions, when combined with either nuclear or echocardiographic imaging, may be useful in patients who cannot exercise. In our institution the immediate availability of stress dobutamine echocardiography has made it an attractive alternative.

Figure 1.

The Ability of Exercise Testing to Predict Events in Unstable Angina

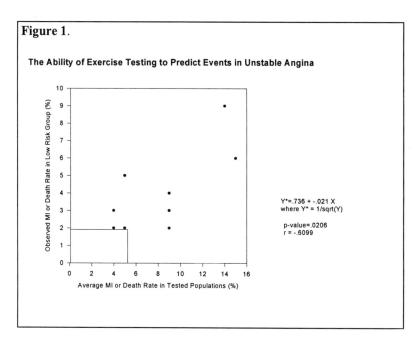

$Y^{*} = .736 + .021 X$
where $Y^{*} = 1/\mathrm{sqrt}(Y)$

p-value=.0206
r = -.6099

The role of stress electrocardiography to prognosticate has been the subject of 2 large trials. The first trial, the Multicenter Myocardial Ischemia Research Group[31] studied 936 patients who had a recent hospitalization for myocardial infarction (70%) or unstable angina (30%). Using a composite endpoint of death, recurrent myocardial infarction or unstable angina during a 23 month follow-up, they determined that the combination of ST depression and an exercise duration < 9 minutes identified patients at a 3.4 fold (< 6 minutes) or 1.9 fold (6-9 minutes) increase in risk of cardiac events. A reversible thallium defect plus increased lung thallium uptake indicated a 2.8 fold increase in risk. A sole reversible thallium defect signified only a 1.2 fold increase in risk.

The second trial, the RISC trial,[32] studied 740 men with unstable angina or non-Q MI also revealed that a combination of ST depression and low workload were independent predictors of 1 year infarct-free survival.

Meta-analysis of studies of stress testing[33-39] (Table 3) reveals that negative results on stress testing confer a 1-9% chance of mortality or of the population tested. The results of studies of the prognostic value of stress testing after acute coronary syndromes where more than 10 events were observed in follow-up[40] shows that the difference between observed event rate in the patients deemed to be at low risk after stress testing (i.e., "post-test" probability) is linearly related to the observed event rate in the entire study population (pre-test probability). By choosing a low risk group for early stress testing, an extremely low post-test probability may be obtained. Hence, the value of a good clinical prediction model (such as ours) is apparent.

Table 3. Noninvasive studies in patients with unstable angina reporting at least 10 cardiac events (cardiac death or myocardial infarction) during follow-up

Study	Inclusion criteria	Low risk	High risk
Moss, Goldstein, Hall et al, 1993[31]	30% unstable angina; 26% Non-Q-wave MI	893	23
Swahn, Areskog, Berglund et al, 1987[37]	All unstable angina	247	145
Severi, Orsini, Marraccini et al, 1988[38]	All unstable angina	199	175
Madsen, Thomsen, Mellemgaard et al, 1988[36]	All unstable angina	118	98
Nyman, Larsson, Areskog et al, 1992[32]	All unstable angina	366	374
Krone, Dwyer, Greenberg et al, 1989[41]	All non-Q wave MI	85	7
Moss, Goldstein, Hall et al, 1993[31]	30% unstable angina; 26% Non-Q wave MI	876	20
Madsen, Thomsen, Mellemgaard et al, 1988[36]	All unstable angina	129	29
Gibson, Beller, Gheorghiade et al, 1989[42]	36% Non-Q-wave MI; 64% MI	133	108
Younis, Byers, Shaw et al, 1989[43]	58% unstable angina, 42% MI	14	54

The AHCPR Guidelines specifically recommend that stress testing be performed within 72 h if patients are being managed conservatively. Our experience[44] suggests that 68% of major cardiac complications actually occur within the first 48 h of presentation. Therefore, we believe stress testing, if used in lower-risk groups of patients, should be considered within 24 h of presentation unless clinical prediction of risk is < 1% (See Chapter 1).

A SUGGESTED CRITICAL PATHWAY FOR UNSTABLE ANGINA

Integrating our knowledge about risk stratification in unstable angina with published guidelines on the evaluation and management of unstable angina, we believe care can be optimized for all patients by the use of the critical pathway which is presented in algorithmic form in Figure 2. Low risk unstable angina patients are evaluated and managed in the emergency room and observation unit using a pathway specific for these patients. This pathway allows for early discharge in low risk patients who have a negative provocative test (stress ECG, stress thallium or stress echo). The choice of stress testing should be consistent with AHCPR guidelines and should be based on patient's resting ECG and his or her physical ability to exercise. Standard ECG stress testing is indicated for patients with normal resting ECG and not taking digoxin. A nanogram proposed by Mark et al[39] can be used to assess risk using the presence of chest pain, amount of ST depression and workload. An imaging modality should be considered for patients with widespread ST depression, ST changes due to digoxin, LVH and conduction abnormalities or pre-excitation syndromes. Pharmacological stress testing is indicated for patients who cannot exercise physically. Patients at higher risk are admitted to either CCU or CSU as outlined in Figure 2. The designation of high risk is based on predictors suggested by AHCPR and our own model. High risk patients should have early angiography considered. All admitted intermediate and high risk patients should receive intensive medical therapy. Invasive evaluation should be completed within 48 hours. Patients selected for conservative strategies should have stress tests completed within 48 hours of being free from angina or heart failure and noninvasive evaluation of ventricular function should be performed. Medical therapy should be consistent with AHCPR guidelines (Tables 4 and 5).

Figure 2. **Clinical Evaluation and Management of Unstable Angina**

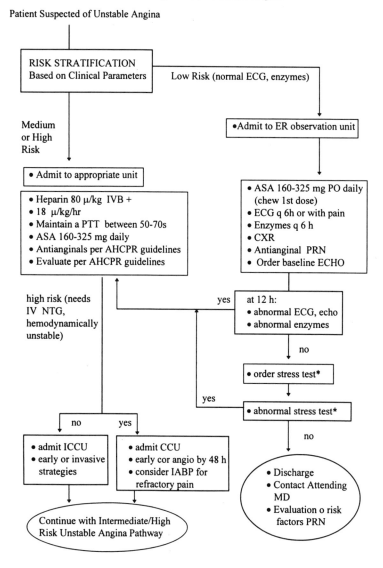

*Standard ECG stress testing is indicated for patients with normal resting ECG and not taking digoxin. An imaging modality should be considered for patients with widespread ST depression, ST changes due to digoxin, LVH and conduction abnormalities or pre-excitation syndromes. Pharmacological stress testing is indicated for patients who cannot exercise physically.

Table 4. Drugs commonly used in intensive medical management of patients with unstable angina

Drug category	Clinical condition	When to avoid[1]
Aspirin[2]	Unstable angina	• Hypersensitivity • Active bleeding • Severe bleeding risk
Heparin	Unstable angina in high-risk category	• Active bleeding • History of heparin-induced thrombocytopenia • Severe bleeding risk • Recent stroke
Nitrates	Symptoms are not fully relieved with three sublingual nitroglycerin tablets and initiation of beta blocker therapy	• Hypotension
Beta blockers [3]	Unstable angina	• PR ECG segment > 0.24 seconds • 2° or 3° atrioventricular (AV) block • Heart rate <60 • Blood pressure < 90 mmHg • Shock • Left ventricular failure with congestive heart failure • Severe reactive airway disease
Calcium channel blockers	Patients already on adequate doses of nitrates and beta blockers or in patients unable to tolerate adequate doses of one or both of these agents or in patients with variant angina	• Pulmonary edema • Evidence of left ventricular dysfunction
Morphine sulfate	Patients whose symptoms are not relieved after three serial sublingual nitroglycerin tablets or whose symptoms recur with adequate anti-ischemic therapy	• Hypotension • Respiratory depression • Confusion • Obtundation

[1]Allergy or prior intolerance contraindication for all categories of drugs listed in this chart.

[2]Patients unstable to take aspirin because of a history of hypersensitivity or major gastrointestinal intolerance should be started on ticlopidine 250 mg twice a day as a substitute.

[3]Choice of the specific agent is not as important as ensuring that appropriate candidates receive this therapy. If there are concerns about patient intolerance due to existing pulmonary disease, especially asthma, left ventricular dysfunction, or risk of hypotension or severe bradycardia, initial selection should favor a short-acting agent, such as propranolol or metoprolol or the ultra short-acting agent, esmolol. Mild wheezing or a history of chronic obstructive pulmonary disease should prompt a trial of a short-acting agent at a reduced dose (e.g., 2.5 mg intravenous metoprolol, 12.5 mg oral metoprolol, or 25 mcg/kg/min esmolol as initial doses) rather than complete avoidance of beta-blocker therapy.

Table 5. Drug Doses

Drug category	Dose
Aspirin[2]	• 324 mg (160-324) daily
Heparin	• 80 units/kg intravenous (IV) bolus • Constant intravenous infusion at 18 units/kg/hr • Titrated to maintain aPTT between 1.5 to 2.5 times control
Nitrates	• 5 to 10 mcg/min by continuous infusion • Titrated up to 75 to 100 mcg/min until relief of symptoms or limiting side-effects (headache or hypotension with a systolic blood pressure <90 mmHg or more than 30 percent below starting mean arterial pressure levels if significant hypertension is present) • Topical, oral, or buccal nitrates are acceptable alternatives for patients without ongoing or refractory symptoms
Beta blockers [3]	• **Metroprolol** • 5 mg increments by slow (over 1 to 2 minutes) intravenous administration • Repeated every 5 minutes for a total initial dose of 15 mg • Followed in 1 to 2 hours by 25 to 50 mg by mouth every 6 hours • If a very conservative regimen is desired, initial dose can be reduced to 1 to 2 mg • **Propranolol** • 0.5 to 1.0 mg intravenous dose • Followed in 1 to 2 hours by 40 to 80 mg by mouth every 6 to 8 hours • **Esmolol** • Starting maintenance dose of 0.1 mg/kg/min intravenously • Titration in increments of 0.05 mg/kg/min every 10 to 15 minutes as tolerated by blood pressure until the desired therapeutic response has been obtained, limiting symptoms develop, or a dose of 0.20 mg/kg/min is reached • Optional loading dose of 0.5 mg/kg may be given by slow intravenous administration (2 to 5 minutes) for more rapid onset of action • **Atenolol** • 5 mg intravenous dose • Followed 5 minutes later by a second 5 mg intravenous dose and then 50 to 100 mg orally every day initiated 1 to 2 hours after the intravenous dose
Calcium channel blockers	• Dependent on specific agent
Morphine sulfate	• 2 to 5 mg intravenous dose • May be repeated every 5 to 30 minutes as needed to relieve symptoms and maintain patient comfort

[2]Patients unstable to take aspirin because of a history of hypersensitivity or major gastrointestinal intolerance should be started on ticlopidine 250 mg twice a day as a substitute.

[3]Choice of the specific agent is not as important as ensuring that appropriate candidates receive this therapy. If there are concerns about patient intolerance due to existing pulmonary disease, especially asthma, left ventricular dysfunction, or risk of hypotension or severe bradycardia, initial selection should favor a short-acting agent, such as propranolol or metoprolol or the ultra short-acting agent, esmolol. Mild wheezing or a history of chronic obstructive pulmonary disease should prompt a trial of a short-acting agent at a reduced dose (e.g., 2.5 mg intravenous metoprolol, 12.5 mg oral metoprolol, or 25 mcg/kg/min esmolol as initial doses) rather than complete avoidance of beta-blocker therapy.

NOTE: Some of the recommendations in this guide suggest the use of agents for purposes or in doses other than those specified by the Food and Drug Administration (FDA). Such recommendations are made after consideration of concerns regarding non approved indications. Where made, such recommendations are based on more recent clinical trials or expert consensus.

Revascularization should be considered as soon as possible after evaluation is completed and promptly scheduled.

Patients in whom medical therapy is chosen should be weaned from intravenous medications, converted to oral antianginals and aspirin and ambulated prior to hospital discharge.

References:

1.   Fineberg HV, Scadden D, Goldman L. Care of patients with a low probability of acute myocardial infarction: Cost effectiveness of alternatives to coronary care unit admission. New England Journal of Medicine 1984; 310:1301-1307.

2.   Fiebach N, Cook E, Lee T, Brand D, Rouan G, Weisberg M, et al. .Outcomes in patients with myocardial infarction who are initially admitted to stepdown unit: data from the multicenter chest pain study. American Journal of Medicine 1990; 89:15-20.

3.   Udvarhelyi I, Goldman L, Komaroff A, Lee T. Determinants of resource utilization for patients admitted for evaluation of acute chest pain. Journal of General Internal Medicine 1992; 7:1-10.

4.   Calvin JE, VandenBerg BJ, Ramirez-Morgen L, Klein L, Parrillo J. Does admission to an intermediate care unit (CICU) influence management strategies or outcomes in unstable angina? Clinical Research 1994; 42(2):248A.

5.   Gaspoz JM, Lee TH, Weinstein MC, Cook EF, Goldman P, Komaroff AL, et al. Cost-effectiveness of a new short-stay unit to "rule out" acute myocardial infarction in low risk patients. Journal of the American College of Cardiology 1994; 24:1249-1259.

6.   Gomez M, Anderson J, Karagounis L, et al. An Emergency Department-Based Protocol for Rapidly Ruling Out Myocardial Ischemia Reduces Hospital Time and Expense: Results of A randomized Study (ROMIO). Journal of American College of Cardiology 1996; 28:25-33.

7.   Pozen M, D'Agostino R, Selker H, Sytkowski P, Hood W, Jr. A predictive instrument to improve coronary-care-unit admission practices in acute ischemic heart disease: a prospective multicenter clinical trial. New England Journal of Medicine 1984; 310:1273-1278.

8.   Aase O, Jonsbu JK, Liestol L et al. Decision support by computer analysis of selected case history variables in the emergency room among patients with acute chest pain. European Heart Journal 1993; 14:433-40.

9.   Baxt W, Skora J. Prospective validation of artificial neural network trained to identify acute myocardial infarction. Lancet 1996; 347:12-15.

10.   Goldman L, Weinberg M, Weisberg M, Olshen R, Cook E . Sargent R.A computer-derived protocol to aid in the diagnoses of emergency room patient with acute chest pain. New England Journal of Medicine 1982; 307:588-596.

11.   Braunwald E. Unstable angina: A classification. Circulation 1989; 80:410-414.

12.   Calvin JE, Klein LW, VandenBerg BJ et al. Risk stratification in unstable angina: prospective validation of the Braunwald Classification. Journal of American Medical Association 1995; 273:136-141.

13.   Lee T, Cook E, Weisberg M, et al. Acute chest pain in the emergency room: identification and examination of low-risk patients. Archives of Internal Medicine 1985; 145:65-69.

14.   Goldman L, Cook EF, Brand DA, Lee TH, Rouan GW, Weisberg MC, et al. A computer protocol to predict myocardial infarction in emergency department patients with chest pain. New England Journal of Medicine 1988; 318:797-803.

15.   Selker H, Griffith J, D'Agostino R. A tool for judging coronary care unit admission appropriateness, valid for both real-time and retrospective use: A time-insensitive predictive instrument (TIPI) for acute cardiac ischemia: A multicenter study. Medical Care 1991; 29:610-627.

16.   Goldman L, Cook F, Johnson P, et al. Prediction of the Need for Intensive Carein Patients who Come to Emergency Departments with Acute Chest Pain. New England Journal of Medicine 1996; 334:1498-504.

17.   Fuchs R, Scheidt S. Improved criteria for admission to cardiac care units. Journal of American Medical Association 1981; 246:2037-2041.

18.   Gheorghiade M, nderson J, Rosman H, Lakier J, Velardo B, Goldberg D, et al. Risk identification at the time of admission to coronary care units in patients with suspected myocardial infarction. American Heart Journal 1988; 116:1212-1217.

19.   Tierney W, Roth B, Psaty B, McHenry R, Fitzgerald J, Stump D, et al. Predictors of myocardial infarction in emergency room patients. Critical Care Medicine 1985; 13:526-531.

20.   Pozen M, D'Agostino R, Mitchell J, Rosenfeld D, Guglielmino J, Schwartz M, et al. The usefulness of a predictive instrument to reduce inappropriate admissions to the coronary care unit. Annals of Internal Medicine 1980; 92 (Part 1):238-242.

21.   Brush J, Jr., Brand D, Acampora D, Chalmer B, Wackers F. Use of the initial electrocardiogram to predict in-hospital complications of acute myocardial infarction. New England Journal of Medicine 1985; 312:1137-1141.

22.   Braunwald E, Mark D, Jones R, et al. Unstable angina: diagnosis and management., in Clinical Practice Guideline, Number 10. AHCPR Publication No. 94-0602. 1994, U.S. Department of Health and Human Services: Rockville.

23.   Katz D, Griffin J, Beshansky J. The use of empiric clinical data in the evaluation of practice guidelines for unstable angina. Journal of American Medical Association 1996; 276(19):1568-1574.

24.   Calvin JE, Klein LW, VandenBerg BJ, Meyer P, Parrillo JE, Rush Medical College Chicago, IL. A Simple, Clinically Useful Method of Triage in Unstable Angina. Circulation 1997; 96 (8):I-618.

25.   Calvin JE, Klein LW, Vandenberg BJ, Meyer P, Parrillo JE. Clinical variables predict costs and resource utilization unstable angina. Journal of the American College of Cardiology 1997; 29 (2):350A.

26.   Weingarten S, Riedinger M, Conner L, Lee T, Hoffman I, Johnson B, et al. Practice guidelines and reminders to reduce duration of hospital stay for patients with chest pain. An interventional trial. Annals of Internal Medicine 1994; 120(4):257-63.

27.   Calvin JE, Klein LW, VandenBerg BJ, Spokas D, Hursey T, Parrillo JE, et al. Guideline reminders facilitate adoption of clinical practice guidelines in medium andhigh risk unstable angina. Circulation 1996; 94(8):005.

28.   Iliadis E, Klein LW, VandenBerg BJ, Parrillo JE, Calvin JE. The influence of clinical practice guideline reminders on outcome in medium and high risk unstable angina. Circulation 1997; 96(8):I-504.

29.   Zhu Y, Chung W, Botvinick E, et al. Dipyridamole perfusion scintigraphy: The experience with the application in one hundred seventy patients with known or suspected unstable angina. American Heart Journal 1991; 121:33-43à.

30.   Tanimoto M, Pai RG, Jintapakorn W, Shah PM. Dobutamine Stress Echocardiography for the Diagnosis and Management of Coronary Artery Disease. Clinical Cardiology 1995; 18:252-260.

31.   Moss A, Goldstein R, Hall W, Bigger J Jr, et al. Detection and significance of myocardial ischemia in stable patients after recovery from an acute coronary event. Journal of American Medical Association 1993; May 12:269(18):2418-2419.

32.   Nyman I, Larsson H, Areskog M, Areskog N, Wallentin L. RISC Study Group. The predictive value of silent ischemia at an exercise test before discharge after an episode of unstable coronary artery disease. American Heart Journal 1992; 123:324-331.

33.   Marmur J, Freeman M, Langer A, Armstrong P. Prognosis in medically stabilized unstable angina: early Holter ST-segment monitoring compared with predischarge exercise thallium tomography. Annals of Internal Medicine 1990; 113:575-579.

34.   Nyman I, Wallentin L, Areskog M, Areskog N, Swahn E   RISC Study Group. Risk stratification by early exercise testing after an episode of unstable coronary artery disease. International Journal of Cardiology 1993; 39:131-142.

35.   Larsson H, Areskog M, Areskog NH et al. Should The Exercise Test (ET) be Performed at Discharge or One Later After an Episode of Unstable Angina or Non-Q wave Myocardial Infarction? International Journal of Cardiology Imaging 1991; 7(1):7-14.

36.   Madsen JK, Thomsen BL, Mellemgaard K, et al. Independent prognostic risk factors for patients referred because of suspected acute myocardial infarction without confirmed diagnosis. prognosis after discharge in relation to medical history and non-invasive investigations. European Heart Journal 1988; 9(6):611-618.

37. Swahn E, Areskog M, Berglund U, Walfridsson H, Wallentin L. Predictive importance of clinical findings and a predischarge exercise test in patients with suspected unstable coronary artery disease. American Journal of Cardiology 1987; 59:208-214.

38. Severi S, Orsini E, Marraccini P, et al. The basal electrocardiogram and exercise stress test in assessing prognosis in patients with unstable angina. European Heart Journal 1988; 9:441-446.

39. Mark D, Shaw L, Harrell F, Hlatky M, Lee K, Bengtson J, et al. Prognostic value of a treadmill exercise score in outpatients with suspected coronary artery disease. New England Journal of Medicine 1991; 325:849-853.

40. Bertolet B, Dinerman J, Hartke R, Conti C. Unstable angina: relationship of clinical presentation, coronary artery pathology, and clinical outcome. Clinical Cardiology 1993; 16:116-122.

41. Krone R, Dwyer E, Greenberg H, Miller J Gillespie J. Risk stratification in patients with first non-Q wave infarction: limited value of the early low level exercise test after uncomplicated infarcts. Journal of the American College of Cardiology 1989; 14:31-37.

42. Gibson R, Beller G, Gheorghiade M. The prevalence and clinical significance of residual myocardial ischemia two weeks after uncomplicated non Q-wave infarction: a prospective natural history study. Circulation 1986; 73(6):1186-1198.

43. Younis LT, Byers S, Shaw L, et al. Prognostic value of intravenous dipyridomole thallium scintigraphy after an acute myocardial ischemic event. American Journal of Cardiology 1989; 64(3):161-166.

44. Oldridge N, G Guyatt, Jones N, et al. Effects of Quality of Life With Comprehensive Rehabilitation After Acute Myocardial Infarction. American Journal of Cardiology 1991; 67:1084-1089.

4
EVIDENCE BASED MANAGEMENT OF ACUTE MYOCARDIAL INFARCTION

James E. Calvin, MD
Rush-Presbyterian-St. Luke's Medical Center, Chicago, IL

MANAGEMENT OF ACUTE MYOCARDIAL INFARCTION
CONVENTIONAL TREATMENT

Prior to the use of thrombolytic therapy, therapy for acute myocardial infarction consisted of pain relief, electrocardiographic and blood pressure monitoring, treatment of ventricular arrhythmias, and the management of acute heart failure. The general measures of treatment are listed in Table 1.

Table 1.

General Measures for the Medical Management of Acute Myocardial Infarction

INDICATION	MEASURE	DOSE
Pain Control	- Nitrates	- 0.3-0.4 mg sublingual - IV 10-200 mcg/min
	- Morphine	- 2-8 mg q 5-15 mins titrated to pain control or evidence of hypotension, vomiting, or respiratory depression
	- O$_2$	- 2-4 l by nasal cannula
Infarction Reduction	- Beta blocker	- Metoprolol 5 mg IV q 15 min for 3 doses - then 50-100 mg daily P.O.
		- 24-36 h with progressive ambulation
	- Bed rest	
Monitoring	- 2-3 lead bedside ECG in CCU	- 24-48 h for low risk patients

These measures continue to be used.   However, the benefits of thrombolytic therapy necessitate rapid clinical assessment including an electrocardiogram performed within 15 minutes of arriving in the emergency room.   Oxygen continues to be used to enhance oxygen transport to the myocardium.   Electrocardiographic monitoring should be instituted immediately to both diagnose serious ventricular dysrhythmias and monitor ST-segment changes.   Intravenous lines should be established for the subsequent administration of thrombolytic agents and other medical therapy.   Most clinicians use sublingual nitroglycerin when first encountering the patient.   If the pain continues, intravenous nitroglycerin, starting at a dose of 5 µg per minutes is initially administered and rapidly titrated to control chest pain.   Morphine sulphate in doses of 4 to 8 mg should also be administered.

THROMBOLYTIC THERAPY

In the 1970s, a great deal of attention was focused on reducing infarction size by afterload reduction, thereby reducing myocardial oxygen demand. Mortality reduction was suggested by one series of patients with low cardiac output states[1] whose mortality was reduced compared to historical controls by the use of afterload reduction.   Later, randomized controls have shown improved survival in heart failure by afterload reduction with ACE inhibitors[2-4] and nitrates and hydralazine, [5] but it was not until very recently that any randomized control trials showed mortality benefit with ACE inhibitors after myocardial infarction.[6, 7]

Because the benefits of afterload reduction were not initial dramatic and the consistent of demonstration of benefits of thrombolytic therapy.   The focus of reducing myocardial infarction size and mortality has switched drastically to an emphasis on restoring coronary perfusion.

Streptokinase was first described in 1933[8] and was first used to treat a patient with acute myocardial infarction in 1958.[9] It is a foreign protein produced by Group C streptococci which combines with circulating plasminogen to form an activator complex.   This complex converts plasminogen to plasmin which then acts in fibrin.[10] This agent is antigenic and can cause anaphylaxis.

Anisoylated Plasminogen-Streptokinase Activator Complex binds directly to fibrin.   It is semi-clot specific at low doses.   Its fibrinolytic activity is longer than streptokinase (90-120 min versus 20-25 minutes).[10]

Tissue-Type Plasminogen Activator is the other naturally occurring plasminogen activator found in blood. It occurs as a one-chain molecule or a degraded two-chain molecule. Both are active enzymes. It is relatively inactive in the absence of fibrin, and fibrin significantly enhances the activation rate of plasminogen. This high affinity for plasminogen in the presence of fibrin allows for its clot selectivity. The half life of tPA is 5 minutes. It is not antigenic. All agents can cause significant bleeding. Their doses and characteristics are summarized in Table 2.

The use of intravenous thrombolytic therapy has been popularized because of the extensive number of large multicenter trials over the past 14 years. Several trials[13-19] demonstrated in patients randomized to either intracoronary streptokinase or placebo that intracoronary streptokinase could lyse intracoronary thrombus, improve ventricular function, and improve mortality. Unfortunately, the logistics of providing intracoronary thrombolytic therapy was so great that attention was swiftly turned toward the use of intravenous thrombolytic therapy. The TIMI Phase I Trial[20, 21] demonstrated in 316 patients randomized to either intravenous tPA or streptokinase that mortality was markedly reduced if the infarct-related artery was opened by 90 minutes by either tPA or streptokinase therapy. Their study also demonstrated that tPA had a higher patency rate than streptokinase at 90 minutes from the time the medication was administered (Table 2 & 3). This improved patency rate of tPA was less dramatic if the observation time was delayed beyond 3 hours. TPA's improvement in patency was confirmed by the European Cooperative Study.[22]

Table 2. Dosing and Characteristics of tPA

	tPA ACCELERATED	tPA STANDARD
Thrombolytic	- 15 mg IV over 1-2 minutes - then 50 mg IV over 30 min - then 35 mg IV over 1 hr	- 60 mg for 1st h - 40 mg over next 2-3 h
Adjunctive Therapy	- ASA 160-325 mg - plus IV heparin	- ASA 160-325 mg - plus IV heparin
Clot Selectivity	- relative	- relative
Patency rate at 90 min	- 85%	- 70-85%
Hypotension	- none	- none
Allergic reactions	- no	- no
Cost/dose	- 2800	- 2800
Noncerebral bleeds	- 5.4%†	- 5.2%*
Stroke	- 1.55†	- 1.39%*

From ISIS-3.[11]; † From GUSTO.[12]

Table 3. Dosing and Characteristics of Streptokinase and APSAC Therapy

	SK	APSAC
Thrombolytic	- 1.5 million units in 250 cc D5W over 1 h	- 30 mg in 5 min
Adjunctive Therapy	- ASA 160-325 mg - IV or S.C. heparin	- 160-325 - no heparin
Clot Selectivity	- none	- minor
Patency rate at 90 min	- 50-60%	- 60%
Hypotension	- yes	- yes
Allergic reactions	- yes	- yes
Cost/dose	- $125	- $1,800
Noncerebral bleeds	- 4.5-6.3%*,†	- 5.4%*
Stroke	- 1.04-1.22% *,†	- 1.26%*

From ISIS-3.[11]; † From GUSTO.[12]

Several large scale clinical trials comparing thrombolytic therapy to placebo were initiated in the early to mid 1980s (Table 4 & 5).[21, 23-31] All trials showed mortality benefits from tPA, streptokinase, or APSAC compared to placebo. In 1986, the first GISSI Trial,[32] randomizing 11,806 patients within 12 hours of the onset of symptoms, demonstrated clear mortality reductions with the use of intravenous streptokinase.

Table 4. Summary of Major Intravenous Thrombolytic Studies in Acute Myocardial Infarction

Study	N	Agents	Protocol
TIMI I	316	- IV SK, tPA	- randomized < 7 hrs
EUROPEAN COOPERATIVE	123	- IV SK, tPA	- randomized < 6 hrs; single blind
GISSI	11,806	- IV SK	- randomized vs P < 12 hrs
ISAM	1,741	- IV SK	- randomized < 6 hrs vs P
AIMS	1,000	- AP	- randomized vs P < 6 hrs
ASSET	4,911	- IV tPA, H	- randomized vs P, < 5 hrs
ISIS 2	17,187	- IV SK, ASA	- randomized ≤ 24 hrs - 4 groups: SK/A/SK&A/None
GISSI 2	12,490	- IV SK, tPA, H - All given atenolol & ASA	- Randomized 2 x 2
ISIS 3	41,299	- IV SK, tPA, AP	- Randomized within 24 h - Also randomized to s.c. H & IV heparin
GUSTO	41,021	- IV tPA, H	- Randomized within 6 h to: - tPA + H - SK + IV H - SK + SC H - SK + tPA + IV H
LATE	5,711	- tPA	- Randomized 6-24 h compared to P
EMERAS	4,534	- IV SK	- Randomized 6-24 h compared to P

tPA = tissue plasminogen activator; SK = Streptokinase; AP = APSAC; ASA = aspirin; H = Heparin; PTCA = Angioplasty; UK = Urokinase; P = Placebo; IC = Intracoronary; IV = Intravenous

Overall, this reduction was 18% with the highest reduction being found within the first hour of the onset of symptoms (47%). The ISIS 2 Trial, randomizing 17,187 patients up to 24 h, demonstrated not only the value in mortality reduction of streptokinase but also the value of aspirin therapy as an adjunctive therapy.[26]

The first trial to compare tPA and streptokinase directly was the GISSI II Trial.[33] While finding no mortality difference between streptokinase and tPA treated patients, this study did demonstrate a benefit of heparin therapy in patients treated with streptokinase. Overall, patients receiving heparin, 12,500 U twice SC daily, subcutaneously had a mortality of 7.9% in the streptokinase treated group compared to 9.2% in those patients who did not receive heparin. In tPA treated patients, the heparin treated group had a mortality of 9.2% compared to 8.7% in patients who did not. The ISIS 3 Trial[11] compared the three thrombolytic agents (streptokinase, tPA, and APSAC) and also attempted to determine whether adding heparin had an additional benefit. It consisted of 41,299 randomized patients from 914 centers in 20 countries. Patients presenting within 24 hours from symptom onset who had suspected or definite acute MI with or without ECG changes were enrolled in the study. Fifty percent of the patients received subcutaneous heparin in a dose of 12,500 international units twice a day for 7 days, and 50% of the patients received no heparin. Aspirin was administered to all patients. The 5-week mortality was similar between all three thrombolytic groups which was consistent with GISSI II (Figure 1).

Although the recurrent infarction rate appeared to be less in tPA treated patients, the higher incidence of cerebral hemorrhage in both tPA and APSAC treated patients negated their potential benefit. In that study, allergic reactions were more common especially in APSAC treated patients.

Table 5. Results: **Summary of Major Intravenous Thrombolytic Studies in Acute Myocardial Infarction**

Study	
TIMI I	- Patency better with T - 56 vs 26% (0) - 62 vs 31% (0-1)
EUROPEAN COOPERATIVE	- Patency better with T - 70 vs 51%
GISSI	- Decreased mortality 10.7% vs 13% (hospital) - Decreased mortality by 50% @ 21 days - Best if < 6 hrs, ant., < 65
ISAM	- No change in mortality; P mortality extremely low
AIMS	- 47% reduction in mortality
ASSET	- 26% reduction in mortality
ISIS 2	- Both SK & AS decreased mortality and were additive
GISSI 2	- No difference in mortality between T & SK (heparin given later)
ISIS 3	- H + ASA: ↑ hemorrhages and hemorrhagic strokes - Mortality: APSAC = SK = TPA - APSAC had more allergic reactors - tPA had more strokes but fewer reinfarction
GUSTO	- Accelerated tPA reduced mortality by 14%, but increased hemorrhagic stroke
LATE	- Treatment < 12 h reduced mortality 25.6%
EMERAS	- Patients treated with SK @ 13-24 h had no benefit

tPA = tissue plasminogen activator; SK = Streptokinase; AP = APSAC;

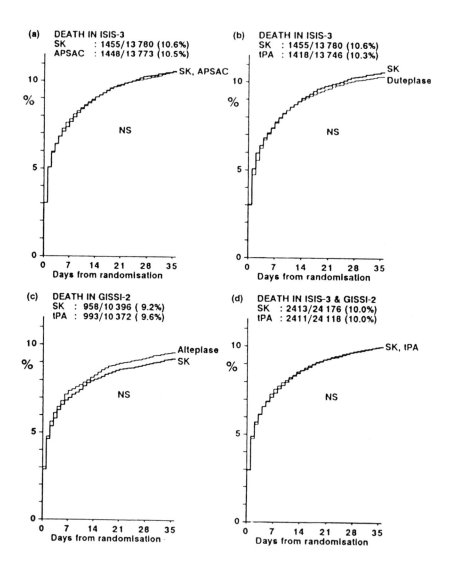

Figure 1. Cumulative percentage dead in days 0-35 in ISIS-3 and in GISSI-2 fibrinolytic comparisons. Panel (a) all patients allocated SK (thicker line) vs all allocated APSAC in ISIS-3 only; Panels (b, c, d): all patients allocated SK vs all allocated tPA in ISIS-3 (b), GISSI-2 (c), and ISIS-3 and GISSI-2 combined (d). (From ISIS-3: ISIS-3: a randomized comparison of streptokinase vs tissue plasminogen activator vs anistreplase and of aspirin plus heparin vs aspirin alone among 41,299 cases of suspected acute myocardial infarction. Lancet 1992; 339:753-770. Reproduced by permission.)

A great deal of controversy arose over these trials because of the heparinization regimen. As discussed below, the HART trial demonstrated that intravenous heparin improved patency after tPA therapy. Because both ISIS 3 and GISSI II used S.C. heparin, another trial was necessary to settle the issue. The GUSTO Trial of 41,021 patients[12] randomized within 6 h of symptom onset specifically asked and answered the question of whether or not the combination of an accelerated dosing regimen, tPA and intravenous heparin therapy, would have a lower mortality than either use of streptokinase combined with intravenous or subcutaneous heparin therapy or a combination of intravenous streptokinase and tPA. An angiographic substudy also asked the question of whether or not preservation of ventricular function was related to patency rate at 90 minutes. This study demonstrated that tPA treated patients had improved mortality at 30 days (14% reduction in mortality compared to either streptokinase group [Figure 2]) and better patency than either streptokinase group, especially when thrombolytic therapy was administered within four hours of the onset of symptoms (Figure 3). This mortality difference was all the more significant because tPA caused more hemorrhage strokes (0.2% more compared to streptokinase). Subgroup analysis also revealed that the mortality reduction with tPA was more marked for patients less than 75 y age and patients treated within 4 h (Figure 3). There was not any difference between the strepokinase/intravenous heparin and streptokinase/subcutaneous heparin groups.

Odds Ratios and 95 Confidence Intervals for Reduction in Mortality and Net Benefit

	Event Rate (%) Strepto-kinase	t-PA	Odds Ratio and 95% CI
30 day mortality			
Streptokinase and SC heparin	7.2	6.3	
Streptokinase and IV heparin	7.4	6.3	
Both streptokinase groups	7.3	6.3	
30 day mortality or disabling stroke			
Streptokinase and SC heparin	7.7	6.9	
Streptokinase and IV heparin	7.9	6.9	
Both streptokinase groups	7.9	6.9	

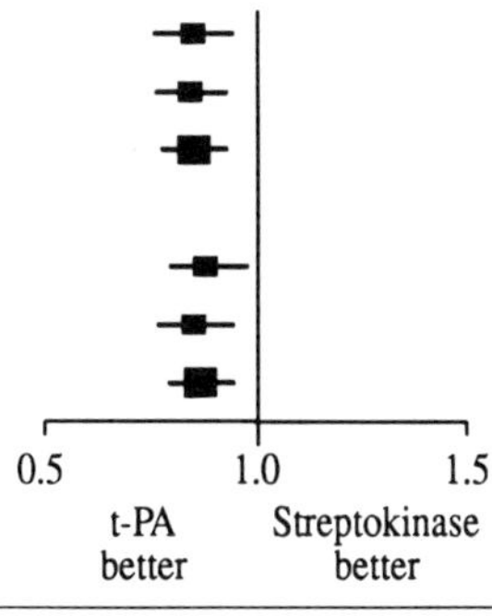

```
        0.5        1.0        1.5
              t-PA     Streptokinase
             better       better
```

Figure 2. Thirty day mortality in four treatment groups (Streptokinase and IV heparin, streptokinase and S.C. heparin, tPA and streptokinase, and accelerated tPA). The group receiving accelerated treatment with tPA had lower mortality than any of the other groups (compared to streptokinase and subcutaneous heparin, p=009; compared to streptokinase plus intravenous heparin, p=.003; and compared to combination therapy with tPA and streptokinase, p=.04). (From The GUSTO Investigators: An international randomized trial comparing four thrombolytic strategies for acute myocardial infarction. N Engl J Med 1993; 329:673-682. Reproduced by Permission.)

The issue of the timing of thrombolytic therapy from the onset of acute myocardial infarction symptoms has been debated. The majority of trials have used relatively short windows for treatment with thrombolytic therapy, i.e., usually < 6 h from symptom onset. However, the ISIS 2 randomized all patients admitted with 24 h and found benefit in the group treated between 6-24 h.

Odds Ratios and 95 Confidence Intervals for 30-day Mortality in Prespecified Subgroups

	% of Patients	Mortality Rate (%) Strepto-kinase	t-PA	Odds Ratio and 95% CI
Age (yr)				
<75	88	5.5	4.4	
>75	12	20.6	19.3	
Infarct location				
Anterior	39	10.5	8.6	
Other	61	5.3	4.7	
Hours to thrombolytic therapy				
0 to 2	27	5.4	4.3	
2 to 4	51	6.7	5.5	
4 to 6	19	9.3	8.9	
>6	4	8.3	10.4	(2.13)

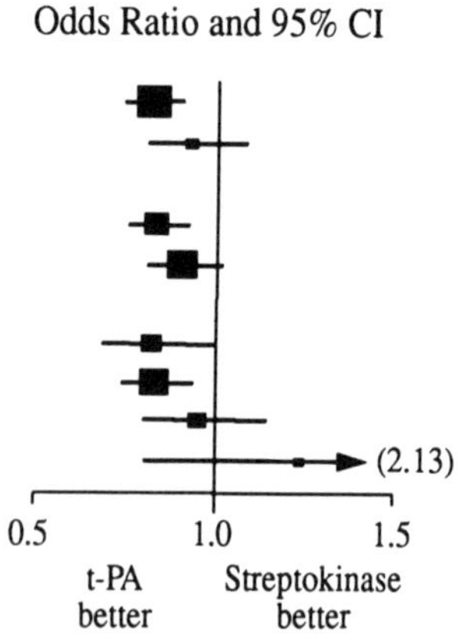

```
        0.5        1.0        1.5
        t-PA       Streptokinase
        better     better
```

Figure 3. Odds ratios and 95 percent confidence intervals (CI) for 30 day mortality in prespecified subgroups defined by age, infarct location, and time to thrombolytic therapy.

To answer the question does therapy initiated after 12 h reduce mortality in Late Assessment of Thrombolytic Efficacy (LATE)[34] study and the EMERAS (Estudio Multicentrico Enstreptoquinasa Republicas de America del Sur).[34] Collaborative group designed trials to determine whether treatment with tPA or streptokinase, respectively, between 6 and 24 h reduced mortality. Both trials failed to show mortality benefits for treatment initiated after 12 h (Figure 4).

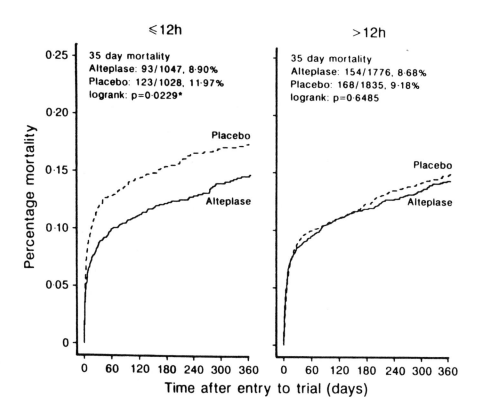

Figure 4. Mortality by time to randomization from onset of acute myocardial infarction. Treatment with alteplase reduced mortality if administered within 12 h of onset. (From LATE Study Group: Late Assessment of thrombolytic efficacy [LATE] study with alteplase 6-24 hours after onset of acute myocardial infarction. Lancet 1993; 342:759-766. Reproduced by permission.)

In 1994, the Fibrinolytic Therapy Trialists (FTT) Collaborative Group[35] reviewed the indications for thrombolytic therapy by evaluating the results from all randomized trials of 1000 or more patients with suspected acute myocardial infarction. The results of 9 trials including 58,600 patients are summarized in Figure 5.

Proportional Effects of Fibrinolytic Therapy on Mortality During Days 0-35 Subdivided by Presentation Features

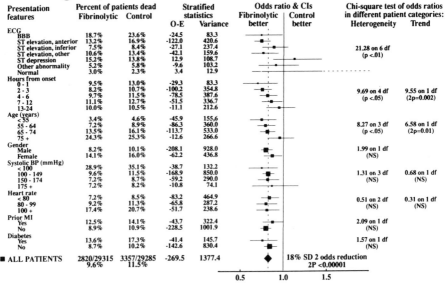

Presentation features	Percent of patients dead		Stratified statistics		Odds ratio & CIs Fibrinolytic better | Control better	Chi-square test of odds ratios in different patient categories:	
	Fibrinolytic	Control	O-E	Variance		Heterogeneity	Trend
ECG							
BBB	18.7%	23.6%	-24.5	83.3			
ST elevation, anterior	13.2%	16.9%	-122.0	420.6			
ST elevation, inferior	7.5%	8.4%	-27.1	237.4		21.28 on 6 df	
ST elevation, other	10.6%	13.4%	-42.1	159.6		(p <.01)	
ST depression	15.2%	13.8%	12.9	108.7			
Other abnormality	5.2%	5.8%	-9.6	103.2			
Normal	3.0%	2.3%	3.4	12.9			
Hours from onset							
0 - 1	9.5%	13.0%	-29.3	83.3			
2 - 3	8.2%	10.7%	-100.2	354.8		9.69 on 4 df	9.55 on 1 df
4 - 6	9.7%	11.5%	-78.5	387.6		(p <.05)	(2p=0.002)
7 - 12	11.1%	12.7%	-51.5	336.7			
13-24	10.0%	10.5%	-11.1	212.6			
Age (years)							
< 55	3.4%	4.6%	-45.9	155.6			
55 - 64	7.2%	8.9%	-86.3	360.0		8.27 on 3 df	6.58 on 1 df
65 - 74	13.5%	16.1%	-113.7	533.0		(p <.05)	(2p=0.01)
75 +	24.3%	25.3%	-12.6	266.6			
Gender							
Male	8.2%	10.1%	-208.1	928.0		1.99 on 1 df	
Female	14.1%	16.0%	-62.2	436.8		(NS)	
Systolic BP (mmHg)							
< 100	28.9%	35.1%	-38.7	132.2			
100 - 149	9.6%	11.5%	-168.9	850.0		1.31 on 3 df	0.68 on 1 df
150 - 174	7.2%	8.7%	-59.2	290.0		(NS)	(NS)
175 +	7.2%	8.2%	-10.8	74.1			
Heart rate							
< 80	7.2%	8.5%	-83.2	464.9			
80 - 99	9.2%	11.3%	-65.8	287.2		0.51 on 2 df	0.31 on 1 df
100 +	17.4%	20.7%	-51.7	238.6		(NS)	(NS)
Prior MI							
Yes	12.5%	14.1%	-43.7	322.4		2.09 on 1 df	
No	8.9%	10.9%	-228.5	1001.9		(NS)	
Diabetes							
Yes	13.6%	17.3%	-41.4	145.7		1.57 on 1 df	
No	8.7%	10.2%	-142.6	830.4		(NS)	
■ **ALL PATIENTS**	2820/29315 9.6%	3357/29285 11.5%	-269.5	1377.4	18% SD 2 odds reduction 2P <0.00001		

0.5   1.0   1.5

Figure 5. Proportional effects of fibrinolytic therapy on mortality during days 0-35 subdivided by presentation features. The data are expressed as odds ratios of death among patient's allocated to fibrinolytic therapy compared to those allocated to control. Odds ratios are depicted by black squares with 95% confidence intervals depicted by the horizontal lines. Diamond figure depicts overall odds ratio. (From Fibrinolytic Therapy Trialists (FTT) Collaborative Group: Indications for fibrinolytic therapy in suspected acute myocardial infarction. Lancet 1994; 343:311-322. Reproduced by permission.)

Clear treatment advantages with fibrinolytic agents exist for patients who have bundle branch block, ST elevation (especially anterior), who are treated under 12 h of onset, and who are younger than 75 y of age (ACC/AHA Class I recommendation).[36-37] Benefits also exist in patients with systolic blood pressure < 100 mmHg or tachycardia. A direct relationship between benefit and hours from symptom onset and treatment is apparent (Figure 6).

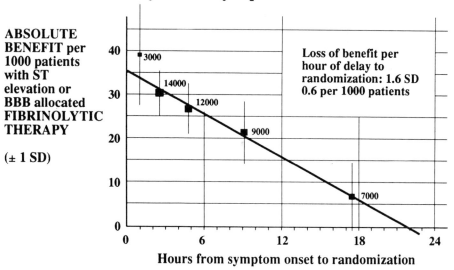

Figure 6. Absolute reduction in 35 day mortality versus delay from symptom onset to randomization among 45,000 patients with ST elevation or BBB.

Contraindication to thrombolytic therapy are summarized in Table 6 and reflect the recommendations of the AHA/ACC Task Force on the early treatment of acute myocardial infarction.

Table 6. Contraindications To Thrombolytic Therapy

Absolute
• Active internal bleeding
   • Suspected aortic dissection
   • History of stroke known to be hemorrhage
   • Recent (within 2 months) intracranial or intraspinal
   surgery or trauma
   • Intracranial neoplasm, arteriovenous malformation, or
   aneurysm
   • Pregnancy
   • Diabetic hemorrhagic retinopathy or other hemorrhagic
   ophthalmic condition
   • Any bleeding disorder
   • Severe uncontrolled hypertension (> 200/120) that
   persists despite acute therapy
   • Trauma or surgery < 2 weeks

Relative
   • Major surgery or trauma > 2 weeks
   • Major invasive procedure within 10 days
   • Current use of anticoagulants
   • High likelihood of left heart thrombus
   • Significant liver dysfunction
   • Acute pericarditis
   • Active pepticular disease
   • History of severe chronic hypertension with or without
   • Drug therapy
   • History of cerebrovascular accident

Prehospital thrombolysis by paramedics has been suggested as a means to preserve LV function and mortality[38]. One double-blind parallel group clinical trial of 311 patients demonstrated that prehospital administration could save approximately 130 minutes and reduce mortality (relative reduction 52% [95% confidence interval 14 to 89%]). However, in the United States the degree of time served and mortality reduction is less conclusive[39]

ADJUNCTIVE THERAPY TO THROMBOLYTICS (< 24 OF SYMPTOM ONSET)

The role of aspirin as adjunctive therapy after thrombolytic therapy is strongly suggested by the Second International Study of Infarct Survival (ISIS-2) where aspirin alone reduced mortality and the combination of streptokinase and aspirin was additive[26] have been suggested by these large trials. The issue of heparin therapy continues to be debated because of the different dosing regimens in many trials and a lack of outcome data.

In a subgroup analysis of the Thrombosi Ventricolare nell' Infarcto Studio Sulla Calciparina nell'angina e rella (SCATI) trial,[40] the only data available to assess the utility of heparin as sole adjunctive therapy, there were 10 deaths in 218 patients treated with subcutaneous heparin, and 19 among 215 patients receiving placebo as adjunctive therapy to streptokinase. Furthermore, intravenous heparin appears to improve patency rates after thrombolytic therapy, especially tPA. The Heparin-Aspirin Reperfusion (H.A.R.T.) Trial[41] demonstrated that the use of intravenous heparin in doses sufficient to increase the APTT to twice normal improved patency rate after tPA therapy at 7-24 h after thrombolytic therapy compared to aspirin in a dose of 80 mg/d. At 7 days, the patency rate for the heparin group was 88% in the heparin group and 95% in the ASA group. The data from GISSI 2 and ISIS 3 suggest that subcutaneous heparin added to ASA does not reduce mortality but increases the risk of important side effects.[11, 33] Furthermore, the Duke University Clinical Cardiology Study (DUCCS)[42] demonstrated that the addition of heparin to APSAC increased adverse bleeding events. In summary, there is strong evidence to recommend aspirin in all patients receiving thrombolytic therapy. There is little evidence to add subcutaneous heparin. The use of intravenous heparin with tPA still requires further study.

The use of intravenous beta blockers in the early hours of acute myocardial infarction has been proven to be efficacious. In ISIS-I[43] atenolol was given in a dose of 5 mg intravenously followed by two additional doses of 5 mg, and then 100 mg per day was started orally (Figure 7). The group receiving atenolol had fewer deaths by the end of day 14. Similarly, metoprolol has been also used and found to be efficacious and should be administered in patients who have no contraindications (Class I ACC/AHA recommendations). [36-37]

Some debate exists as to the value of prophylactive magnesium sulphate administration in reducing mortality. Of 7 studies published by 1992, only 2 showed benefit although metaanalyses suggested a significant reduction in mortality.[44] The LIMIT 2 Study (Leicester Intravenous Magnesium Intervention Trial) demonstrated a 24% reduction in 28 day mortality. This benefit was greatest in patients who were not treated with beta blockers and may be related to the frequency of sinus bradycardia that was observed in this study.[45] In contrast, the ISIS 4 trial did not show any mortality benefit from magnesium.[46] At present, magnesium should be used for magnesium deficiency, refractory ventricular dysrhythmia, and torsades des points (Class IIa/ACC/AHA recommendation).[36-37]

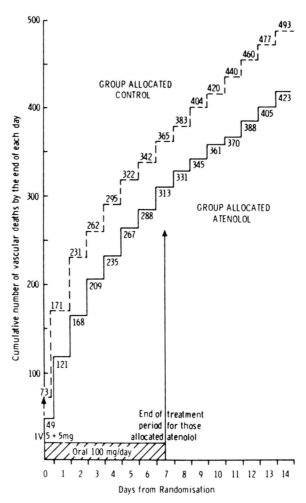

Figure 7. Vascular mortality during scheduled treatment period (days 0-7) and immediately after (to day 14) in myocardial patients treated with atenolol or placebo. (From ISIS-1 Collaborative Group: Randomised trial of intravenous atenolol among 16 027 cases of suspected acute myocardial infarction. <u>Lancet</u> 1986; 8498:57-65. Reproduced by permission.)

The GISSI-3[6] trial of 19,394 patients investigated the effects of lisinopril and transdermal glyceryl trinitrate found mortality reduction at 6 weeks (odds ratio = 0.88; 95% confidence internal = 0.79-0.99) with lisinopril started within 24 h but not with nitrates (Figure 8). Although metaanalyses of intravenous nitrates had suggested benefit, this trial which used intravenous nitrates for 24 h and then transdermal nitrates did not. On the basis of this study ACE inhibition has a Class I indication for acute MI with ST segment elevation in anterior leads or with heart failure.

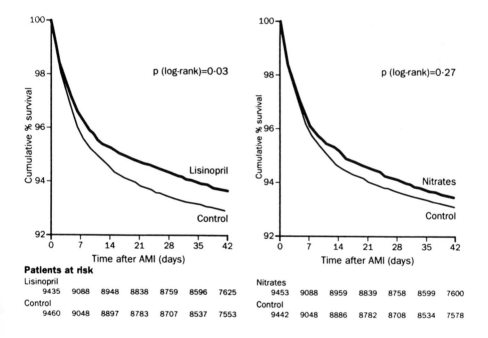

Figure 8. Six week survival in lisinopril, nitrate, and respective control groups. (From Gruppo Italiano per to Studio della sopravvivenza nell'infarto Miocardico: GISSI-3: effects of lisinopril and transdermal glyceryl trinitrate singly and together on 6-week mortality and ventricular function after acute myocardial infarction. Reproduced by permission.)

Adjunctive therapy with beta blockers[43] and aspirin[26, 47] should be considered in all patients without contraindication. Intravenous heparin therapy should be used following tPA therapy and in patients with ST depression.[26, 41]

PERCUTANEOUS TRANSLUMINAL CORONARY ANGIOPLASTY IN ACUTE MYOCARDIAL

The role of angioplasty in the early treatment of acute myocardial infarction has sparked some controversy. Many authors have suggested that both patency and TIMI Grade 3 flow affect subsequent ventricular function and prognosis.[48, 49] Nonetheless, aggressive protocols randomizing patients to early coronary angiography and angioplasty for significant residual lesions after thrombolytic therapy have failed to demonstrate efficacy[50-52]

At the present time, immediate angioplasty after thrombolytic therapy is not recommended in the routine case,[50-52] However, in patients who clinically fail to reperfuse, rescue angioplasty may be helpful.[21, 51, 53] In contrast to early angioplasty after thrombolytic therapy, angioplasty as a primary reperfusion therapy appears promising.

In 1993, three important trials were published that looked at the role of primary percutaneous transluminal coronary angioplasty to treat acute myocardial infarction.[53-55] These studies demonstrated that the use of primary PTCA could result in a low mortality. Unfortunately, this form of therapy is limited to institutions that have cardiac catheterization facilities available 24 hours a day and may not be a practical choice in must patients. Nonetheless, the superior results of direct PTCA over thrombolytic therapy, especially in large anterior infarctions and cardiogenic shock without apparently increasing the cost of care,[56] suggests that its role as definitive therapy in at least select patients will continue to emerge. Presently, primary PTCA has a Class I indication for early reperfusion at centers who do more than 200 PTCAs per year and by operators who perform more than 75 PTCAs per year.

In an attempt to facilitate early diagnosis and treatment, an algorithms is depicted in Figure 9. Patients in whom the diagnosis of acute myocardial infarction is suspected should have an electrocardiogram (EKG) with 5 minutes and read within 10 minutes of initial triage. Patients in whom alternate diagnosis are suspected will require more definitive investigation. Figure 9 depicts the decision tree for the management of acute myocardial infarction of the EKG shows evidence of ST elevation $\geq$ 1 mm in 2 contiguous leads on LBBB configuration. This decision tree serves as a guide but takes into account the latest information on reperfusion therapy. All patients with 6 hours of onset should receive either thrombolytic therapy or PTCA with the later preferred if contraindications to thrombolytic therapy exist and if the infarction is associated with severe heart failure or shock.

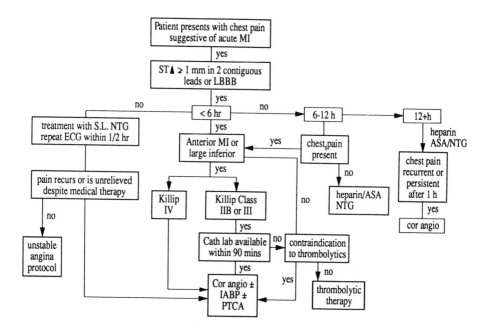

Figure 9. Management algorithm for acute myocardial infarction based on the results of randomized control trials. Patients with diagnostic electrocardiograms presenting within 6 h should receive thrombolytic therapy. If the patient is having a large anterior wall infarction (Killip Class IIb or III), large inferior infarction (associated with precordial ST depression or ST elevation in VR), or cardiogenic shock, PTCA should be considered. Patients presenting between 6-12 h who are continuing to have chest pain should also receive reperfusion therapy. Patients with late presentation (12+ h) with ongoing pain should be considered for coronary angiography.

Patients presenting between 6-12 h who still have pain should also receive reperfusion therapy. Patients with chest pain beyond 12 h should receive heparin and ASA and have coronary angiography if pain persists or recurs. Beta blockers should be routinely administered except in the presence of contraindications such as:

1)   heart rate < 60 beats/min
2)   systolic blood pressure < 100 mmHg
3)   moderate to severe left ventricular failure
4)   signs of peripheral hypoperfusion
5)   AV condition abnormalities such as PR > .22, Type I and II AV block, or complete heart block
6)   severe chronic obstructive pulmonary disease
7)   asthma
8)   severe peripheral vascular disease
9)   difficult diabetes

THE MANAGEMENT OF THE POST MYOCARDIAL INFARCTION PATIENTS

The subsequent management of the patient after myocardial infarction is largely based on the assessment of risk. The assessment of risk is predicated largely on three factors: 1) degree of left ventricular dysfunction,[57] 2) the presence and severity of residual ischemia, and 3) the propensity for life threatening arrhythmias (i.e., sudden cardiac death).[57-60]

Stress testing [61-69] in any of several forms is the most common type of risk stratification. The results of conventional stress ECG testing using a variety of protocols are summarized using likelihood ratios in Table 7& 8.

Table 7. Likelihood Ratios of Exercise Testing to Predict Mortality after MI

Study	Follow-up Mo.	Exercise Protocol	Indicator
Theroux et al[67]	12	Naughton: 70% of PHR	0.1 mV ST depression
Weld et al[68]	12	9 min; 4 mets	Duration; VPB
Krone et al[64, 65]	12	9 min; 4 mets	Peak BP < 110 ex. time < 9 min pulmonary congestion
DeFeyter et al[61]	28	Bruce	Duration < 10 min
DeBusk et al[62]	6	Naughton	2 mV, ST depression, and HR < 135 bpm
Williams et al[69]	12	Bruce	Duration < 6 min
Fioretti et al[63]	12	symptom limited bicycle	Systolic BP increase $\leq$ 30 mm Hg
Madsen et al[66]	12	Variable	$\leq$ 4 mets

PHR = peak heart rate; Ex. time = exercise time; BP = blood pressure

Table 8. Likelihood Ratios of Exercise Testing to Predict Mortality after MI (continued)

Study	Endpoint	LR (+)	LR (-)
Theroux et al[67]	Death, MI	2.09	.61
Weld et al[68]	Death	2.04	.09
Krone et al[64, 65]	Death	1.91	0
DeFeyter et al[61]	Death, MI	1.5	.12
DeBusk et al[62]	Death, MI	2.1	.87
Williams et al[69]	Death, MI	1.14	.74
Fioretti et al[63]	Death	2.64	.40
Madsen et al[66]	Death, MI	3.16	.28

MI = Myocardial infarction; LR(+) = likelihood ratio of observing endpoint in a patient with a (+) test response; LR(-) = likelihood ratio of observing endpoint in a patient with a negative test response; HR = heart rate.

The likelihood ratio represents the odds of observing the cardiac end point of interest in a patient with either a positive or negative test response. The pretest likelihood (probability/1- probability) can be multiplied by the likelihood ratio of the test result to compute a post-test odds and probability (odds/1+ odds). A test with good discrimination when positive has a likelihood ratio in excess of 2 and when negative a likelihood ratio of 0.20 or less. Excellent discrimination for positive test response is $\geq$ 10. In this regard, negative stress tests are extremely useful in that such patients have a mortality rate of only 2% in the first year. Positive test responses confer a greater likelihood of events in the first year but the range is quite variable, anywhere from 3-20 times higher than that of patients without this abnormality. This translates into an infarction rate of 5-15%.

Thallium studies (Table 9) can increase the sensitivity for detecting myocardial ischemia.[70-76] Myocardial ischemia also predicts subsequent mortality. Recent studies suggest that symptom limited stress testing with Thallium imaging can be performed safely before hospital discharge at approximately 5-10 days.[77-79]

Table 9. Frequency of Exercise-Induced Ischemia after Acute Myocardial Infarction*

Study	Year	Patients, N	Time of Testing	St Depression N(%)	Thallium-201 N(%)	P
				DETECTION METHOD		
Buda, et al.[70]	1982	26	3wk	6 (35)	18(69)	0.050
Gibson, et al.[72]	1983	140	10d	47(34)	71(59)	0.004
Hung, et al.[73]	1984	51	3wk	14(27)	30(59)	0.050
Hung, et al.[74]	1984	117	3wk	32(27)	65(57)†	0.001
Gibson, et al.[71]	1986	241	10d	77(32)	143(59)	0.001
Wilson, et al.[76]	1988	97	10d	47(27)	45(46)†	0.001
Tilkemeier, et al.[75]	1990	171	10d	47(27)	96(56)	0.001
Pooled data		843		247(29)	468(57)	0.001

Adapted from Gibson and Watson; with permission. † Numbers reflect only patients with infarct zone by thallium-201 (i.e., transient perfusion defect). MI = myocardial infarction.

Persantine Thallium has ACC/AHA Class IIa indications for patients who cannot exercise. It has been shown to have similar sensitivity than submaximal stress testing to detect ischemia.[80, 81] However, other important predictors such as exercise capacity, blood pressure response, and heart rate response cannot be assessed by this method. The role of persantine Thallium in detecting reversible left ventricular dysfunction has not been established, but a 24 h reinjection of Thallium should be used for the purpose. Persantine thallium is not recommended for patients who have post-infarctional angina.

Newer studies such as dobutamine echocardiography,[82] rest-redistribution Thallium imaging,[83] and late redistribution (24 h reinjection)[83] Thallium imaging all have been shown to be useful to detect viable myocardium suggestive of either myocardial hibernation or stunning. Many of these reports represent small sample sizes and variable predictive accuracies have been observed. As well, their predictive value shortly after myocardial infarction has not been established. At this point no single test is recommended by any peer reviewed organization, and the choice rests with the patient's own status, physician preference and test availability. Because of the current unavailability of PET scanning, stress Thallium with delayed (24 h) re-injection of Thallium currently is the preferred method to determine reversible dysfunction and the potential value of a revascularization procedure in this institution. However, dobutamine echo[84] has been shown to have equivalent sensitivity to stress Thallium to detect ischemia and reversible ventricular dysfunction and can be considered in patients who cannot exercise or who have received recent radiopharmaceuticals. PET scanning is an alternative where it is available.

Stress cardiolyte has better resolution than stress Thallium for ischemia detection and may be preferable in obese patients.[85] Its ability to determine reversible LV function is still controversial.[82, 83, 86] Some reports have suggested it has less sensitivity than 24 h reinjection Thallium.

A great deal of debate has surrounded the issue of noninvasive stress testing and has been specially addressed by the American College of Cardiology and American Heart Association Task Force on the Management of Acute Myocardial Infarction.[87] Both the SWIFT (Should we intervene following thrombolysis?) trial[88] and TIMI II[89] have demonstrated that a conservative strategy for assessing the risk of patients results in similar outcomes at one year (Figure 10). Using the following grading system for indicating for procedures, test and interventions where:

Class I	=	usually indicated, always acceptable and considered useful/effective
Class IIa	=	acceptable, of uncertain efficacy and may be controversial weight of evidence in favor of usefulness/ efficacy
IIb	=	not well established by evidence, can be helpful and probably not harmful
Class III	=	not indicated, may be harmful

They recommended that:

1) Stress ECG has the following ACC/AHA Class I indications for stable patients without recurrent angina or heart failure:

    a) submaximal stress at 6-10 days[67] (McNaughton protocol, target heart rate = 75% of predicted maximal heart rate (PMHR))

        or

    b) symptom limited (Bruce protocol target heart rate = 85% PMHR) at 10-14 days

        or

    c) at 3 weeks

        or

    d) at 3-8 weeks if submaximal stress test was negative

        or

    e) stress Thallium if ECG baseline abnormalities preclude interpretation

2) Stress Thallium has ACC/AHA Class IIa indications for:

    a) submaximal predischarge

        or

    b) maximal at 10-14 days

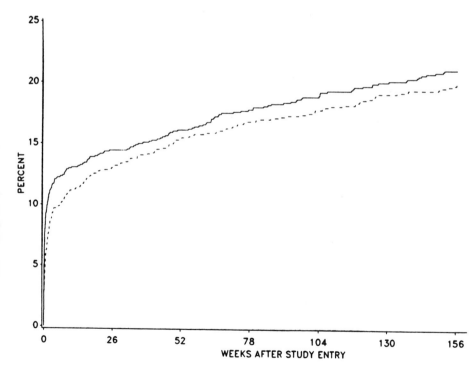

Figure 10. Three year cumulative rates of death or myocardial infarction in the Thrombolysis in Myocardial Infarction Trial, Phase II. Solid curve = invasive strategy, dashed curve = conservative strategy. (From Terrin ML, Williams DO, Kleiman NS, et al: Two- and three-year results of the thrombolysis in myocardial infarction (TIMI) Phase II Clinical Trial. *Reproduced by permission.*

Resting MUGA scanning currently has an ACC/AHA Class I indication for predischarge risk assessment, an ejection fraction < .40 increase mortality at one year after myocardial infarction.[60] Resting two-dimensional echo has a Class I indication for detecting mechanical complications of infarction and a IIa indication for predicting low risk patients. Ross, et al[90] has demonstrated that patients with EF between .20 and .40 may benefit from coronary angiography. Therefore, assessments of ventricular function can be considered either as a preliminary screening test or as an adjunctive test in patients who cannot exercise. Patients with depressed ventricular function are at significant risk for sudden cardiac death. This risk is raised even further in the presence of ventricular ectopy[60] or an abnormal signal-averaged ECG.[91]

An abnormal signal averaged ECG at 7-10 days following myocardial infarction identifies a group with a 17-27% chance of an electrical event in the first year following myocardial infarction and may warrant further evaluation (EPS) particularly if the LVEF < 40%, and nonsustained VT, or complex ventricular ectopy are present.[91] A normal signal averaged ECG in this group has a high negative predictive value (<4% chance of an electrical event at one year) in the presence of an inferior myocardial infarction but may not be as benign in the presence of an anterior myocardial infarction. Further evaluation with electrophysiology study should be considered if other non-invasive risk factors are present, i.e., complex ventricular ectopy or nonsustained VT, in the anterior infarction cohort.

The presence of nonsustained VT on Holter at 4-10 days following myocardial infarction in the presence of an LVEF <40% identifies a cohort with a 2 fold increased risk of sudden cardiac death and should be considered for further risk stratification (signal averaged ECG and/or electrophysiology study).[57, 92]

Holter monitoring has a Class IIa indication for patients with moderate to severe ventricular dysfunction or significant ventricular dysrhythmia. Signal averaged ECG has no definite ACC/AHA guidelines. The correct algorithm for using signal averaged ECG, Holter monitoring, left ventricular ejection fraction and electrophysiology study for stratification of sudden death or ventricular tachycardia risk following myocardial infarction requires further investigation.

Table 10 & 11 outlines a variety of clinical noninvasive and invasive test results that can aid in stratifying patients into high, medium, and low risk.

High risk patients can be identified clinically on the basis of recurrent angina at rest or at low levels of ambulation, the presence of heart failure,[60, 93, 94] the presence of ventricular tachycardia or fibrillation especially after 48 h, the occurrence of a new bundle branch block, and previous myocardial infarction. In patients with a non-Q-wave myocardial infarction, anterior location or persistent ST depression denote higher risk patients.[95-98] High risk patients who do not fulfill these clinical criteria can be identified on stress EKG by a low work load, ST depression > 2 mm, hypotension, and angina at a low workload. Multiple reversible defects on stress scintigraphy also indicate a higher risk for future ischemia events. Echocardiographic or nuclear evidence of depressed LV function, especially an EF < .40, also indicates high risk.

Table 10

Clinical Risk Stratification			
	High Risk	**Medium Risk**	**Low Risk**
Clinical[87] features:	- recurrent angina - pump failure (Killip III, IV) - VT/VF - mechanical defects - new BBB - previous MI - anterior non Q wave MI - persistent ST depression	- ventricular ectopic - activity - Killip II	- uncomplicated clinical course

Signal averaged ECG evidence of after potentials and Holter monitor evidence of nonsustained ventricular tachycardia or excessive ventricular ectopy is especially helpful in identifying patients at risk for malignant cardiac arrhythmias. Angiographic evidence of an occluded infarct related artery, especially when it supplies a large amount of myocardium, is associated with more cardiac events, ventricular dysfunction, and ventricular ectopy.[20, 48, 49, 99, 100] The presence of left main or triple vessel disease identifies patients who benefit from coronary revascularization.

Low risk patients have uncomplicated clinical courses, excellent exercise tolerance and a lack of ischemia or subsequent exercise testing, preserved left ventricular function, and no evidence of ventricular irritability. Coronary angiography reveals patient infarct related criteria with either TIMI Grade III flow or collaterals.[48, 49, 99, 101, 102] As might be expected, medium risk patients or collaterals have intermediate test results.

Table 11.

Noinvasive and Invasive Test Results (Continued)			
Form of Evaluation	**High Risk**	**Medium Risk**	**Low Risk**
Stress ECG[87]	- low work load < 6.5 mets - ST depression > 2mm - hypotension - angina a low workload	- 6.5 - 3-8 mets - ST > 1mm - No hypotension - Angina at medium workload	- > 10 mets - no ST - no hypotension - no angina
Stress Thallium	- reversible defect - multiple defects	- Fixed defect	- no defect
Echocardiogram[60] or MUGA	- EF < .40	- EF > .40 - regional wall motion abnormality - aneurysm of false aneurysm	- EF > .50 - minimal wall motion abnormality - No intracavitary thrombus - No cavitary dilatation
SAECG	- after potentials		- no after potentials
Holter monitor	- NSVT - > 100 VPB's/hr	- > 10 VPB's/hr	- no VPB's
Coronary angiography	- occluded artery - EF < .50		- patent artery $\leq$ 50% stenosis - TIMI grade III flow - LVEF > .50

In an attempt to aid the clinician in the optimal choice of diagnostic testing, a clinical evaluation is shown in Figure 11. This algorithm provides for early coronary angiography in all patients with class I or Ia ACC/AHA indication and other high risk groups. It provides both the options of an invasive strategy or any of 4 noninvasive strategies that can be performed before discharge. Each strategy assesses ischemia, employs stress testing, and functional (Echo or MUGA), assessments in patients with depressed ventricular function, assessments of coronary anatomy, myocardial ischemia, or viability should be first performed. If there is no evidence of ischemia or reversible dysfunction, arrhythmic stratification should be considered.

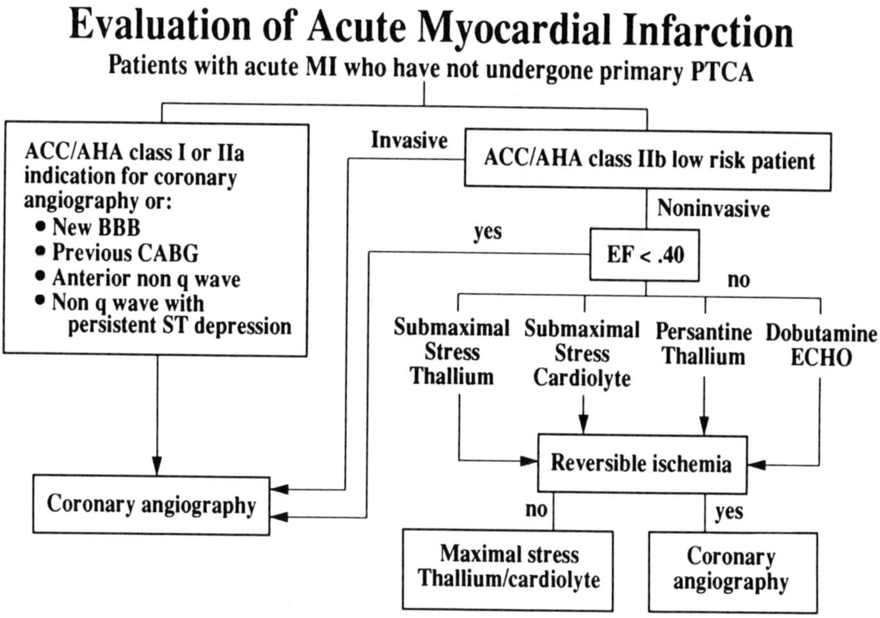

Evaluation of Acute Myocardial Infarction
Patients with acute MI who have not undergone primary PTCA

Figure 11. Evaluation of Acute Myocardial Infarction. High risk patients have an ACC/AHA Class I or IIa for coronary angiography. Low risk patients can be evaluated with either a conservative or invasive strategy. A noninvasive approach requires an assessment of LV function and an assessment of myocardial ischemia using submaximal stress testing (while in hospital), or persantine thallium or dobutamine echo in patients who cannot exercise. An alternative would be maximal stress testing at 2 weeks or more. A normal submaximal stress testing result needs further evaluation with maximal stress testing after discharge. The addition of nuclear imaging to stress ECG increases sensitivity for the detection of myocardial infarction.

For patients who undergo direct PTCA for the early treatment of acute myocardial infarction, an alternative algorithm is outlined in Figure 12. At the present time no clear guideline exists for the management of patients with a poor angiographic result of PTCA (i.e., residual stenosis $\geq$ 50%, intimal dissection or flap, or poor flow grade). The management needs to be individualized by the attending physicians. Recurrent angina will have a Class I indication for coronary angiography. Patients with ventricular tachycardia or fibrillation should have a formal electrophysiological evaluation. Patients with depressed EF (<.40) should be considered for either Holter monitoring or signal averaged ECG. Asymptomatic patients do not require predischarge exercise testing (in fact, the false positive rate may be high), but should be considered for late stress testing between 8-12 weeks to screen for restenosis.

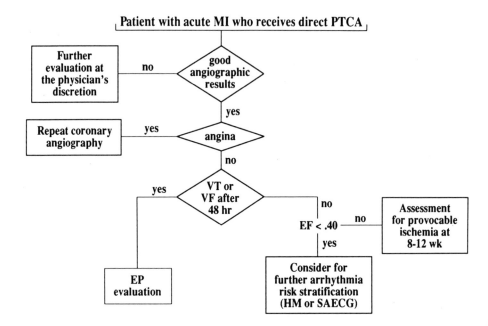

Figure 12. Evaluation of patients who receive direct or primary angioplasty. In-hospital evaluation is directed towards coronary angiography if angina is present or a poor angiographic result is obtained. There is no need of early stress testing in patients with good angiographic results. Further evaluation is directed towards assessment of risk of sudden cardiac death (early VT, VF, or depressed ventricular function).

MEDICAL MANAGEMENT AFTER ACUTE MYOCARDIAL INFARCTION SECONDARY PREVENTION

Beta blockers are now well established as being efficacious for the secondary prevention after a primary myocardial infarction. The BHAT Trial[103] was the first study that demonstrated a significant mortality reduction of approximately 20% with the use of propanolol (Figure 13). Other beta blockers which do not have any intrinsic sympathomimic activity have also been demonstrated to confer a mortality reduction after acute MI.[104-107]

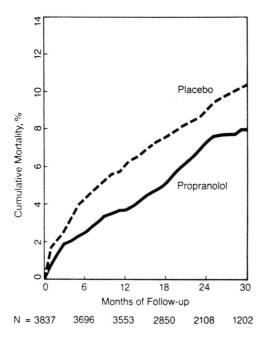

Figure 13. Cumulative mortality curves for patients with MI treated with either propanolol or placebo; N = total number of patients followed up through each time point.
From β-blocker Heart Attack Study Group: β-blocker heart attack trial among. JAMA 1981; 246:2073-2074. Reproduced by permission.

Beta blockers should be considered in all but low risk patients who do not have a clear contraindication for secondary prevention in patients without myocardial revascularization (ACC/AHA Class I, strength of evidence = A). Low risk patients have a Class IIa indication.

Calcium channel blockers have not yet been demonstrated to have a consistent benefit.[104, 108, 109] Diltiazem in the case of non-Q-wave MI has been demonstrated to have a mortality reduction, but its use in all patients with acute MI is mixed. Patients who have pulmonary congestion actually have the higher event rate with the use of Diltiazem. In patients who do not have any evidence of pulmonary congestion, Diltiazem was actually associated with fewer event rates at approximately three years compared to placebo treated patients (Figure 14). Therefore, in Q-wave myocardial infarction their use is indicated for angina. Diltiazem has a Class IIa indication in non Q-wave myocardial infarction (strength of evidence = A) based on a lower infarction rate in treated patients observed in the Multicenter Diltiazem Postinfarction Trial Research Group.[108]

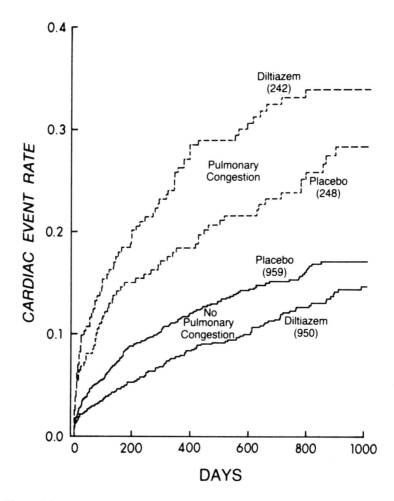

Figure 14. Cumulative rate of first recurrent cardiac events according to treatment with either diltiazem or placebo in patients with or without pulmonary congestion. Diltiazem treated patients with pulmonary congestion had a higher rate of recurrent events than patients receiving placebo; in patients without pulmonary congestion, the reverse was the case. Numbers in parentheses refer to numbers of patients. *From Multicenter Diltiazem Postinfarction Trial Research Group: The effect of diltiazem on mortality and reinfarction after myocardial infarction. N Engl J Med 1988; 319:385-392. Reproduced by permission.*

Recently, ACE inhibitors have been demonstrated to confer reduction in death from all cardiovascular causes including recurrent myocardial infarction or heart failure in patients who have ejection fractions less than 40% (Figure 15). One recent study has also shown benefits in mortality reduction with lisinopril.[6] In contrast, early therapy with enalapril (< 24h) does not improve long-term survival.[110]

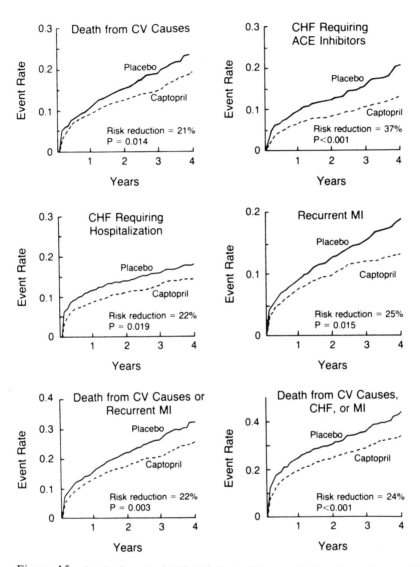

Figure 15. Results from the SAVE trial Captopril improved all cardiovascular mortality, reduced hospitalization for heart failure and recurrent myocardial infarction (FromPfeffer MA, Braunwald E, Moye LA, et al: Effect of captopril or mortality and morbidity in patients with left ventricular dysfunction after myocardial infarction. N Engl J Med 1992; 327:669-677).

ACE inhibitors should be considered in patients who have been found to have an ejection fraction < .40 (strength of evidence = A). Captopril, in a dose of 6.25-50 mg P.O. did, is supported by the results of the SAVE trial.

References:

1.   Chatterjee K, Swan H, Kaushik V, et al. Effects of vasodilator therapy for severe pump failure in acute myocardial infarction on short-term and late prognosis.Circulation 1976; 53(5): 797-802.

2.   Cohn J, Johnson G, Ziesche S, et al. A comparison of Enalapril with Hydralazine-Isosorbide Dinitrate in the treatment of chronic congestive heart failure.New England Journal of Medicine 1991; 325:303-310.

3.   Consensus Trial Study Group. Effects of enalapril on mortality in severe congestive heart failure. Results of the Cooperative North Scandinavian Enalapril Survival Study.New England Journal of Medicine 1987; 316:1429-1435.

4.   SOLVD Investigators. Effect of enalapril on survival in patients with reduced left ventricular ejection fractions and congestive heart failure. New England Journal of Medicine 1991; 325:293-302.

5.   Cohn J, Archibald D, Phil M, et al. Effect of vasodilator therapy on mortality in chronic congestive heart failure. Results of a Veterans Administration Cooperative Study.New England Journal of Medicine 1986; 314:1547-1552.

6.   GISSI-3. Effects of lisinopril and transdermal glyceryl trinitrate singly and together on 6-week mortality and ventricular function after acute myocardial infarction. Gruppo Italiano per to Studio della Soprawivenza nell'Infarto Miocardico. Lancet 1994; 343:1115-1122.

7.   Pfeffer M, Braunwald E, Moye L, et al. Effect of captopril on mortality and morbidity in patients with left ventricular dysfunction after myocardial infarction. Results of the Survival and Ventricular Enlargement trial. New England Journal of Medicine 1992; 327:669-677.

8.   Tillet W, Garner R. The fibrinolytic activity of streptococci.J Exp Med 1933; 58:485.

9.   Fletcher A, Sherry S, Alkjaersig M, et al. The treatment of patients suffering from early myocardial infarction with massive and prolonged streptokinase therapy. Trans Assoc Am Physicians 1958; 71:287.

10.   Wasserman A, Ross A. Coronary thrombolysis. Current Problems in Cardiology 1989 XIV: 1-54.

11.   ISIS-3. A randomised comparison of streptokinase vs tissue plasminogen activator vs anistreplase and of aspirin plus heparin vs aspirin alone among 41,299 cases of suspected acute myocardial infarction. ISIS-3 (Third International Study of Infarct Survival). Lancet 1992; 339:753-770.

12.   GUSTO Investigators. An international randomized trial comparing fourthrombolytic strategies for acute myocardial infarction.New England Journal of Medicine 1993; 329:673-682.

13.   Anderson J, Marshall H, Bray B. A randomized trial of intracoronary streptokinase in the treatment of acute myocardial infarction.New England Journal of Medicine 1983; 308:1312.

14.   Chapman RA. Control of cardiac contractility at the cellular level. American Journal of Physiology 1983; 245:H535-H552.

15.   Furberg C. Clinical value of intracoronary streptokinase. American Journal of Cardiology 1984; 53:626.

16.   Ganz W, Buchbinder N, Marcus H, et al. Intracoronary thrombolysis in evolving myocardial infarction. American Heart J 1981; 101:4.

17.   Kennedy J, Gensini G, Timmis G, Maynard C. Acute myocardial infarction treated with intracoronary streptokinase A report of the society for cardiac angiography.American Journal of Cardiology 1985; 55:871-877.

18.   Kennedy J, Ritchie J, Davis K, et al. Western Washington randomized trial of intracoronary streptokinase in acute myocardial infarction.New England Journal of Medicine 1983; 309:1477.

19.   Leiboff R, Katz R, Wasserman A, et al. A randomized trial of intracoronary streptokinase in the treatment of acute myocardial infarction.American Journal of Cardiology 1984; 53:404.

20.   Dalen J, Gore J, Braunwald E, et al. Six- and twelve-month follow-up of the Phase I Thrombolysis in Myocardial Infarction (TIMI) Trial. American Journal of Cardiology 1988; 62:179-185.

21.   White H, Rivers J, Maslowski A, et al. Effect of intravenous streptokinase as compared with that of tissue plasminogen activator on left ventricular function after first myocardial infarction. New England Journal of Medicine 1989; 320:817-821.

22.   Verstraete M, Bernard B, Bory M, et al. Randomized trial of intravenous recombinant tissue-type plasminogen activator versus intravenous streptokinase in acute myocardial infarction Report from the European Cooperative Study Group for Recombinant Tissue-type Plasminogen Activator. Lancet 1985; 1:842.

23.   Anderson J, Rothbard R, Hackworthy R. Multicenter reperfusion trial of intravenous anisoylated plasminogen streptokinase activator complex APSAC in acute myocardial infarction Controlled comparison with intracoronary streptokinase.J Am Coll Cardiol 1988; 11:1153.

24.   APSAC Multicenter Investigators. Multicenter Reperfusion Trial of intravenous anisoylated plasminogen streptokinase activator complex (APSAC) in acute myocardial infarction controlled comparison with intracoronary streptokinase.J Am Coll Cardiol 1988; 11:1153-1163.

25.   GISSI. Long-term effects of intravenous thrombolysis in acute myocardial infarction final report of the GISSI study. Lancet 1987; 2:871-874.

26.   ISIS. Randomised trial of intravenous streptokinase, oral aspirin, both, or neither among 17187 cases of suspected acute myocardial infarction: ISIS-2. Lancet 1988; 2 (1)349-360.

27.   Serruys P, Simoons M, Suryappanata H, et al. Preservation of global and regional left ventricular function after early thrombolysis in acute myocardial infarction.J Am Coll Cardiol 1986; 7:729-742.

28.   Timmis A, Griffin B, Crick J, et al. Anisoylated plasminogen streptokinase activator complex in acute myocardial infarction A placebo-controlled arteriographic coronary recanalization study. J Am Coll Cardiol 1987; 10:205.

29.   Verstraete M, Bernard R, Bory M, et al. Randomized trial of intravenous recombinant tissue-type plasminogen activator versus intravenous streptokinase in acute myocardial infarction. Lancet 1985; 2:965.

30.   White H, Norris R, Brown M, et al. Effect of intravenous streptokinase on left ventricular function and early survival after acute myocardial infarction.New England Journal of Medicine 1987; 317:850-855.

31.   Wilcox R, Lippe GVD, Olsson C, et al. Trial of tissue plasminogen activator for mortality reduction in acute myocardial infarction (Anglo-Scandinavian Study of Early Thrombolysis [ASSET]). Lancet 1988; 2:525-530.

32.   GISSI. Effectiveness of intravenous thrombolytic treatment in acute myocardial infarction. Lancet 1986; 1:397-401.

33.   GISSI-2: A factorial randomised trial of alteplase versus streptokinase and heparin versus no heparin among 12,490 patients with acute myocardial infarction.Lancet 1990; 336:65-71.

34.   EMERAS Collaborative Group. Randomised trial of late thrombolysis in patients with suspected acute myocardial infarction.Lancet 1993; 342:767-772.

35.   Fibrinolytic Therapy Trailists (FTT) Collaborative Group. Indications for fibrinolytic therapy in suspected acute myocardial infarction Collaborative overview of early mortality and major morbidity results from all randomised trials of more than 1000 patients. Lancet 1994 343:311-322.

36.   Ryan TJ, Anderson JL, Antman EM, Braniff BA, et al. ACC/AHA guidelines for the management of patients with aucte myocardial infarction: Executvie summary. Circulation 1996; 94:2341-2350.

37.   Ryan TJ, Anderson JL, Antman EM, Braniff BA, et al. ACC/AHA guidelines for the management of patients with aucte myocardial infarction. JACC 1996: 28 (5): 1328-428.

38.   Bouten M, Simoons M, Hartman J, et al. Prehospital thrombolysis with alteplase (rt-PA) in acute myocardial infarction. European Heart Journal 1992 13:925-931.

39.   Weaver J, Cerqueira M, Hallstrom P, et al. Prehospital-initiated vs hospital-initiated thrombolytic therapy. Journal of American Medical Association 1993 270:1211-1216.

40.   SCATI Group. Randomised controlled trial of subcutaneous calcium-heparin in acute myocardial infarction. Lancet 1989, 2:182-186.

41. Hsia J, Hamilton W, Kleiman N, et al. A comparison between heparin and low-dose aspirin as adjunctive therapy with tissue plasminogen activator for acute myocardial infarction. New England Journal of Medicine 1990; 323:1436-1437.

42. O'Connor C, Meese R, Carneyl R. A randomized trial of intravenous heparin in conjunction with anistreplase (anisoylated plasminogen streptokinase activator complex) in acute myocardial infarction: The Duke University Clinical Cardiology Study (DUCCS) 1. J Am Coll Cardiol 1994; 23:11-18.

43. ISIS-1 Collaborative Group. Randomised trial of intravenous atenolol among 16 027 cases of suspected acute myocardial infarction: ISIS-1. Lancet 1986; 8498:57-66.

44. Horner S. Efficacy of intravenous magnesium in acute myocardial infarction in reducing arrhythmias and mortality: Meta-analysis of magnesium in acute myocardial infarction. Circulation 1992; 86:774-779.

45. Woods K, Fletcher S, Roffe C, Haider Y. Intravenous magnesium sulphate in suspected acute myocardial infarction: Results of the second Leicester Intravenous Magnesium Intervention Trial (LIMIT-2). Lancet 1992; 339:1553-1558.

46. ISIS-4 Collaborative Group. Randomised study of intravenous magnesium in over 50,000 patients with suspected acute myocardial infarction, abstracted. Circulation 1993; 88 (Suppl I):I-292.

47. Ridker P, Hebert P, Fuster V, Hennekens C. Are both aspirin and heparin justified as adjuncts to thrombolytic therapy for acute myocardial infarction? Lancet 1993; 341:1574-1577.

48. Jeremy R, Hackworthy R, Bautovich G, et al. Infarct artery perfusion and changes in left ventricular volume in the month after acute myocardial infarction. J Am Coll Cardiol 1987; 9:989-995.

49. White H, Cross D, Elliott J, et al. Long-term prognostic importance of patency of the infarct-related coronary artery after thrombolytic therapy for acute myocardial infarction. Circulation 1994; 89:59-67.

50. Guerci A, Gerstenblith G, Brinker J, et al. A randomized trial of intravenous tissue plasminogen activator for acute myocardial infarction with subsequent randomization to elective coronary angioplasty. New England Journal of Medicine 1987; 317:1613-1618.

51. Topol E. Coronary angioplasty for acute myocardial infarction. Annals of Internal Medicine 1988; 109:970-980.

52. Topol E, Califf R, George B, et al. Thrombolysis and Angioplasty in Myocardial Infarction Study Group. A randomized trial of immediate versus delayed elective angioplasty after intravenous tissue plasminogen activator in acute myocardial infarction. New England Journal of Medicine 1987; 317 (10)581-588.

53. Grines C, Browne K, Marco J, et al. A comparison of immediate angioplasty withthombolytic therapy for acute myocardial infarction. New England Journal of Medicine 1993; 328:673-679.

54. Gibbons R, Holmes D, Reeder G, et al. Immediate angioplasty compared with the administration of a thrombolytic agent followed by conservative treatment for myocardial infarction. New England Journal of Medicine 1993; 328:685-691.

55. Zijlstra F, Boer JD, Hoorntje C, et al. A comparison of immediate coronary angioplasty with intravenous streptokinase in acute myocardial infarction. New England Journal of Medicine 1993; 328:680-684.

56. Reeder G, Bailey K, Gersh B, et al. Cost comparison of immediate angioplasty versus thrombolysis followed by conservative therapy for acute myocardial infarction A randomized prospective trial. Mayo Clinical Proceedings 1994; 69:5-12.

57. Bigger JT, Fleiss JL, Kleiger R, et al. The relationship among ventricular arrhythmias, left ventricular dysfunction, and mortality in the 2 years after myocardial infarction. Circulation 1984; 69:250-258.

58. Bigger Jr J, Fleiss J, Rolnitzky L, Multicenter Post-Infarction Research Group. Prevalence, characteristics and significance of ventricular tachycardia detected by 24-hour continuous electrocardiographic recordings in the late hospital phase of acute myocardial infarction. American Journal of Cardiology 1986; 58:1151-1160.

59.   Hallstrom A, Bigger J, Roden D, et al. Prognostic significance of ventricular premature depolarizations measured 1 year after myocardial infarction in patients with early postinfarction asymptomatic ventricular arrhythmia. J Am Coll Cardiol 1992; 20:259-264.
60.   Multicenter Postinfarction Research Group. Risk stratification and survival after myocardial infarction. New England Journal of Medicine 1983 309:331-336.
61.   De Feyter P, VanFenige M, Dighten D. Prognostic value of exercise testing, coronary angiography and left ventriculography six to eight weeks after myocardial infarction. Circulation 1982; 66:527-536.
62.   DeBusk R. Evaluation of patients after recent acute myocardial infarction. Annals of Internal Medicine 1989; 110:485-488.
63.   Fioretti P, Brower R, Simmons M, et al. Prediction of mortality during the first year after acute myocardial infarction from clinical variables and stress test at hospital discharge. American Journal of Cardiology 1985 55:1313-1318.
64.   Krone R, Dwyer E, Greenberg H, et al. Risk stratification in patients with first non-q wave infarction: limited value of the early low level exercise test after uncomplicated infarcts. J Am Coll Cardiol 1989; 14:31-37.
65.   Krone R, Gillespie J, Weld F, et al. Low-level exercise testing after myocardial infarction: usefulness in enhancing clinical risk stratification. Circulation 1985 71:80-89.
66.   Madsen E, Gilpin E, Ahnvee S. Prediction of functional capacity and use of exercise testing for predicting risk after acute myocardial infarction. American Journal of Cardiology 1985 56:839-845.
67.   Theroux P, Waters D, Halphen C, et al. Prognostic value of exercise testing soon after myocardial infarction. New England Journal of Medicine 1979 301:341-345.
68.   Weld F, Chu K, Bigger J, Rolnitzky L. Risk stratification with low level exercise testing 2 weeks after acute myocardial infarction. Circulation 1981; 64:306-314.
69.   Williams W, Nair R, Higginson L, et al. Comparison of clinical and treadmill variables for the prediction of outcome after myocardial infarction. J Am Coll Cardiol 1984; 4:477-486.
70.   Buda A, Dubbin J, MacDonald I, et al. Spontaneous changes in thallium-201 myocardial perfusion imaging after myocardial infarction. American Journal of Cardiology 1982 50:1271-1278.
71.   Gibson R, Beller G, Gheorghiade M. The prevalence and clinical significance of residual myocardial ischemia two weeks after uncomplicated non Q-wave infarction A prospective natural history study. Circulation 1986; 73(6)1186-1198.
72.   Gibson R, Watson D, Graddock G, et al. Prediction of cardiac events after uncomplicated myocardial infarction: A prospective study comparing predischarge exercise thallium-201 scintigraphy and coronary angiography. Circulation 1983 68:321-336.
73.   Hung J, Gordon E, Houston N, et al. Changes in rest and exercise myocardial perfusion and left ventricular function 3 to 26 weeks after clinically uncomplicated acute myocardial infarction. American Journal of Cardiology 1984 54:943-950.
74.   Hung J, Goris M, Nash E, et al. Comparative value of maximal treadmill testing, exercise thallium myocardial perfusion scintigraphy and exercise radionuclide ventriculography for distinguishing high- and low-risk patients soon after acute myocardial infarction. American Journal of Cardiology 1984 53:1221-1227.
75.   Tilkemeier P, Guiney T, LaRaia P, Boucher C. Prognostic value of predischarge low-level exercise thallium testing after thrombolytic treatment of acute myocardial infarction. American Journal of Cardiology 1990 66:1203-1207.
76.   Wilson W, Gibson R, Nygaard T. Acute myocardial infarction associated with single vessel coronary artery disease: An analysis of clinical outcome and the prognostic importance of vessel patency and residual ischemia myocardium. J Am Coll Cardiol 1988; 11:223-234.
77.   Hamm L, Crow R, Stuli G et al. Safety and characteristics of exercise testing early after acute myocardial infarction. American Journal of Cardiology 1989 63:1193-1197.
78.   Jain A, Myers H, Sapin P, O'Rourke R. Superiority and safety of maximal exercise testing early after myocardial infarction. J Am Coll Cardiol 1993; 21 (suppl A:98A.

79.   Juneau M, Colles P , Theroux P. Symptom-limited versus low level exercise testing before hospital discharge after myocardial infarction. J AmColl Cardiol 1992; 20:927-933.

80.   Botvinick E, Dae M. Dipyridamole perfusion scintigraphy. Semin Nucl Med 1991; XXI:242-265.

81.   Gimple L, Hutter A, Guiney T, Boucher C. Prognostic utility of predischarge dipyridamole-thallium imaging compared to predischarge submaximal exercise electrocardiography and maximal exercise thallium imaging after uncomplicated acute myocardial infarction. American Journal of Cardiology 1989; 64:1243-1248.

82.   Marzullo P, Parodi O, Reisenhofer B, et al. Value of rest thallium-201/technetium-99m sestamibi scans and dobutamine echocardiography for detecting myocardial viability. American Journal of Cardiology 1993; 71:166-172.

83.   Dilsizian V, Bonow R. Current diagnostic techniques of assessing myocardial viability in patients with hibernating and stunned myocardium. Circulation 1993 87:1-20.

84.   Barilla F, Gheorghiade M, Alam M, et al. Low-dose dobutamine in patients with acute myocardial infarction identifies viable but not contractile myocardium and predicts the magnitude of improvement in wall motion abnormalities in response to coronary revascularization. American Heart J 1991; 122:1522-1531.

85.   Berman D, Kiat H, Van Train K, et al. Technetium 99m sestamibi in the assessment of chronic coronary artery disease. Seminars in Nuclear Medicine 1991; 21:190-212.

86.   Cuocolo A, Pace L, Ricciardelli B, et al. Identification of viable myocardium in patients with chronic coronary artery disease Comparison of thallium-201 scintigraphy with reinjection and technetium-99m-methoxyisobutyl isonitrile. Journal of Nuclear Medicine 1992 33:505-511.

87.   ACC/AHA Task Force. Guidelines for the early management of patients with acute myocardial infarction: A report of the American College of Cardiology/American Heart Association Task Force on assessment of diagnostic and therapeutic cardiovascular procedures (subcommittee to develop guidelines for the early management of patients with acute myocardial infarction). Journal of the American College of Cardiology 1990 16:249-292.

88.   SWIFT Trial Study Group. SWIFT trial of delayed elective intervention vs conservative treatment after thrombolysis with anistreplase in acute myocardial infarction. British Medical Journal 1991; 302:555-560.

89.   TIMI II Investigators. Selective versus routine predischarge coronary arteriography after therapy with recombinant tissue-type plasminogen activator, heparin and aspirin for acute myocardial infarction. J Am Coll Cardiol 1991; 17:1007-1016.

90.   Ross R, Gilpin E, Madsen E, et al. A decision scheme for coronary angiography after acute myocardial infarction. Circulation 1989, 79:292-303.

91.   Shenasa M, Fetsch T, Martinez-Rubio A, et al. Signal averaging in patients with coronary artery disease: How helpful is it? Journal of Cardiovascular Electrophysiology 1993 4:609-626.

92.   O'Quin R, Marini JJ. Pulmonary artery occlusion pressure Clinical physiology, measurement and interpretation. American Revision Respiratory Disease 1983 128:319-326.

93.   Moss A, DeCamilla J, Davis H. Cardiac death in the first 6 months after myocardial infarction Potential for mortality reduction in the early post-hospital period. American Journal of Cardiology 1977; 39:816-820.

94.   Mukharji J, Rude R, Pool W. Risk factors for sudden death after acute myocardial infarction Two year follow-up. American Journal of Cardiology 1984 54:31-36.

95.   Hutter A, DeSanctis R, Flynn T, Yeatman L. Nontransmural myocardial infarction A comparison of hospital and late clinical course of patients with that of matched patients with transmural anterior and transmural inferior myocardial infarction. American Journal of Cardiology 1981; 48:595-602.

96.   Kao W, Khaja F, Goldstein S, Gheorghlade M. Cardiac event rate after non-q-wave acute myocardial infarction and the significance of its anterior location. American Journal of Cardiology 1989, 64:1236-1242.

97.   Schechtman K, Capone R, Kleiger R, et al. Risk stratification of patients with non-Q wave myocardial infarction. The critical role of ST segment depression. Circulation 1989 80:1148-1158.

98.   Schechtman K, Kleiger R, Boden W, et al. The relationship between 1-year mortality and infarct location in patients with non-Q wave myocardial infarction. American Heart J 1992 123:1175-1181.

99.   Anderson J, Karagounis L, Becker L, et al. TIMI perfusion Grade 3 but not Grade 2 results in improved outcome after thrombolysis for myocardial infarction: Ventriculographic, enzymatic, and electrocardiographic evidence from the TEAM-3 Study. Circulation 1993 87:1829-1839.

100.   Vogt A, Essen RV, Tobbe U, et al. Impact of early perfusion status of the infarct-related artery on short-term mortality after thrombolysis for acute myocardial infarction Retrospective analysis of four German multicenter studies. J AmColl Cardiol 1993; 21:1391-1395.

101.   Gohike H, Heim E ,Roskamm H. Prognostic importance of collateral flow and residual coronary stenosis of the myocardial infarction artery after anterior wall Q-wave acute myocardial infarction. American Journal of Cardiology 1991 67:1165-1169.

102.   Rogers W, Hood W, Mantle J, et al. Return of left ventricular function after reperfusion in patients with myocardial infarction Importance of subtotal stenoses or intact collaterals. Circulation 1984; 69:33.

103.   β-blocker Heart Attack Research Group. A randomized trial of propranololin patients with acute myocardial infarction. Journal of American Medical Association 1982 247:1707-1714.

104.   Hampton J. Secondary prevention of acute myocardial infarction with beta-blocking agents and calcium antagonists. American Journal of Cardiology 1990 66:3C-8C.

105.   Hjalmarson A, Elmfeldt D, Herlitz J, et al. Effect on mortality of metroprolol in acute myocardial infarction: A double-blind randomised trial. Lancet 1981; 2:823.

106.   Norwegian Multicenter Study Group. Timolol-induced reduction in mortality and reinfarction in patients surviving acute myocardial infarction. New England Journal of Medicine 1981 304:801-807.

107.   Yusuf S, Peto R, Lewis J et al. Betablockade during and after myocardial infarction An overview of the randomized trials. Prog Cardiovasc Dis 1985; 27:335-371.

108.   Multicenter Diltiazem Post-Infarction Research Group. The effect of diltiazem on mortality and reinfarction after acute myocardial infarction. New England Journal of Medicine 1988 319:385-392.

109.   (SPRINT) Secondary Prevention Reinfarction Nifedipine Trial. A randomized intervention trial of nifedipine in patients with acute myocardial infarction. European Heart Journal 1988 9:354-364.

110.   Swedberg K, Held P, Kjekshus J, et al. Effects of the early administration of enalapril on mortality in patients with acute myocardial infarction. Results of the cooperative new Scandinavian enalapril survival study II (Consensus II). New England Journal of Medicine 1992 327:678-684.

5

PLATELET GLYCOPROTEIN IIB/IIIA INTEGRIN INHIBITION IN ACUTE MYOCARDIAL INFARCTION

Conor O'Shea, MD
James E. Tcheng, MD
Duke University Medical Center, Durham, NC

INTRODUCTION:

The initial cascade of events responsible for acute (ST segment elevation) myocardial infarction is now well elucidated. The vast majority of cases are precipitated by spontaneous plaque rupture resulting in platelet adhesion, activation, and aggregation, and finally thrombosis (1,2). The initial thrombus produces a hemostatic plug that limits blood flow to varying degrees, with most cases of acute infarction being the result of complete thrombotic occlusion of the coronary artery (3).

The two therapeutic approaches to the initial treatment of acute myocardial infarction, direct angioplasty and thrombolytic therapy, share the same goal: rapid and sustained reperfusion to improve long-term clinical outcomes. While both approaches have greatly reduced mortality, each has limitations that might be further improved through the aggressive management of thrombus. With direct angioplasty, dealing with coronary thrombus during the intervention can prove problematic; procedural complications of thrombosis including distal embolization, the no-reflow phenomenon, thrombus propagation, and rethrombosis are poorly addressed with mechanical technologies (4). Longer-term issues include vessel restonsis or reocclusion, which can be silent, result in signs or symptoms of ischemia, or cause a second acute infarction (5). Thrombolysis is associated with a somewhat different but parallel set of issues related to thrombus management. Despite advances in thrombolytic strategies, normal TIMI (Thrombolysis in Myocardial Infarction) (6) grade 3 flow will be restored in only about half of patients within 90 minutes of treatment (7,8). In addition, a ceiling of reperfusion around 80% is well recognized (9). Inadequate coronary perfusion is associated with a doubling in the 30 day mortality from roughly 4% to 8% (7). Reengineered thrombolytics have only marginally augmented the proportion of patients achieving reperfusion without reducing cardiac mortality (10,11). Even with successful reperfusion, a substantial proportion of patients develop recurrent ischemia or vessel occlusion due to continued instability of the infarct-related artery (12-14). Overall, only about 1 in 4 patients receiving thrombolytic therapy for myocardial infarction achieve optimal reperfusion (12).

A greater appreciation of the role of the platelet in the pathophysiology of thrombosis has suggested that potent inhibition of platelet aggregation might improve outcomes following acute myocardial infarction. Aspirin, which prevents platelet aggregation by inhibiting the formation of thromboxane A_2, is known to enhance the efficacy of thrombolytic therapy (15) and is a critical adjunct to coronary intervention. However, aspirin has only a limited anti-platelet effect, inhibiting only one of the myriad of pathways leading to platelet activation. (16,17). Recent investigations have therefore focused on inhibitors of platelet aggregation, namely the platelet glycoprotein (GP) IIb/IIIa integrin blockers, as more potent antagonists of overall platelet function. The GP IIb/IIIa receptor is the final common pathway leading to platelet aggregation, facilitating thrombus formation by its role as the platelet membrane surface receptor for the binding of dimeric adhesive proteins including von Willebrand factor, fibrinogen, and fibrinonectin (17). This integrin recognizes an Arg-Gly-Asp (RGD) sequence as well as a Lys-Gln-Ala-Gly-Asp-Val sequence on the fibrinogen molecule (18). These two regions serve as the binding sites for fibrinogen with GP IIb/IIIa (19).

The groundwork for the clinical investigation of GP IIb/IIIa inhibition in acute myocardial infarction was pioneered by Gold and colleagues. Using the Folts model (in dogs) of coronary artery thrombosis and reperfusion, Gold and colleagues demonstrated the potential of m7E3 (a monoclonal antibody to GP IIb/IIIa) to improve patency kinetics and prevent vessel reocclusion (20) (Figure 1). While the early large scale investigations of the GP IIb/IIIa antagonists have focused on coronary intervention and unstable angina / non-Q-wave myocardial infarction (21-23), more recently attention has turned to acute myocardial infarction. A number of parenteral GP IIb/IIIa receptor blockers are now undergoing clinical investigation (Table 1).

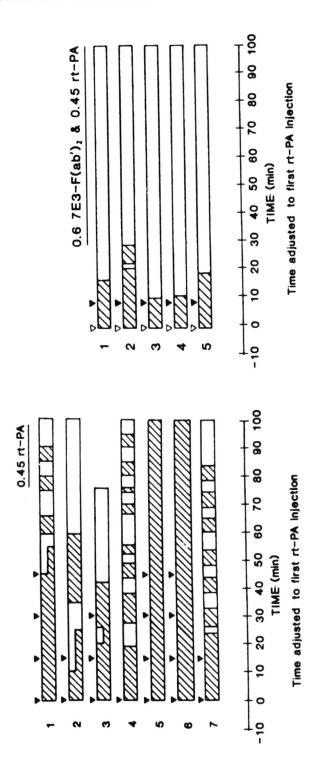

Figure 1. Schematic representation of coronary artery reperfusion/reocclusion cycles in dogs receiving boluses of rt-PA and of 7E3-F(ab')2 alone or in combination. $\triangledown$ =7E3-F(ab')2 injection; $\blacktriangledown$ = rt-PA injection; hatched bar = occlusion; open bar = reperfusion.

Table 1

Trial	N	GP IIb/IIIa Antagonist	Study Design	Primary endpoint
Adjunct to thrombolysis				
IMPACT-AMI	180	eptifibatide	tPA/phase II	TIMI 3 flow at 90 min.
PARADIGM	353	lamifiban	tPA, SK/phase II	30 day Death, MI, TVR
Integrilin with SK	181	eptifibatide	SK/phase II	TIMI 3 flow at 90 min
TIMI 14A	450	abciximab	tPA, SK/phase II	TIMI 3 flow at 90 min
SPEED	350	abciximab	rPA/phase II	TIMI 3 flow at 60 min
Adjunct to direct PTCA				
GRAPE	41	abciximab	direct PTCA/phase II	TIMI 3 flow at 45 min.
RAPPORT	483	abciximab	direct PTCA/phase III	6 month Death, MI, TVR
TAMI 8	70	m7E3	tPA/phase II (non-randomized)	Recurrent ischemia
CADILLAC	2000	abciximab	PTCA/primary stenting (ACS Multilink)/phase III	6 month Death, MI, Stroke, TVR

N: number of patients enrolled; TVR: target vessel revascularization: tPA: tissue plasminogen activator; SK: streptokinase; rPA: recombinant plasminogen activator; min: minutes.

Parenteral Glycoprotein IIb/IIIa Receptor Inhibitors

The first agent approved for clinical use was abciximab (ReoPro™; Centocor, Malvern, PA/Eli Lilly, Indianapolis, IN), a chimeric human-mouse monoclonal antibody Fab fragment. The high affinity binding and slow dissociation of abciximab from GP IIb/IIIa causes its effects to persist long after infusion of the antibody is discontinued (24). Other properties of the agent are that it binds to the $\alpha_v\beta3$ (vitronectin) and MAC-1 receptors, decreases the production of PAI-1, inhibits clot retraction, and can cause "dethrombosis", or dissolution, of fresh thrombus (25). Abciximab has also been shown to be immunogenic, most likely because of its large molecular size and protein composition (26).

Several small molecule GP IIb/IIIa inhibitors are also under scrutiny in the clinical setting. In contrast to abciximab, these agents have competitive pharmacodynamic profiles, with platelet blockade essentially being a function of plasma concentration. These inhibitors have relatively rapid dissociation and clearance parameters that permit restoration of platelet function and normal hemostasis within hours of discontinuation. Eptifibatide (Integrilin™; COR Therapeutics, South San Francisco, CA / Schering-Plough, Kenilworth, NJ) is a synthetic, cyclic heptapeptide approved for the treatment of unstable angina / non-Q-wave myocardial infarction and as an adjunct to coronary intervention. It is fashioned after the structure of the integrin antagonist barbourin (27), a small protein inhibitor of GP IIb/IIIa isolated from the venom of the Southeastern pygmy rattlesnake *Sistrurus m barbouri*. The specificity and stability of eptifibatide for GP IIb/IIIa are enhanced compared to linear RGD based peptides by its cyclic structure and a single amino acid substitution of lysine for arginine (28; 29). In large clinical trials, an antibody response to eptifbatide has not been detected; this may be important in patients requiring repeat administration of a GP IIb/IIIa inhibitor. Other representative agents include lamifiban (Hoffman-La Roche, Basel, Switzerland), and the tyrosine derivative tirofiban (MK-383, or Aggrastat™, Merck Research Laboratories, West Point, Pennsylvania). These synthetic, highly specific, short acting, non-peptide (but peptidomimetic) inhibitors of glycoprotein IIb/IIIa were also designed to avert some of the problems of the linear peptides, namely instability and short survival times in the circulation.

Clinical Trials of GP IIb/IIIa Inhibition with Thrombolytic Therapy

TAMI-8

The first clinical trial combining GP IIb/IIIa inhibition with thrombolysis was reported by the Thrombolysis and Angioplasty in Myocardial Infarction (TAMI) group (30). The TAMI-8 study evaluated m7E3 in a dose-ranging study of m7E3 given after administration of recombinant tissue plasminogen activator (t-PA). A total of 70 patients were enrolled, with trial regimens including bolus injections of m7E3 in ascending doses (0.1-1.25 mg/kg) at 3, 6 or 15 hours after the initiation of t-PA. As opposed to current investigations, in this first experience thrombolytic and GP IIb/IIIa inhibitor therapies were not given concurrently because of the unknown and unexplored potential for serious bleeding. The outcome trends all favored m7E3 treatment. Recurrent ischemia occurred in fewer patients (13% versus 20% in the control group). Delayed follow-up angiography (performed late in the hospital course in a limited number of patients) demonstrated patency (TIMI grade 2 or 3 flow) in 92% of m7E3 treated patients as opposed to 56% of controls. Major bleeding and transfusions occurred at a similar rate in both groups. This first study thus suggested that adjunctive GP IIb/IIIa inhibition could help maintain vascular patency and prevent reocclusion following thrombolysis.

IMPACT-AMI

The Integrelin to Manage Platelet Aggregation to Prevent Coronary Thrombosis in Acute Myocardial Infarction (IMPACT-AMI) study was the first trial to evaluate the effects of glycoprotein IIb/IIIa inhibition given concurrently with thrombolytic therapy. IMPACT-AMI was a randomized, blinded, dose-ranging trial of eptifibatide with full-dose, accelerated regimen tPA (31. Patients presenting within 6 hours of an acute myocardial infarction were randomized to placebo (n=55) or ascending doses of eptifibatide, given as a bolus plus 24 hour infusion, in addition to front loaded t-PA, heparin and aspirin. The primary endpoint, TIMI grade 3 flow at 90-minute coronary angiography, improved from 39% in the control group to 66% of those receiving the highest dose of eptifibatide (p=0.006). A secondary endpoint, time to recovery of ST segment elevation per continuous electrocardiography, also improved with treatment. The median time from t-PA administration to recovery of ST-segment elevation was significantly shorter in those receiving the highest dose of eptifibatide compared to placebo (65 vs 116 minutes; p = 0.05) and was intermediate for all eptifibatide treated patients. Clinical outcomes, however, were no different. The incidence of death or reinfarction was 7.3% with placebo treatment, 8.0% for all patients randomized to eptifibatide, and 7.8% for those on the highest dose of eptifibatide. Finally, the incidences of bleeding were similar among groups. Mild bleeding, mostly at the femoral access site, occurred in more than 60% of cases. Moderate and severe bleeding occurred in 14% and 2% of the eptifibatide-treated and 9% and 5% of placebo-treated patients, respectively. There was one hemorrhagic stroke in the eptifibatide-treated group and none in the control group. In summary, IMPACT-AMI suggested that GP IIb/IIIa inhibition would improve both the proportion of patients achieving reperfusion as well as the kinetics of reperfusion. Unknown was whether or not reduced dose thrombolytic therapy might achieve similar outcomes while improving bleeding profiles.

PARADIGM

The next trial to be completed was the Platelet Aggregation receptor Antagonist Dose Investigation for Reperfusion Gain in Myocardial Infarction (PARADIGM) trial. In PARADIGM, 353 patients presenting within 24 hours of acute myocardial infarction received either lamifiban as a bolus plus infusion or placebo in combination with streptokinase or t-PA (32). All subjects were given aspirin. The initial goal of PARADIGM was to identify a dose of lamifiban that would produce greater than 80% inhibition of ADP-induced platelet aggregation; to this end, the first 30 patients received lamifiban as an open label drug. The remaining study patients were randomized in a 2:1 fashion to lamifiban or placebo (33). There was no significant difference in the primary composite clinical end-point (death, reinfarction, ischemia requiring urgent revascularization, or the absence of TIMI grade 3 flow at angiography). However, continuous electrocardiography suggested improvement in 90-minute infarct artery patency (from 56% to 76% with lamifiban, P= 0.019) and reduced recurrent ischemia during the first 24 hours (33% versus 69%, P=0.001). In summary, while the surrogate endpoints appeared promising, PARADIGM failed to document any significant reduction in harder clinical end-points.

Integrilin in Streptokinase Trial

Recently, Simoons and colleagues reported the results of a study using a combination of Integrilin as a 180µg/kg bolus followed by an infusion of 0.75, 1.33 or 2.0 µg/kg/min with 1.5 million units of streptokinase in 181 patients with acute myocardial infarction (34). The combined therapy yielded only a modest increase in early 90 minutes TIMI grade 3 flow (53%-integrilin 180/0.75) compared with streptokinase with placebo (38%).The highest dose arm was discontinued when an increased bleeding rate was observed. Coupled with the PARADIGM trial results, these findings are obviously disappointing, particularly with respect to the potentiation of thrombolysis by streptokinase. These data would suggest an intrinsic difference in the ability of GP IIb/IIIa blockade to enhance thrombolytic potency with streptokinase vis á vis the more selective thrombolytic agents such as t-PA and r-PA.

TIMI 14a

To date, the largest and most provocative study of the combination of GP IIb/IIIa inhibition with reduced dose thrombolytic therapy during acute myocardial infarction was the TIMI 14a study (35). TIMI 14a was a dose-ranging study that evaluated full-dose abciximab inhibition in 14 different treatment regimens (including abciximab alone) in over 450 patients as a prelude to larger scale investigation. Both t-PA and streptokinase were studied. As presented by Antman and colleagues, a summary of the findings are included in Figure 2. With the combination of full-dose abciximab and a 15 mg bolus of t-PA followed by a 35 mg

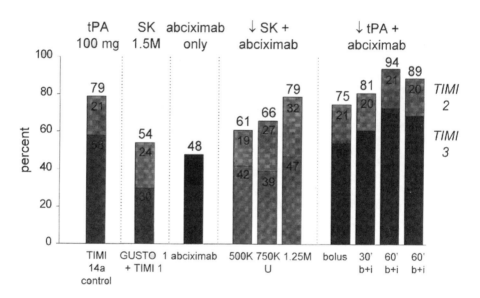

Figure 2. Angiographic Results of the TIMI 14A Trial. A total of 14 different combinations of tissue plasminogen activator or streptokinase with abciximab were investigated; results observed with seven of the combinations, as well as the t-PA alone and abciximab alone controls. For comparison purposes, the results with streptokinase alone as observed in the GUSTO 1 and TIMI 1 trials is included. The right most bar in the graph are the results with an increased bolus dose (0.3 mg/kg) of abciximab. Adapted from Antman E et al., J Am Coll Cardiol 1998; 31:191A (abstract). TIMI: Thrombolysis in Myocardial Infarction; t-PA: tissue plasminogen activator; SK: streptokinase; GUSTO: Global Use of Strategies To Open Occluded Coronary Arteries; U: units; b: bolus; i: infusion.

infusion of t-PA over 1 hour, TIMI 3 flow in the infarct-related artery was improved from 45% to 67% at 60 minutes and from 58% to 73% at 90 minutes (P=0.02 for the 90 minute comparison). Consistent with the observations of the PARADIGM and the Integrilin with Streptokinase trials, combinations of abciximab with streptokinase failed to achieve patency rates observed even with t-PA alone and were associated with unacceptable bleeding. Bleeding rates were not increased among the t-PA plus abciximab regimens. In summary, TIMI 14a suggests that rates of reperfusion and patency kinetics can be further augmented by combining abciximab with lower dose t-PA (but not streptokinase). These results have provided the impetus and justification for moving forward to TIMI 14b, a study which will build upon the findings of TIMI 14a by comparing front-loaded t-PA versus the best 50 mg t-PA plus abciximab treatment strategy in a blinded, controlled, randomized study enrolling a large number of patients.

SPEED

Abciximab is also being studied in conjunction with r-PA. As a precursor to the planned GUSTO 4 trial, the SPEED trial is evaluating varying doses of r-PA, with 60 and 90 minute angiography defining the primary end-point (36). Patients are currently being recruited into the SPEED trial. The intent is to leverage the findings of SPEED to optimize the potential for identification of a beneficial regimen in the pivotal GUSTO 4 trial. As currently projected, enrollment into GUSTO 4 will begin sometime in 1998.

Clinical Trials of GP IIb/IIIa Inhibition with Direct Coronary Intervention

RAPPORT

As of this writing, the largest randomized, multicenter trial of GP IIb/IIIa inhibition as an adjunct to direct angioplasty during acute myocardial infarction has been the RAPPORT study (Reopro in Acute myocardial infarction and Primary PTCA Organization Randomized Trial) (37). The GRAPE trial (Glycoprotein Receptor Antagonist Receptor Evaluation) (38), has also been completed recently with findings similar to RAPPORT. In RAPPORT, 483 patients were randomized in the emergency department or the catheterization suite to abciximab bolus plus infusion or placebo treatment. All patients received aspirin and full-dose heparin to achieve an activated clotting time of greater than 300 seconds. The patients then underwent diagnostic catheterization with the intent to perform a coronary intervention. Stent implantation was actively discouraged. As presented by Brener and colleagues, at 30 days, a significant 62% reduction in the composite endpoint of death, reinfarction, or urgent revascularization was observed among the 409 patients receiving any study drug and undergoing angioplasty (12.0% vs. 4.6% for the treated patient analysis, P=0.005). By the intention to treat analysis (inclusive of all 483 patients), the difference remained significant (11.2% vs. 5.8%, P=0.038). However, the primary endpoint of death, reinfarction, or any target vessel revascularization at 6 months was no different between groups. In addition, rates of bleeding were higher with abciximab treatment. RAPPORT thus suggests that abrupt closure following direct angioplasty can be reduced with abciximab treatment; however, no restenosis benefit should be anticipated. Now that we are in the stent era, the next obvious question becomes the role of combining stent implantation with adjunctive GP IIb/IIIa inhibition in acute myocardial infarction. The CADILLAC trial (Controlled Abciximab and Device Investigation to Lower Late Angioplasty Complications), a study of nearly 2,000 patients, will address this question through a factorial randomization (stent vs. no stent and abciximab vs. no abciximab) (39). With reductions in abrupt closure expected with both stent implantation and GP IIb/IIIa inhibition, another novel concept being tested in CADILLAC is the safety of early (within 2-3 days) hospital discharge, particularly with regard to overall resource consumption.

DISCUSSION:

Studies of glycoprotein IIb/IIIa inhibition in combination with thrombolytic therapy have the potential to address the remaining limitations of standalone thrombolytic therapy: failure to achieve reperfusion in half of patients, suboptimal reperfusion kinetics, vessel reclosure, and catastrophic bleeding. Findings to date support the hypothesis that platelet activity remains a key component explaining the limitations of thrombolytic therapy. All of the pilot trials have demonstrated trends consistent with improved restoration of coronary perfusion, although this has not translated into improved clinical outcomes. Large-scale phase III trials will be required to determine if the angiographic findings correlate with reduced mortality. Interestingly, while one might expect to see reductions in *cardiac* mortality, in fact there is an equal chance that mortality will be reduced by eliminating intracranial hemorrhage secondary to high dose thrombolytic therapy. Finally, the role of GP IIb/IIIa antagonism is still undefined as an adjunct to direct coronary intervention. The hope is that adjunctive GP IIb/IIIa inhibition will improve procedural outcomes, reduce subacute closure, and permit the earlier discharge home of patients than is practiced today.

References:

1.   Fuster V, Badimon L, Badimon JJ, Chesebro JH. The pathogenesis of coronary artery disease and the acute coronary syndromes (1). *N Engl J Med* 1992; 326: 242-250.

2.   Fuster V, Badimon L, Badimon JJ, Chesebro JH. The pathogenesis of coronary artery disease and the acute coronary syndromes (2). *N Engl J Med* 1992; 326: 310-318.

3.   DeWood MA, Spores J, Notske R, Mouser LT, Burroughs R, Golden MS, Lang HT. Prevalence of total coronary occlusion during the early hours of transmural myocardial infarction. *N Engl J Med* 1980; 303: 897-902.

4.   Landau C, Glamann DB, Willard JE, Hillis LD, Lange RA. Coronary angioplasty in the patient with acute myocardial infarction. *Am J Med* 1994; 96: 536-543.

5.   Califf RM, Abdelmeguid AE, Kuntz RE et al. Myonecrosis after revascularisation procedures. *J Am Coll Cardiol* 1998; 31: 242-251.

6.   Chesebro JH, Knatterud G, Roberts R, et al. Thrombolysis in Myocardial Infarction (TIMI) Trial, Phase I: a comparison between intravenous tissue plasminogen activator and intravenous streptokinase. *Circulation* 1987; 76: 142-154.

7.   The GUSTO angiographic investigators. The effects of tissue plasminogen activator, streptokinase, or both on coronary artery patency, ventricular function, and survival after myocardial infarction. *N Engl J Med* 1993; 329: 1615-1622.

8.   Smalling RW, Bode C, Kalbfleisch J, et al. The Rapid Investigators. More rapid, complete, and stable coronary thrombolysis with bolus administration of reteplase compared with alteplase infusion in acute myocardial infarction. *Circulation* 1995; 91: 2725-2732.

9.   International Society and Federation of Cardiology and World Health Organization task force on myocardial reperfusion. Reperfusion in acute myocardial infarction. International Society and Federation of Cardiology and World Health Organization task force on myocardial reperfusion. *Circulation* 1994; 90: 2091-2102.

10.   Bode C, Smalling RW, Berg G, et al. Randomized comparison of coronary thrombolysis achieved with double-bolus reteplase (recombinant plasminogen activator) and frontloaded , accelerated alteplase (recombinant tissue plasminogen activator) in patients with acute myocardial infarction. *Circulation* 1996; 94: 891-898.

11.   Cannon CP, McCabe CH, Gibson CM, et al. The TIMI 10A Investigators. TNK-tissue plasminogen activator in acute myocardial infarction. Results of the Thrombolysis in Myocardial Infarction (TIMI) 10A dose-ranging trial. *Circulation* 1997; 95: 351-356.

12.   Grainger CB, Califf RM, Topol EJ. Thrombolytic therapy for acute myocardial infarction. *Drugs* 1992; 44: 293-325.

13   Ohman EM, Califf RM, Topol EJ, et al. Consequences of reocclusion after successful reperfusion therapy in acute myocardial infarction. *Circulation* 1990; 82: 781-791.

14   Lincoff AM, Topol EJ. Illusion of reperfusion: does anyone achieve optimal reperfusion during acute myocardial infarction? *Circulation* 1993; 87: 1792-1805.

15.   ISIS-2 (Second International Study of Infarct Survival)Colaborative Group. Randomized trial of intravenous streptokinase, oral aspirin, both, or neither among 17, 187 cases of suspected myocardial infarction; ISIS-2. *Lancet* 1988; II: 349-360.

16.   Coller BS. The role of platelets in arterial thrombosis and the rationale for blockade of GP IIb/IIIa receptors as antithrombotic therapy. *Eur Heart J* 1995; 16 (Suppl L): 11-15.

17.   Lefkovits J, Plow EF, Topol EJ. Platelet glycoprotein IIb/IIIa receptors in cardiovascular medicine. *N Engl J Med* 1995; 332: 1553-1559.

18.   Pytela R, Pierschbacher MD, Ginsberg MH, Plow EF, Ruoslahti E. Platelet membrane glycoprotein IIb/IIIa: a member of a family of Arg-Gly-Asp-specific adhesion receptors. *Science* 1986; 231: 1559-1562.

19   Mustard JF, Kinlough-Rathbone RL, Packham MA. Comparison of fibrinogen association with normal and thrombasthenic platelets on exposure to ADP or Chymotrypsin*Blood* 1979; 54: 987-993.

20   Gold HK, Coller BS, Yasuda T, et al. Rapid and sustaianed coronary recanalization with combined bolus injection of recombinant tissue-type plasminogen activator and monoclonal antiplatelet glycoprotein IIb/IIIa antibody in a canine preparation.*Circulation* 1988; 77: 670-677.

21   The EPIC investigators. Use of a monoclonal antibody directed against the platelet glycoprotein IIb/IIIa receptor in high risk coronary angioplasty. *N Engl J Med* 1994; 330: 956-961.

22   Tcheng JE, Harrington RA, Kottke-Marchant K, et al. Multicenter, randomized, double-blind, placebo-controlled trial of the platelet integrin glycoprotein IIb/IIIa blocker Integrelin in elective coronary intervention. *Circulation* 1995; 76: 2151-2157

23   Tcheng JE, Lincoff AM, Sigmon KN et al. for The IMPACT II Investigators. Randomized placebo-controlled trial of effect of eptifibatide on complications of percutaneous coronary intervention: IMPACT II. *Lancet* 1997; 349: 1422-1428.

24.   Tcheng JE. Platelet integrin glycoprotein IIb/IIIa inhibitors: opportunities and challenges.*J Invas Cardiol* 1996; 8 (Suppl B): 8-14.

25.   Tcheng JE. Dosing and administration of Reopo (c7E3 Fab). *J Invas Cardiol.* 1994;6(suppl) 29-33A

26.   Faulds D, Sorkin EM. Abciximab (c7E3 Fab): a review of its pharmacology and therapeutic potential in ischaemic heart disease. *Drugs* 1994; 48: 583-598.

27.   Scarborough RM, Rose JW, Hsu MA. Barbourin. A GPIIb/IIIa-specific integrin antagonist from the venom of *Sistrurus m barbouri*. *J Biol Chem* 1991; 266: 9359-9362.

28.   Scarborough RM, Naughton MA,Teng W. Design of potent and specific integrin antagonists with high specificity for glycoprotein IIb/IIIa. *J Biol Chem* 1993; 268: 1066-1073.

29.   Charo IF, Scarborough RM, Du Mee CP et al. Therapeutics I: Pharmacodynamics of the glycoprotein IIb/IIIa antagonist integrelin: Phase 1 clinical studies in normal healthy volunteers. *Circulation* 1992; 86 (Suppl I): I-260.

30.   Kleiman NS, Ohman EM, Califf RM, et al. Profound inhibition of platelet aggregation with monoclonal antibody 7E3 Fab after thrombolytic therapy: Results of the Thrombolysis and Angioplasty in Myocardial Infarction (TAMI) 8 Pilot Study. *J Am Coll Cardiol* 1993, 22: 381-389.

31.   Ohman EM, Kleiman NS, Gacioch G, et al. for the IMPACT-AMI Investigators. Combined accelerated tissue-plasminogen activator and glycoprotein IIb/IIIa integrin receptor blockade with Integrelin in acute myocardial infarction: results of a randomized, placebo-controlled dose ranging trial. *Circulation*. 1997; 95: 846-854.

32.   Moliterno DJ, Harrington RA, Krucoff MW, et al. for the PARIDIGM Investigators. Randomized, placebo-controlled study of Lamifiban with thrombolytic therapy for the treatment of acute myocardial infarction: rational and design for the Platelet Aggregation Receptor Antagonist Dose Investigation and reperfusion Gain in Myocardial infarction (PARIDIGM) study. *J Throm Thrombol* 1995; 2: 165-169.

33   Moliterno DJ, Harrington RA, Krucoff MW, et al. for the PARIDIGM Investigators. More complete and stable reperfusion with platelet IIb/IIIa antagonism plus thrombolysis for AMI: The PARIDIGM Trial [abstract]. *Circulation* 1996; 94(Suppl): I-553.

34.   Ronner E, Van Kerteren HA, Zijnen P et al. Combined therapy with Streptokinase and Integrilin. *J Am Coll Cardiol*. 1998; 31(suppl A): 191A.

35.   Antman EM, Giugliano RP, McCabe CH, et al. For the TIMI investigators. Abciximab (Reopro) potentiates thrombolysis in ST elevation myocardial infarction: Results of the TIMI 14 trial. *J Am Coll Cardiol*. 1998; 31(suppl A): 191A.

36.   Madan M, Tcheng JE. Platelet glycoprotein IIb/IIIa Integrin blockade: Focus on acute myocardial infarction. *J Invas Cardiol*. 1998;10(suppl): 27-32A

37.   Brener SJ, Barr LA, Burchenal J, et al. A randomized placebo controlled trial of abciximab with primary angioplasty for acute myocardial infarction. The RAPPORT trial. *Circulation* 1997; 96(suppl I): I-473.

38.   Merkhof-Van Den L, Liem A. Zijlstra F, et al. Early coronary patency evaluation of a glycoprotein receptor antagonist (abciximab) in primary PTCA: The GRAPE pilot study. *Circulation* 1997; 96(suppl I): I-474.

39.   Stone G. Stenting in Acute myocardial infarction: Observational studies and randomized trials - 1998. *J Invas Cardiol*. 1998;10(suppl) 16-26A

6

RISK FACTOR MODIFICATION

Robert S. Rosenson, MD
Lynne T. Braun, PhD, RN
Preventive Cardiology Center, Section of Cardiology
Rush University College of Nursing
Rush Presbyterian-St. Luke's Medical Center, Chicago, IL

INTRODUCTION

Risk factor modification in patients with established coronary heart disease (CHD) is intended to slow progression of atherosclerotic vascular disease and, more importantly, prevent recurrent coronary and other vascular events. This chapter will present an overview of risk factor modification in patients with established CHD and provide a template for the implementation of preventive strategies based on randomized clinical trials and new concepts in the pathophysiology of acute coronary syndromes.

Assessment of Cardiac Risk

The presence of coronary atherosclerosis identifies a high-risk population with susceptibility to the disease process that is independent of a specific risk factor.[1] (Figure 1).[1] Thus, risk factor modification in patients with established CHD is more likely to yield benefit from a specific intervention than a corresponding population without apparent atherosclerotic vascular disease.

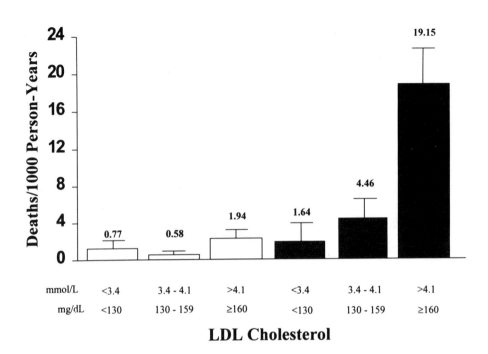

Age-adjusted rates CHD deaths per 1000 person-years of follow-up, according
to LDL cholesterol in men with and men without cardiovascular disease at baseline.

Men without cardiovascular disease at baseline are represented by open bars, and men with evidence of
cardiovascular disease by shaded bars. The T bars indicate the standard errors.

Hypertension

The relationship between the level of blood pressure and cardiovascular risk is
strong, continuous, and graded for individuals with CHD.[2] Hypertensive patients
with CHD have increased risk for cardiovascular morbidity and mortality. Blood
pressure is categorized as high-normal (130-139/85-89 mmHg), Stage 1
hypertension (140-159/90-99 mmHg), Stage 2 hypertension (160-179/100-109
mmHg), or Stage 3 hypertension (≥180 / ≥110 mmHg).[3] When systolic and
diastolic blood pressures fall into different categories, the higher category is used to
describe a patient's blood pressure status. Furthermore, in the presence of clinical
cardiovascular disease, blood pressure levels at or above the high-normal range
place the patient in the highest risk category.[3] (Table 1).[3]

Table 1. Risk Stratification and Treatment (4)*

Blood Pressure Stages (mm Hg)	Risk Group A (No Risk Factors No TOD/CCD) †	Risk Group B (At Least 1 Risk Factor, Not Including Diabetes; No TOD/CCD)	Risk Group C (TOD/CCD And/or Diabetes With or Without Other Risk Factors)
High-normal (130-139/85-89)	Lifestyle modification	Lifestyle modification	Drug Therapy§
Stage 1 (140-159/90-99)	Lifestyle modification (up to 12 months)	Lifestyle modification‡ (up to 6 months)	Drug Therapy
Stages 2 and 3 (≥160/≥100)	Drug Therapy	Drug Therapy	Drug Therapy

* Lifestyle modification should be adjunctive therapy for all patients recommended for pharmacologic therapy.

† TOD/CCD indicates target organ disease/clinical cardiovascular disease.

‡ For patients with multiple risk factors, clinicians should consider drugs as initial therapy plus lifestyle modifications.

§ For those with heart failure, renal insufficiency, or diabetes.

Dyslipidemia

Lipid abnormalities are arbitrarily defined as age- and gender-adjusted levels of low density lipoprotein (LDL) cholesterol, total triglycerides or lipoprotein (a) that exceed the 90th percentile or high-density lipoprotein (HDL) cholesterol levels that are below the 10th percentile.[5] In patients with angiographically documented coronary stenoses prior to ages 55 to 60 years, 80% to 88% of patients are diagnosed with a major lipid abnormality. Although hypercholesterolemia is present in 20-25% of patients, other lipid abnormalities are commonly diagnosed. (Figure 2).[4] Thus far, clinical trials of lipid altering therapy have predominantly focused on LDL lowering, and these trials have established that lower levels of LDL cholesterol are beneficial for CHD patients.

+CAD (%)

LDL + TG (3.4)   LDL (12.1)   Normal (12.5)

LDL + HDL (3.7)   HTG (9.7)

LDL + TG + HDL (3.1)

TG + HDL (9.7)   HyperapoB (10.7)

Low HDL (19.3)

Lp(a) excess (15.8)

Screening for hyperlipidemia during unstable angina pectoris, acute myocardial infarction or surgical trauma may be fraught with spurious results from an acute phase illness.[5] Plasma lipids remain stable for 24 to 48 hours after an acute myocardial infarction, then total, LDL and HDL cholesterol falls by 47, 48 and 32% respectively at 4 to 7 days, and these levels return to baseline 2 months later. (Figure 3).[5] Thus, a low LDL cholesterol concentration (e.g. < 130 mg/dL, 3.36 mmol/L) may be due to acute phase changes and a repeat lipid profile should be obtained at 2 months. Conversely, plasma triglycerides increase by 58% in the days subsequent to an acute myocardial infarction. Furthermore, the hospitalization process itself, independent of the acute phase response, has been associated with significantly reduced levels of HDL cholesterol compared to outpatient values. As a result, lipoprotein analysis may be obtained on the first overnight fast, but lipid analysis will be most accurate if obtained in the outpatient setting after the 2 month acute phase period has elapsed.

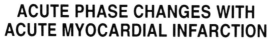

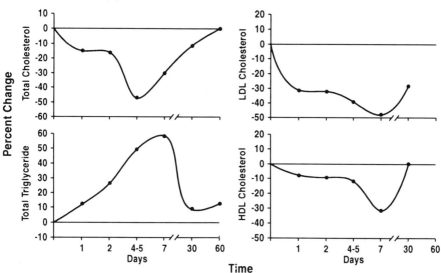

Cigarette Smoking

Smoking produces a variety of harmful cardiovascular effects that may be mitigated or even reversed by smoking cessation.[6] Smoking increases the rate of atherogenesis and may directly cause vascular endothelial injury, increases platelet adhesiveness and plasma fibrinogen levels, and decreases high density lipoprotein cholesterol levels.

Diabetes Mellitus

Diabetes mellitus, types 1 and 2, are a major risk factor for CHD, with higher CHD prevalence rates for female and older diabetics.[7] Atherosclerosis is responsible for approximately 80% of all deaths from diabetes mellitus, of which 75% are from CHD and 25% from either cerebrovascular or peripheral vascular disease.[7] Individuals with non-insulin dependent diabetes mellitus develop CHD at a younger age, and are more likely to have diffuse multivessel disease with reduced vasodilatory reserve, and have congestive heart failure. Furthermore, the risk of CHD is increased even in the newly diagnosed patient with type 2 diabetes mellitus probably as a consequence to the long latent period that precedes the diagnosis, and exposure to atherogenic risk factors.

The criteria for the diagnosis of diabetes mellitus has been recently revised, particularly as they relate to fasting plasma glucose (FPG) levels.[8] Diabetes mellitus is diagnosed in one of three ways: symptoms of diabetes mellitus (polyuria, polydipsia, unexplained weight loss) plus random plasma glucose concentration $\geq$ 200 mg/dL (11.1 mmol/L); FPG $\geq$ 126 mg/dL (7.0 mmol/L); or 2-hour plasma glucose $\geq$ 200 mg/dL (11.1 mmol/L) during an oral glucose tolerance test (75 g). Each criteria must be confirmed on repeat testing.

Postmenopausal Status

CHD risk increases as women age, with the largest gains in morbidity occurring between the ages of 45 and 64 years. With the onset of menopause women lose estrogen-mediated resistance to CHD (cardioprotection), and CHD risk more than doubles irrespective of age or type of menopause (surgical versus natural).[11] Postmenopausal is defined as: amenorrheic for a minimum of 1 year and/or serum FSH concentration > 40 mIU/ml, or having had a prior hysterectomy and bilateral oophorectomy.

Physical Inactivity

Currently, more than 60% of adults in the United States do not engage in regular physical activity, and 25% of the adult population is not active at all.[9] Population studies have shown an inverse association between physical activity/fitness and CHD incidence and mortality. Sedentary individuals have almost a twofold increase in CHD risk (relative risk 1.9), which is comparable to the relative risks associated with elevated systolic blood pressure (relative risk 2.1), cigarette smoking (relative risk 2.5), and hypercholesterolemia (relative risk 2.4).[10] Although comprehensive cardiac rehabilitation must focus on intensive health-behavior change directed at cardiovascular risk reduction, exercise is a key component of the standard of care for secondary prevention of CHD. Randomized clinical trials confirmed that comprehensive cardiac rehabilitation services reduces the risk of total mortality, cardiovascular mortality, and fatal reinfarction by 20-25%.[11]

IMPLEMENTATION OF SECONDARY PREVENTIVE THERAPY

The secondary prevention of CHD requires implementation of proven myocardial infarction strategies that include anti-platelet agents, beta-adrenergic blockers, angiotensin converting enzyme inhibitors followed by a comprehensive risk factor analysis. **(Table 2)**. This section will emphasize treatment strategies for hypertension, hypercholesterolemia, physical inactivity, cigarette smoking, and discuss the putative benefits of hormone replacement therapy for post-menopausal women.

Antiplatelet Agents

Antiplatelet agents are beneficial in myocardial infarction and for other patients with atherosclerotic vascular disease. The clinical benefit of aspirin appears to be independent of dose with no difference in the magnitude of the treatment effect seen at low dose (<160 mg/day), intermediate dose (160 to 325 mg/day) and high dose (500 to 1500 mg/day).[12] Most recently, lower dose aspirin (75 mg/day) reduced major cardiovascular events (15%, p=0.03) and all myocardial infarction (36%, p=0.002) with no effect on stroke in 18,790 treated hypertensive patients.[13]

The CAPRIE trial compared aspirin (325 mg/day) to clopidogrel (75 mg/day) in patients with myocardial infarction, ischemic stroke or peripheral vascular disease.[14] Clopidogrel reduced the annual incidence of first ischemic stroke, myocardial infarction or vascular death from 5.83% to 5.32% or a relative risk reduction of 8.7%, p=0.043

Hypertension

Blood pressure should be lowered to the usual target parameters (less than 140/90 mmHg). However, rapid lowering of blood pressure and sympathetic nervous system activation, particularly in the acute setting should be avoided.[3]

Unless contraindicated, the drugs of choice for blood pressure control in CHD patients are beta blockers (without intrinsic sympathomimetic activity) and ACE inhibitors.[15] In addition to lowering arterial pressure, beta blockers reduce heart rate and contractility. Therefore, these agents protect the ischemic myocardium by reducing myocardial oxygen requirements. Meta-analyses of clinical trials indicate that beta blocker therapy after myocardial infarction grants significant reductions in all-cause mortality, cardiovascular mortality, nonfatal cardiac arrest and sudden death, cardiac rupture, ventricular fibrillation, and myocardial infarction.[16] Furthermore, numerous clinical trials of antihypertensive drug efficacy with beta blockers have shown decreased CHD events and mortality. Although beta blockers may have adverse effects on the lipid profile (increased triglycerides and decreased HDL), the cardioprotective benefit conferred by these agents outweighs the risk by a ratio of 10:1.

Table 2

TIME	INTERVENTION IN PATIENTS WITH ACUTE CORONARY SYNDROMES	ADDITIONAL RESOURCES
Admission	Aspirin or other anti-platelet therapy Beta-adrenergic blocker Thrombolytic therapy Acute PTCA	
Day 1	ACE-Inhibitor Fasting lipid profile →	
Day 2	LDL-C ≥ 125 mg/dL + TG ≤ 400 mg/dL → [HMG-CoA reductase inhibitor] → LDL < 125 mg/dL + TG ≤ 400 mg/dL LDL <125 mg/dL + TG 400 - 1000 mg/dL { [Potential acute phase response] → LDL < 125 mg/dL + TG > 1000 mg/dL → [Fibric acid derivative] →	Diet assessment Nutrition counseling Physical activity management (Phase I cardiac rehabilitation) Smoking cessation
Discharge Plan	Schedule repeat fasting lipid profile, LFT's, and other biochemical studies in 2 months. Follow-up visit for cardiac risk factor interventions.	Nutrition counseling Phase II cardiac rehabilitation Smoking cessation

ACE inhibitors improve left ventricular dysfunction, slow the progression to heart failure, and reduce mortality in the immediate and convalescent phase after myocardial infarction. ACE inhibitors have a greater benefit in patients with congestive heart failure, anterior infarction, and left ventricular ejection fraction less than 40%.[15]

Dyslipidemia Management

An increasing number of clinical trials have shown an improvement in clinical outcomes with cholesterol lowering therapy. This includes a reduction in recurrent myocardial infarction, CHD death, stroke and all-cause mortality.[17-19] Several angiographic-based studies of atherosclerosis disease progression have shown that cholesterol lowering therapy can retard or reverse coronary stenoses and reduce the need for revascularization procedures.[20] Current National Cholesterol Education Program Adult Treatment Panel II guidelines for patients with existing CHD recommend cholesterol lowering therapy with diet or medication for patients with LDL cholesterol levels that exceed 130 mg/dL (3.36 mmol/L).[21] The clinical trials of LDL cholesterol lowering have evaluated patients at different risk as determined by baseline LDL cholesterol level and the use of adjunctive therapies.

In general, lipid-lowering drugs are required, since dietary modification alone is relatively ineffective.[21-23] Lifestyle modifications should be initiated during the hospitalization. Early use of pharmacological therapy for hypercholesterolemia does not diminish the importance of lifestyle modification, instead, this approach recognizes a paradigm shift in understanding the importance of vulnerable atherosclerotic plaques in acute coronary syndromes and the contribution of thrombus to the severity of the clinical event.[24]

The secondary prevention trials of LDL lowering have demonstrated that aggressive treatment of borderline-high LDL-cholesterol levels (>125 mg/dL) can reduce fatal and non-fatal myocardial infarctions, stroke and the need for revascularization procedures.[19] Coronary and all-cause mortality has been shown to be reduced in patients with higher LDL cholesterol levels (≥150 mg/dL).[17,18] The most potent drugs for lowering LDL-cholesterol levels are the HMG-CoA reductase inhibitors. The clinical trials employing these agents have demonstrated safety, tolerability, and improved adherence compared with other LDL lowering agents.

A summary of the major clinical trials of cholesterol lowering therapy is presented. The baseline characteristics of the study population are described in **Table 3**. The Scandinavian Simvastatin Survival Study (4S) evaluated 4444 patients with established CHD who were treated with a lipid lowering diet, and then randomly assigned to therapy with placebo or simvastatin in an attempt to reduce the level of total cholesterol below 200 mg/dL (5.2 mmol/L).[17] At the end of 5.4 years, there was a reduction in total mortality in patients treated with simvastatin (8 versus 12 % with placebo). There were also highly statistically significant reductions in major coronary events (19% versus 28%), CHD deaths (42% reduction), revascularization procedures (CABG or coronary angioplasty, 37%), and fatal plus nonfatal cerebrovascular events (2.7% versus 4.3%).

Table 3

Trial	Agent/ Dosage	LDL Cholesterol Mean Level [(mg/dL) (mmol/L)]	Annualized MI Event Rate in Placebo Treated Subjects*	Aspirin (%)	ß-blocker (%)	Revascularization Procedures (%)
4S	Simvastatin 20-40 mg	188 (4.87)	0.053	37	57	8
LIPID	Pravastatin 40 mg	150 (3.89)	0.017	83	46	41
CARE	Pravastatin 40 mg	139 (3.60)	0.026	83	40	54

* Fatal or Nonfatal MI

The Long-Term Intervention with Pravastatin in Ischemic Heart Disease (LIPID) Study evaluated 9,014 men and women with prior myocardial infarction (64%) or unstable angina pectoris (36%) and randomly assigned them to therapy with placebo or pravastatin (40 mg nightly) after a minimum of three months following the acute event.[18] The entry criteria include levels of total cholesterol less than 240 mg/dL and total triglycerides less than 445 mg/dL (mmol/L). After 6 years, pravastatin treated patients had a significant 24% reduction in CHD mortality, the primary endpoint (p=0.0004), and a 23% reduction in all-cause mortality (p=0.00002). There were also highly significant reductions in fatal plus nonfatal myocardial infarction (-23%, p=0.000002), and stroke (-20%, p=0.022). LIPID demonstrated a survival benefit in a lower risk patient group than 4S.

The CARE (Cholesterol and Recurrent Events) Trial also found benefits with lipid-altering therapy among patients with borderline-high LDL cholesterol levels.[19] This study included 4,159 patients with a history of a myocardial infarction in the previous two years who had cholesterol levels < 240 mg/dL (6.21 mmol/L). At five years, benefits with pravastatin treatment (40 mg before sleep) compared to placebo included significant reductions in the combined incidence of coronary death and nonfatal MI (10.2 versus 13.2%, p = 0.003), the need for revascularization with CABG or PTCA (14.1 versus 18.8%, p<0.001) and the development of stroke (2.6 versus 3.8%, p = 0.03). As mentioned earlier, the benefits were seen only in patients with LDL cholesterol levels above 125 mg/dL (3.2 mmol/L). They were more apparent among those with higher pretreatment levels of LDL, women, and older patients (above age 60).

The Post Coronary Artery Bypass Graft Trial evaluated 1351 patients with LDL cholesterol levels between 130 and 175 mg/dL (3.4 to 4.5 mmol/L) and at least one patent vein graft documented on angiography performed one to 11 years after CABG.[20] Patients were randomized to receive aggressive therapy with lovastatin and if needed cholestyramine to reduce LDL cholesterol to less than 93-97 mg/dL (2.41-2.51 mmol/L) or moderate therapy which resulted in levels of approximately 134 mg/dL (3.5 mmol/L) and with low dose warfarin (INR = 1.4) or placebo. Angiography was repeated an average of 4.3 years. Aggressive compared to moderate therapy was associated with a lower percentage of grafts showing progression of atherosclerosis (27 versus 39%, p<0.001), a lower rate of revascularization (CABG or PTCA) (6.5 versus 9.2%, p = 0.03), and a reduction in the need for repeat revascularization procedures.

Several factors have been thought to contribute to the cardiovascular benefit in these trials that include plaque stabilization, improvement in endothelium-dependent coronary vasomotion, a reduction in the prothrombotic state induced by changes in fibrinogen, plasma viscosity and tissue factor inhibitor, and by inhibition of platelet thrombus formation at the site of plaque rupture.[24] Data from the REGRESS trial, show that statins reduce the number of episodes of transient myocardial ischemia, duration of ischemia, and improve coronary blood flow, vasodilatory response, and myocardial perfusion.

Lipid lowering therapy for secondary prevention in survivors of acute MI has been reported in a few studies. The Heart and Estrogen/Progestin Replacement Study is a clinical trial of HRT in postmenopausal women with prior myocardial infarction.[25] The use of lipid lowering therapy was evaluated according to baseline LDL cholesterol levels **(Table 4)**.[25] The use of lipid lowering medications in postmenopausal women with LDL cholesterol levels ≥ 220 mg/dL (5.7 mmol/L) was only 35.5%. The use of lipid lowering agents was also evaluated in a multicenter 13 hospital-based cardiac rehabilitation program in Massachusetts (1995) which prospectively examined patients with myocardial infarction, coronary artery surgery, angioplasty and angina.[26] The use of these lipid lowering medications was more likely to be prescribed by cardiologists (37.7%) and internists than family physicians and general practitioners (17.6%) than other physicians (15.0%, p<0.001).[27] Cardiologists screen for hypercholesterolemia and treat more patients for hyperlipidemia than internists, but adoption of National Cholesterol Education Program guidelines remains low even for patients at high risk.

Table 4   Distribution of LDL-C Level and Use of Lipid-Lowering Drugs*

LDL-C, mmol/L (mg/dL)	No. (%)	No. (%) on Drugs†
<2.6 (<100)	262 (9.5)	165 (62.9)
2.6-3.3 (100-129)	745 (27.1)	437 (58.7)
3.4-4.1 (130-159)	901 (32.7)	388 (43.1)
4.1-4.9 (160-189)	526 (19.1)	188 (35.7)
4.9-5.7 (190-219)	225 (8.2)	72 (32.0)
≥5.7 (≥220)	93 (3.4)	33 (35.5)
Total	2752 (100)	1283 (46.6)

* Lipid-lowering drugs included HMG-CoA reductase inhibitors, bile acid sequestrants, niacin, fibrate, and fish oil. LDL-C indicates low-density lipoprotein cholesterol.
† Percentages are of persons with specified LDL-C level receiving lipid drug therapy.

Diabetes Mellitus

An analysis of the diabetic patients with CHD (N=202) in the Scandinavian Simvastatin Study (4S) showed that simvastatin treatment produced changes in lipids similar to those observed in nondiabetic patients.[28] The relative risks of major endpoints were as follows: total mortality 0.57, P=.087; major CHD events 0.45, P=.002; and any atherosclerotic event 0.63, P=.018. The Kaplan-Meier 6-year probability of survival for non-diabetics was 88.4% in the placebo group and 91.6% in the simvastatin group. For diabetic patients, it was 68.8% in the placebo group and 84.0% in the simvastatin group. The proportion of non-diabetic patients without a CHD event in 6 years was 71.3% in the placebo group and 79.8% in the simvastatin group. For diabetic patients, it was 50.7% in the placebo group and 75.1% in the simvastatin group. Therefore, 4S provides evidence that treatment with simvastatin is clearly associated with a reduction in risk of CHD death and nonfatal myocardial infarction in patients with diabetes.

In the Cholesterol and Recurrent Events (CARE) trial, patients treated with pravastatin had a 24% lower incidence of fatal CHD or confirmed myocardial infarction during 5 years of follow-up. The presence of diabetes did not alter the effect of pravastatin on the rate of major coronary events.[19]

The American Diabetes Association reinforces the NCEP guidelines for acceptable lipid levels: total cholesterol < 200 mg/dL; LDL cholesterol < 130 mg/dL; triglycerides < 200 mg/dL.[29] Diabetic patients with lipid values that exceed these parameters should receive aggressive therapy with diet and medication.

Hormone Replacement Therapy

There is evidence from prospective cohort studies that estrogen replacement therapy (ERT) may have a role in secondary prevention by reducing the risk of cardiovascular disease and improving survival in women with known or suspected CHD.[30,31] In postmenopausal women with more than a 70% coronary stenosis, estrogen use was associated with an increase in 10-year survival that was observed in women without coronary disease.[30] This benefit may also extend to postmenopausal women with CHD in whom percutaneous transluminal angioplasty was performed.[31] This observational data must be interpreted cautiously until completion of clinical trials of HRT.

Cardiac Rehabilitation

Exercise training reduces CHD risk through hemodynamic, metabolic, and hemostatic mechanisms. Aerobic exercise increases physical work capacity and reduces myocardial oxygen demands by lowering resting and submaximal heart rates, facilitating loss of excess weight and reducing blood pressure. In symptomatic CHD patients, exercise training can delay the onset of angina. The metabolic actions of aerobic exercise include improved glycemic control and favorable lipoprotein changes (reduction in triglycerides and increase in HDL). Furthermore, exercise decreases platelet aggregation and increases fibrinolysis.

Equally important as exercise training, comprehensive cardiac rehabilitation includes multidisciplinary services designed to meet individual patient needs, i.e., education and counseling about coronary risk reduction, return to work, medical surveillance and emergency support, and interventions to improve psychosocial functioning.

Cardiac rehabilitation services are initiated upon hospital admission and continue throughout recovery of the CHD patient. Unless the patient is hemodynamically unstable after myocardial infarction, prolonged bedrest is avoided to prevent the physiological effects of deconditioning. For approximately 12 hours, activity is limited to the use of bedside commode and assisted bathing. The inpatient phase, or Phase I, consists of early graded mobilization of the stable patient to the level of activity required to perform simple household tasks. Phase I rehabilitation includes deep breathing and range-of-motion exercises, progressive ambulation, and stair-climbing. In addition, risk factor assessment is performed and risk factor modification is initiated by implementing a heart-healthy diet, blood pressure control, smoking cessation, a home-walking program, and stress management.

Outpatient cardiac rehabilitation, or Phase II, begins with risk stratification to determine a patient's prognosis based on clinical course and current status, the need for further diagnostic evaluations, and the degree of supervision required during exercise. The traditional Phase II program consists of 8 to 12 weeks of ECG-monitored exercise sessions and educational programs. The goals of these sessions are to develop and teach an individualized, safe, and effective exercise prescription, to continue interventions aimed at reducing risk factors, and to identify and manage psychosocial problems. Phase III, or maintenance phase of cardiac rehabilitation, consists of home- or gymnasium-based exercise with the goal of continuing risk factor modification and exercise program learned in Phase II. All phases of cardiac rehabilitation are physician-directed and implemented by exercise physiologists, physical therapists, or nurses with specialized training.

Smoking Cessation

Smoking cessation is accompanied by a decreased incidence of recurrent ischemic events and cardiovascular deaths in subjects with clinically manifest ischemic heart disease. In high risk post-myocardial infarction survivors who quit smoking, all-cause mortality and arrhythmic death is decreased. Approximately 20 to 60% of long-term smokers are motivated by AMI to stop smoking, but without intervention, most who quit, relapse within 6 months. A meta-analysis of 39 smoking intervention trials found that the most effective cessation resulted from multiple treatment modalities and providers (physician and non-physician).[33] Taylor et al.[34] showed that when the primary physician provides a firm, unequivocal stop smoking message in the coronary care unit, and subsequently nurse counseling using combined motivational and skill-oriented interventions with personal follow-up are carried out, the cessation rate is 61% in the intervention group as compared to 32% of the usual care group of smokers recovering from AMI.

Cost Effectiveness of Cholesterol Lowering Therapies

The cost effectiveness of cholesterol lowering therapies has been evaluated in several clinical endpoint trails. The 4S study[35] evaluated the effect of simvastatin on health care resource use and estimated cost savings by a cost-minimization analysis. Hospitalizations for acute events (myocardial infarction, angina, left ventricular failure) were reduced by 32% and revascularization procedures by 26% in patients treated with simvastatin. The estimated reduction in costs over the 5.4 year trial with simvastatin is $3,872 per patient.

The cost-effectiveness was also analyzed in the PLAC I and PLAC II studies.[36] The estimated cost per life-year saved with pravastatin therapy was $7,124 to $12,665, depending on the patient-risk profile.

Tosteson et al.[37] estimated the cost effectiveness of a population-wide program to reduce serum cholesterol levels by using media campaigns and direct education. Based on a cost of $4.95 per person per year and an average 2% reduction in serum cholesterol levels, the estimated cost was $3,200 per year of life saved.

Cost of Cholesterol Lowering Drugs

Table 5[38] lists the monthly cost of cholesterol-lowering medications for usual daily dosages. Table 6[38] includes the cost in relation to LDL lowering for the HMG-CoA reductase inhibitors.

Table 5

Drug	Daily Dosage	Cost in U.S. Dollars*
Cholestyramine	16 grams, divided	$ 113.70
Colestipol	20 grams, divided	$ 110.06
Gemfibrozil	1200 mg in two doses	$ 10.80
Fenofibrate	201 mg	$ 61.88
Niacin (generic price)	1 gram three times a day	$ 5.98
Niacor	1 gram three times a day	$ 56.34
Niaspan	1500 mg	$ 45.00
Lovastatin	20 mg once a day	$ 69.85
Pravastatin	20 mg once a day	$ 61.86
Simvastatin	10 mg once a day	$ 62.99
Fluvastatin	20 mg once a day	$ 37.70
Atorvastatin	20 mg once a day	$ 84.60
Cerivastatin	0.3 mg once a day	$ 44.00

*Cost to the pharmacist for 30 days' treatment based on average wholesale price listings in Drug Topics Red Book 1998, pg.3.

Table 6

Drug	Dosage	Wholesale Cost*	% LDL Lowering at Specified Dose	Monthly Cost per 1% LDL Lowering
Lovastatin	20 mg	$ 69.85	27%	$ 2.59
	40 mg	$ 125.74	31%	$ 4.06
Pravastatin	20 mg	$ 61.86	32%	$ 1.93
	40 mg	$ 101.68	34%	$ 2.99
Simvastatin	10 mg	$ 62.99	33%	$ 1.91
	40 mg	$ 109.88	40%	$ 2.75
Fluvastatin	20 mg	$ 37.70	22%	$ 1.71
	40 mg	$ 42.15	24%	$ 1.76
Atorvastatin	20 mg	$ 84.60	43%	$ 1.96
	40 mg	$ 101.88	50%	$ 2.04
Cerivastatin	0.2 mg	$ 44.00	25%	$ 1.76
	0.3 mg	$ 44.00	28%	$ 1.57

*For 30 days' treatment, according to average wholesale price listings in Drug Topics. Red Book 1998.

Although direct costs of medications are important considerations for physician and patient, the efficacy of cholesterol-lowering therapy in cardiovascular disease prevention can be determined only from clinical trials due to the pleiotropic anti-atherothrombotic properties of the various agents.[24]

ADHERENCE TO THERAPY

In addition, since CHD risk factors (e.g., lipid abnormalities, smoking, hypertension, diabetes mellitus) are additive, nonadherence to medical or behavioral treatment of any individual risk factor maintains a higher level of risk. Furthermore, nonadherence to one part of the medical regimen may increase the likelihood of nonadherence to other components.

The importance of compliance with lipid-altering medications in patients with dyslipidemia was demonstrated in a post-hoc analysis of data from the West of Scotland Coronary Prevention Study (WOSCOPS).[39] In this primary prevention study of men with hypercholesterolemia, pravastatin therapy was shown to decrease cardiovascular morbidity and mortality. The mean adherence for the entire group was 70%. Those patients with more than 75% adherence had the following benefits: fewer definite coronary events (risk reduction of 38% versus 31% for patients treated with placebo), and lower cardiovascular mortality (risk reduction of 37% versus 32%). Other benefits of adherence to drug therapy may include decreased utilization of medical services, better quality of life, and reduced social costs such as lost productivity.

SUMMARY

Risk factor modification is an essential component of the CHD patient. The proven strategies for secondary preventive care includes anti-hypertensive therapy with beta-adrenergic blockers and ACE-inhibitors, LDL cholesterol, and physical fitness. Other risk factors associated with an increase in recurrent CHD events include post menopausal state and diabetes mellitus. Thus far, there are no randomized clinical trials that demonstrate improved outcome achieved through modification of those risk factors. Nevertheless, improved glucose control in diabetes mellitus has proven benefits for retinopathy.

The onset of acute coronary syndromes is unpredictable, and the vast majority of acute myocardial infarctions arise from non-flow limiting stenosis. Thus, risk factor modification must be initiated promptly since the presence of CHD is a harbinger of future events.

Notes

1. Pekkanen J, Linn S, Heiss G, Suchindran CM, Leon A, Rifkind BM, Tyroler HA. Ten-year mortality from cardiovascular disease in relation to cholesterol level among men with and without preexisting cardiovascular disease. N Eng. J Med. 1990;322:1700-1707.

2. Flack JM, Neaton J, Grimm R, et al. for the Multiple Risk Factor Intervention Trial Research Group. Blood pressure and mortality among men with prior myocardial infarction. Circulation. 1995;92:2437-2445.

3. National Institutes of Health. The Sixth Report of the Joint National Committee on Prevention, Detection, Evaluation, and Treatment of High Blood Pressure. NIH Publication No. 98-4080, November, 1997.

4. Rosenson RS. Beyond low-density lipoprotein cholesterol: a perspective on low high-density lipoprotein disorders and Lp(a) lipoprotein excess. Arch Intern Med. 1996;156:1278-1284.

5. Rosenson RS. Myocardial injury, the acute phase response and lipoprotein metabolism. J Am Coll Cardiol 1993;22:933-940.

6. U.S. Department of Health and Human Services. The Health Benefits of Smoking Cessation: A Report of the Surgeon General. Washington (DC): Public Health Service, Centers for Disease Control, Publication No. (CDC)90-8416, 1990.

7. Webster MWI, Scott R. What cardiologists need to know about diabetes. Lancet. 1997;350 (suppl 1):23-28.

8. Zinman B. Guidelines for the management of type 2 diabetes. Current Approaches to the Management of Type 2 Diabetes: A Practical Monograph. pg. 19-22.

9. Department of Health and Human Services. Physical activity and health: a report of the Surgeon General. Atlanta, GA: U.S. Department of Health and Human Services, Centers for Disease Control and Prevention, National Center for Chronic Disease Prevention and Health Promotion, 1996.

10. Centers for Disease Control and Prevention. Public Health Focus: physical activity and the prevention of coronary heart disease. MMWR . 1993;43:669-672.

11. O'Connor GT, Buring JE, Yusuf S, et al. An overview of randomized trials of rehabilitation with exercise after myocardial infarction. Circulation. 1989;80:234-244.

12. Antiplatelet Trialists' Collaboration. Collaborative overview of randomised trials of antiplatelet therapy - I: Prevention of death, myocardial infarction, and stroke by prolonged antiplatelet therapy in various categories of patients. BMJ 1994;308:81.

13. Hansson L, Zanchetti A, Carruthers GS, Dahlöf B, Elmfeldt D, Julius S, et al. for the HOT Study Group. Effects of intensive blood-pressure lowering and low-dose aspirin in patients with hypertension: principal results of the Hypertension Optimal Treatment (HOT) randomised trial. Lancet 1998;351:1755-1762.

14. CAPRIE Steering Committee. A randomised, blinded, trial of clopidogrel versus aspirin in patients at risk for ischaemic events (CAPRIE). Lancet 1996;348:1329.

15. Ryan TJ, Anderson JL, Antman EM, Braniff BA, Brooks NH, Califf RM, Hillis LD, Hiratzka LF, Rapaport E, Riegel BJ, Russell RO, Smith EE III, Weaver WD. ACC/AHA guidelines for the management of patients with acute myocardial infarction: a report of the American College of Cardiology/American Heart Association Task Force on Practice Guidelines (Committee on Management of Acute Myocardial Infarction). J Am Coll Cardiol. 1996;28:1328-1428.

16. Kennedy HL, Rosenson RS. Physicians' use of beta-adrenergic blocking therapy: a changing perspective. J Am Coll Cardiol. 1995;26:547-552.

17. Scandinavian Simvastatin Survival Study Group. Randomized trial of cholesterol lowering in 4444 patients with coronary heart disease: The Scandinavian Simvastatin Survival Study (4S). Lancet 1994;344:1383.

18. Long-Term Intervention with Pravastatin in Ischemic Disease (LIPID). Presented at the 70th Scientific Sessions of the American Heart Association on November 12, 1997.

19. Sachs FM, Pfeffer MA, Move LA, et al, for the cholesterol and Recurrent Events Trial Investigators. The effect of pravastatin on coronary events after myocardial infarction in patients with average cholesterol levels. N Engl J Med 1996;335:1001.

20. The Post Coronary Artery Bypass Graft Trial Investigators. The effect of aggressive lowering of low density lipoprotein cholesterol levels and low-dose anticoagulation on obstructive changes in saphenous-vein coronary artery bypass grafts. N Engl J Med 1997;336:153.

21. The Expert Panel on Detection, Evaluation, and Treatment of High Blood Cholesterol in Adults. Summary of the second reports of the national cholesterol education program (NCEP) expert panel on detection, evaluation, and treatment of high blood cholesterol in adults (Adult treatment Panel II). JAMA. 1993;269:3015-3023.

22. Rosenson RS. Reversing coronary artery disease: Diet-based strategies. Physic Sports Med. 1992;22:59-64.

23. Hunninghake DB, Stein EA, Dujovne CA, Harris WS, Feldman EB, Miller VT, Tobert JA, Laskarzewski PM, Quiter E. Held J, et al. The efficacy of intensive dietary therapy alone or combined with lovastatin in outpatients with hypercholesterolemia. N Engl J Med. 1993;328:1213-9.

24. Rosenson RS, Tangney CC. Anti-atherothrombotic properties of statins: implications for cardiovascular event reduction. JAMA. 1998;279:1643-1650.

25. Schrott HG, Bittner V, Vittinghoff E, Herrington DM, Hulley S. Adherence to National Cholesterol Education Program Treatment goals in postmenopausal women with heart disease. The Heart and Estrogen/Progestin Replacement Study (HERS). JAMA. 1997;277:1281-1286.

26. Balady GJ, Jette D, Scheer J, and the Massachusetts Association of Cardiovascular and Pulmonary Rehabilitation Database Co-investigators. Changes in exercise capacity following cardiac rehabilitation in patients stratified according to age and gender. J Cardiopulmonary Rehab. 1996;16:38-46.

27. Stafford RS, Blumenthal D, Pasternak RC. Variations in cholesterol management practices of U.S. physicians. J Am Coll Cardiol. 1997;29:139-146.

28. Pylora K, Pedersen TR, Kjekshus J, Faergeman O, Olsson AG, Thorgeirsson G. Cholesterol lowering with simvastatin improves prognosis of diabetic patients with coronary heart disease. A subgroup analysis of the Scandinavian Simvastatin Survival Study (4S). Diabetes Care. 1997;20:614-20.

29. American Diabetes Association. Standards of medical care for patients with diabetes mellitus. Diabetes Care. 1997;20(Suppl 1):S5-513.

30. Sullivan JM, Vander Zwaag R, Hughes JP, et al. Estrogen replacement and coronary artery disease: effect on survival in postmenopausal women. Arch Intern Med. 1990;150:2557.

31. O'Keefe JH, Kim SC, Hall RR, et al. Estrogen replacement therapy after coronary angioplasty in women. J Am Coll Cardiol. 1997;29:1.

32. Schwartz JL. Review and Evaluation of Smoking Cessation Methods. Bethesda (MD): National Cancer Institute, 1987.

33. Kottke TE, Battsta RN, DeFriese GH, et al. Attributes of successful smoking cessation interventions in medical practice: a meta-analysis of 39 controlled trials. JAMA. 1988;259:2883-2889.

34. Taylor B, Houston-Miller N, Killen J, DeBusk RF. Smoking cessation after acute myocardial infarction: effects of a nurse-managed intervention. Ann Intern Med. 1990;113:118-123.

35. Pedersen TR, Kjekshus J, Berg K, Olsson AG, Wilhelmsen L, Wedel H, Pyorala K, Miettinen T, Haghfelt T, Faergeman O, Thorgeirsson G, Jonsson B, Schwartz JS. Cholesterol lowering and the use of healthcare resources. Results of the Scandinavian Simvastatin Survival Study. Circulation. 1996;93:1796-802.

36. Ashraf T, Hay JW, Pitt B, Wittels E, Crouse J, Davidson M, Furberg CD, Radican L. Cost-effectiveness of pravastatin in secondary prevention of coronary artery disease. Am J Cardiol. 1996;78:409-14.

37. Tosteson AN, Weinstein MC, Hunink MG, Mittleman MA, Williams LW, Goldman PA, Goldman L. Cost-effectiveness of population-wide educational approaches to reduce serum cholesterol levels. Circulation. 1997; 95:24-30.

38. 1998 Drug Topics Red Book, Medical Economics Company. Montvale, NJ, 1998. pg.3.

39. Shepherd J. The West of Scotland Coronary Prevention Study (WOSCOPS): Benefits of pravastatin therapy in compliant subjects. Circulation. 1996; 94(Suppl):I-539.

7

HYPERTENSION – DIAGNOSIS AND TREATMENT

Philip R. Liebson, MD
Henry R. Black, MD
Rush-Presbyterian-St. Luke's Medical Center, Chicago, IL

INTRODUCTION

The appropriate utilization of resources in the diagnosis and treatment of hypertension may appear deceptively easy - establish that the blood pressure is elevated, and treat it with nutritional-hygienic intervention augmented, if necessary, by appropriate antihypertensive therapy, and bolstered by very few laboratory examinations such as serum electrolytes, glucose, creatinine, an electrocardiogram, and rarely an echocardiogram. The establishment of periodic guidelines, most recently the Joint National Committee (JNC) VI guidelines, provides a framework which can be easily utilized by the physician caring for a broad range of patients with hypertension [1,2].

Closer investigation of the subject of hypertension reveals intricacies that require more than what may appear to be a simplistic approach to antihypertensive therapy. In this chapter we will provide a comprehensive discussion of the conditions which must be met for adequate treatment of the wide spectrum of hypertensives. The challenges to physicians caring for hypertensive patients at present include improving control of hypertension to at least a blood pressure below 140/90 mm Hg while reducing or eliminating other cardiovascular risks such as obesity, elevated lipids and smoking, and recognizing and intervening in patients with high normal blood pressure when target organ damage is present.

BLOOD PRESSURE MEASUREMENT AND CLINICAL EVALUATION

The accurate determination of blood pressure is essential for diagnosis and assessment of treatment. The most recent JNC guidelines (VI) outline the stages of blood pressure and recommend treatment at each stage on the basis of presence or absence of target organ damage or established cardiovascular disease [2]. In addition to the blood pressure reading (Table 1), the evaluation should include establishing the presence of cardiovascular disease, target organ damage, and other cardiovascular risk factors (Table 2).

Table 1. Classification of Blood Pressures
JNC VI (1997)

	Systolic Pressure (mm Hg)		Diastolic Pressure (mm Hg)
Hypertension			
Stage 3	≥180	or	≥110
Stage 2	160-179 or		100-109
Stage 1	140-159 or		90-99
High Normal	130-139 or		85-89
Normal	120-129 and		80-84
Optimal	<120	and	<80
Categorization by the highest (systolic or diastolic) average BP reading of 2 or more determinations			

Table 2. Hypertension Relevant History, Physical Examination, and Laboratory Studies

Given an average BP ≥ 130 systolic and/ or 85-89 Diastolic

History: Earliest diagnosis of hypertension (or high normal BP)
    Drug treatment
    Dietary assessment: sodium, alcohol, saturated fat, caffeine, licorice
    Illicit and over the counter drugs, herbal remedies.
    Cardiac disease: coronary artery disease, valvular heart disease, cardiomyopathy, congenital heart disease.
    Stroke or TIA
    Renal Disease
    Intermittent claudication of lower extremities.
    Diabetes, smoking, hyperlipidemia, recent weight change,activity status, family history of premature CAD
    Psychosocial and environmental: work status, family, educational level.

Physical Examination:
    Residua of cerebrovascular disease
    Funduscopic examination for retinopathy
    Lungs: Crackles or wheezes
    Heart: Apex beat, intensity of P2, presence of S4 or S3, murmurs
    Palpation of carotid and peripheral pulses, auscultation of carotid bruits
    Trophic changes in lower extremities
    Evidence for hyperlipidemic changes: xanthelesma, arcus, lipemia retinalis, tuberous or tendinous xanthomas

Laboratory Studies:
    Urinalysis [creatinine clearance, microalbuminuria, 24 hour protein]
    Electrocardiogram [limited echocardiogram for LV mass, ambulatory 24 hour BP]
    CBC
    Creatinine, electrolytes, fasting blood sugar, lipid profile [blood calcium, uric acid, glycosylated hemoglobin, TSH]

[ ] = optional, relevant to other clinical findings.

The history should therefore determine the time of first diagnosis of hypertension and whether and what type of drug treatment was used. Cardiovascular disease includes the presence of coronary artery disease, valvular heart disease, cardiomyopathy or congenital heart disease, all of which can lead to heart failure. Whether there has been a previous stroke or transient ischemic attack (TIA), and intermittent claudication should also be established. Other risk factors to be sought include a history of diabetes, smoking, hyperlipidemia, sedentary life style, and family history of premature cardiovascular disease.

The physical examination should be directed at establishing evidence for cerebrovascular disease, the presence of abnormal cardiac findings such as rales or peripheral edema, retinopathy, carotid and femoral bruits, absence of arterial pulses, and trophic changes in the feet and lower legs.

Laboratory studies include baseline electrolytes, creatinine, urinalysis (check for microalbuminuria in diabetics), fasting blood sugar, lipid profile, electrocardiogram, and in some patients a limited or complete echocardiogram and 24 hour ambulatory BP monitoring.

Special diagnostic findings and laboratory studies when secondary hypertension is suspected will be discussed below.

SELF–MEASURMENT OF BLOOD PRESSURE AMBULATORY BP MONITORING

Most patients have higher blood pressures in the office setting than at home. Frequently, the elevated blood pressure in the clinic is normal at home (white coat hypertension)[3] Also, target organ damage such as left ventricular hypertrophy (LVH) appears to correlate more closely with 24 hour BP readings and blood pressures at work than the casual blood pressure obtained in the physician's office. For these reasons, self measurement of blood pressure or ambulatory blood pressure monitoring may be of value in diagnosing hypertension and in following the effects of antihypertensive therapy. (Table 3).

Table 3. Ambulatory 24 Hr Blood Pressure

• Determines averages and peaks of BP over entire 24 hour period.
• Provides measures of systolic and diastolic pressure load.
• Determines sleep patterns of BP variation (dipper vs. non dipper or extreme dipper)
• Closer correlation with echo LV mass and other target organ damage than casual office BP.
• Determines effect of activity on BP.
• May be helpful after therapy in determining drug resistance, hypotensive episodes, and autonomic dysfunction.

IDENTIFIABLE CAUSES OF HYPERTENSION (SECONDARY HYPERTENSION)

It is unusual for patients to have an identifiable specific cause for their hypertension. In most physician's practices, approximately 95% of hypertension is primary (essential hypertension). Nonetheless, there are many easily obtainable clinical and laboratory clues which suggest a secondary or specific cause.

Information from the history of newly evaluated patients may point the way toward an identifiable secondary cause of hypertension . Such symptoms as headaches, diaphoresis, and palpitations, may suggest pheochromocytoma and weakness or nocturia may suggest hypokalemia due to an primary aldosteronism. Clearly, these symptoms are non-specific and so for the most part, the clues to diagnosis of secondary hypertension are discovered during the physical examination, with the addition of a few routine and special laboratory studies. Evidence of increased BP in patients with previously controlled hypertension or newly established hypertension in a previously normotensive individual is the most compelling historical information to lead the clinician to look for a specific cause for that patient's hypertension.

The physical findings which should suggest secondary hypertension are usually determined during the routine evaluation of the patient with an elevated blood pressure. For example, the astute clinician may observe weak femoral pulses, and then check the timing of radial and femoral pulses (radial pulse palpated before femoral pulse is abnormal).This finding, in association with bruits over the lower portion of the ribs posteriorly suggest coarctation of the aorta. In this case, popliteal blood pressure lower than arm blood pressures strongly suggests that diagnosis. Abdominal or flank bruits, especially in diastole, suggest renal artery stenosis and renovascular hypertension. Abdominal masses suggest polycystic kidneys in the young or middle aged hypertensive. The physical habitus of Cushing's syndrome or disease is usually obvious.

Certain abnormalities detected during routine laboratory studies may suggest secondary hypertension. A low serum K^+, especially below 3.2 mEq/L in a patient not taking diuretics, suggests hyperaldosteronism, and an increased serum creatinine may indicate primary renal disease, especially if associated with proteinuria and/or hematuria.

Additional tests which are performed to establish secondary causes of hypertension include (1) echocardiography or angiography, for coarctation; (2) a plasma renin/aldosterone ratio for primary aldosteronism; (3) assay of 24 hour urinary catecholamines,vanillyl mandelic acid (VMA) or metanephrines, for pheochromocytoma; (4) a renal scan after captopril or duplex ultrasound, for renovascular disease; and (5) abdominal ultrasound, for polycystic kidney disease. These tests are only indicated in hypertensives where there is a reasonably strong suspicion after the history, physical examination, and routine laboratory tests, to suspect one of these specific causes of hypertension.

Creatinine clearance and evaluation of the level of urinary protein excretion may be of assistance in serial evaluation of diabetics and patients with parenchymal renal disease to monitor effective blood pressure control, since current guidelines suggest lower target blood pressures to be reached in patients with these conditions than in hypertensives in general (Table 4).

Table 4. Clues to Secondary Hypertension

General

- Sudden onset of hypertension
- Stage 3 hypertension
- Poor BP response to antihypertensive therapy
- Previously well controlled hypertension with BP increase

Specific Clues to Etiology

- Pheochromocytoma: labile hypertension, pallor, palpitations, headache
- Coarctation of Aorta: delayed femoral pulses, bruits over ribs, rib notching
- Polycystic kidneys: flank masses
- Renovascular Hypertension: lateralizing abdominal and/or flank bruits
- Primary Aldosteronism: persistently low K^+ - especially if not on diuretics.
- Cushing's Syndrome: truncal obesity, abdominal striae
- Hyperparathyroidism: hypercalcemia
- Parenchymal Renal Disease: elevated creatinine, proteinuria
- Specific Drug Use: estrogen, cocaine, licorice, MAO oxidase inhibitors + cheese, NSAID

Specific Confirming Tests

- Pheochromocytoma: urinary catecholamines,vanillyl mandelic acid(VMA), metanephrine, abdominal CT or MRI
- Coarctation of Aorta: echocardiography, angiography
- Polycystic Kidneys: abdominal CT, ultrasound
- Renovascular Hypertension: renal arteriogram, captopril renogram, duplex ultrasound
- Primary Aldosteronism: plasma renin/aldosterone ratio, urinary aldosterone elevated despite volume expansion, adrenal CT or MRI,
- Cushing's Syndrome: dexamethasone suppression test, abdominal CT or MRI
- Hyperparathyroidism: calcium and phosphate, parathyroid hormone
- Parenchymal Renal Disease:renal function testing

RISK STRATIFICATION

Determination of risk for cardiovascular consequences of hypertension depends upon (1) the blood pressure level; (2) evidence for other cardiovascular risk factors; (3) presence of target organ damage itself such as retinopathy, coronary artery disease, cerebrovascular disease, peripheral vascular disease, or other arterial pathology (Table 5). While heart failure is obviously evidence for target organ damage, the recent JNC VI also lists left ventricular hypertrophy (LVH) as target organ damage. Recent

Table 5. Risk Stratification *[Modified from (2)]*

High Risk (Use Antihypertensive Therapy Once Diagnosis is Established)

- BP ≥130-159 mm Hg systolic or ≥85-99 mm Hg diastolic
      and
- Target Organ Damage or Clinical cardiovascular disease or Diabetes Mellitus or Multiple Major Risk Factors
      Or
- BP≥160 mm Hg systolic or ≥100 mm Hg diastolic

- Intermediate Risk (Try Lifestyle Modification Alone for 6-12 Months before starting drug therapy)

- BP 149-159 mm Hg systolic or 90-99 mm Hg diastolic with no target organ damage or clinical cardiovascular disease

    Low Risk (Lifestyle Modification Alone – Drug Therapy Not Suggested)

- BP 130-139 mm Hg systolic or 85-89 mm Hg diastolic with no target organ damage or clinical cardiovascular disease

Major Risk Factors	High Risk Categories (Any of Each)
Age older than 60 years	* Diabetes Mellitus
Sex (men and postmenopausal women)	or
Family History of early cardiovascular Disease	* Target Organ Damage
	(Any one):
Dyslipidemia	
Smoking	Left ventricular hypertrophy
	Nephropathy
	Retinopathy
	Or
	*Clinical cardiovascular Disease (Any One):
	Angina/prior MI
	Prior coronary revascularization
	Heart failure
	Stroke or TIA
	Peripheral arterial disease

evidence suggest that of those with LVH and established hypertension, there is a 15-fold increase in 10 year cardiovascular mortality compared with those hypertensives without   LVH on echocardiography[4]. Because of this consideration, a limited echocardiogram for m-mode calculations of LV mass has been recommended (Table 6). Although this technique may be relatively easy to perform, measurements may be deceptive since the expected error of this technique may be as high as 60 g even under optimal conditions. Although LVH is defined by values above the 97th percentile for LV mass indexed by height or body surface area in a normal population of men or women, the Framingham data indicate increases in cardiovascular risk even in those subjects with echo LV mass indices between the 50th and 97th percentile, compared with those below the 50th percentile[6].

Table 6. Values and Limitations of Limited Echocardiogram and 24 Hour Ambulatory BP Monitoring

Limited Echocardiogram
• Gold standard for diagnosis of LVH on basis of indexed LV mass. • Requires meticulous technique in acquisition of wall thickness and chamber dimension, and measurement of at least 3 end diastolic values. • May provide prognostic significance on basis of wall thickness/chamber radius ratio [relative wall thickness]. • Excludes evaluation of LV wall motion and diastolic function, other cardiac chambers, all valves, Doppler studies of valvular regurgitation, appearance of proximal aorta, pulmonary artery, and proximal inferior vena cava.

It is by no means clear than routine screening with an ECG will provide clearcut evidence for LVH. First, on using echocardiography to determine LV mass , ECG is relatively insensitive, in that only 20% of those with echo LVH will have ECG LVH. Second, there are various criteria for ECG LVH, and even the criteria which have been derived to increase sensitivity by comparison with echocardiography do no better than 50-60% sensitivity. A useful screening test must be highly sensitive even if it is not highly specific. There is little rationale for performing a screening test if a large number of those individuals with the condition being evaluated will not be discovered.

To date, there has still been no prospective study to demonstrate that regression of LVH per se, independent of effective treatment of hypertension, will improve prognosis, although retrospective analyses of some clinical studies suggest these possibilities. However, meta-analyses [7] and two recently published large clinical trials of hypertensive subjects [8-10] indicate that all of the major classes of agents (diuretics, beta-blockers, calcium antagonists, alpha-1 blockers, ACE inhibitors or angiotensin receptor blockers, and central alpha-2 agents) are associated with regression of LVH when administered to hypertensive individuals. If a specific class or classes of antihypertensive agents reduced LV mass better than others, the value of echocardiographic screening to detect those individuals with LVH would be justifiable. Since all effective agents except direct vasodilators (hydralazine and minoxidil), which are no longer given as monotherapy , have been demonstrated to regress LV mass. Routine screening by echo to guide therapy is not now warranted.Nor is followup echocardiographic study recommended unless major echocardiographic abnormalities (severe valvular dysfunction, LV wall motion abnormalities) other than LVH are present. In addition, specific followup study for regression of LVH in an individual, if present, is fraught with difficulties relating to test-retest reliability.

PREVENTION OF HYPERTENSION

Although this chapter focuses on intervention in established hypertension, recent guidelines recommend treatment even with high normal blood pressure. This is especially the case when target organ damage is present, either causally related to blood pressure variations, or associated with other causes. There is clear evidence from several epidemiologic studies that target organ damage such as LVH may precede elevations of blood pressure into the hypertensive range [11,12].

It is prudent in subjects with mean blood pressures between 120/80 mm Hg and 139/89 mm Hg to recommend life style changes. These focus on weight reduction, increased physical activity, moderation of alcohol intake, and moderation of dietary sodium[Table 7]. There is no harm in any of these intervention providing appropriate monitoring is conducted (especially with increased physical activity in men over 45 years of age or women over 55 years of age). At any blood pressure level, attention to weight reduction, lipid levels, and smoking cessation are valuable strategies for cardiovascular disease prevention.

Table 7.   Primary Prevention of Hypertension

▪ Limitation of salt intake to 2.4 or 6 g sodium chloride daily
▪ Maintain normal weight or >15% ideal weight
▪ Limit alcohol ingestion to 2 or fewer drinks/day [<1oz ethanol]
▪ Regular physical activity
▪ Maintain adequate potassium intake [approx 90 mmol/day]

TREATMENT OF HYPERTENSION

Evidence Base for Treatment

Since the mid 1940's, the development of antihypertensive drug therapy and results of clinical trials have shown that effective treatment of hypertension is associated with decreased morbidity and mortality [13] Based upon large scale studies over periods of years, the latest guidelines recommend that, in some cases, for those with heart failure, renal insufficiency, or diabetes, drug treatment should begin once blood pressure is above 130/85 mm Hg, and that with evidence for renal disease with 1 gm proteinuria or more, in 24 hours, target blood pressures as low as 125/75 mm Hg should be achieved [2]

CLINICAL TRIAL RESULTS

Most of the clinical trials in hypertension do not mimic the conditions of usual patient care. These clinical trials are efficacy studies in which a nonrepresentational cohort is treated in a carefully controlled manner [14]. Effectiveness studies, in which patients are treated in conditions that resemble practice, often without a placebo group, are now being accomplished more frequently. In circumstances in which the morbidity and mortality of hypertension were so great that effects of treatment were soon apparent, such as in the early studies of antihypertensive therapy in malignant hypertension, in which very small sample sizes and only brief periods of observation were needed to unequivocally demonstrate benefit. This has not been possible in clinical trials of Stage 1 hypertension, in which outcome events are much less common and so large cohorts of participants have been followed for long periods of time before benefits were shown. These trials have indicated that effective lowering of hypertensive levels of blood pressure will decrease the incidence of stroke, heart failure, and coronary artery disease.

PRINCIPLES OF LIFESTYLE MODIFICATION

Is lifestyle modification necessary if antihypertensive agents are used? The Treatment of Mild Hypertension Study (TOMHS) demonstrated that in Stage I hypertension, lifestyle modification, including physical activity, salt intake, weight reduction, and limitation of alcohol intake, reduced blood pressure effectively and decreased LV mass [9]. When the results of all drug treated groups who also received lifestyle modification were compared to those given nutritional-hygienic measures and placebo, the rate of events was lower in the group receiving both drugs and lifestyle modification. Aside from direct effects on blood pressure, life style modification may decrease the doses needed to reach goal blood pressure and may limit drug side effects such as hypokalemia when thiazide diuretics are utilized. An additional benefit of sodium restriction, for example, is reduction of urinary calcium excretion, thereby protecting against osteoporosis and renal stones.

Lifestyle modification should begin with the first patient visit. No matter what the blood pressure, the following findings should lead to lifestyle intervention: (1) a body mass index (Quetelet index) over 27 [wt (kg)/height (m^2)]; and (2) alcohol intake greater than 2-3 drinks a day; (3) sedentary life style; and (4) high sodium intake ($\exists$2.4 g/day). Dietary evaluation independent of blood pressure should assure adequate dietary calcium, potassium, and magnesium for general health. Deficiency of these minerals may impact on blood pressure and its treatment. Finally, dietary lipid modification is expected in those individuals with elevated low density lipoprotein (LDL) cholesterol and/or triglycerides, no matter what blood pressure is recorded, and smoking cessation should be pursued independent of blood pressure.

Antihypertensive agents are categorized by common drug classes. Principles of antihypertensive therapy include (1) once-daily dosing of a single drug if possible; (2) if a high dose of a drug is needed to reach target blood pressure, once daily dosing of drug combinations with lower dosing for each agent may be more effective by minimizing side effects of each drug; (3) demographics are usually not a major consideration for specific drug therapy efficacy, although diuretic or calcium antagonist monotherapy may produce a greater number of responders in African-Americans and the elderly, while ACE inhibitor, angiotensin receptor blockers, or beta-blocker therapy may work better in the young and in whites or Asians [15], (4) concomitant conditions and therapies should be considered in initiating therapy; (5) treatment costs should be considered; (6) adherence to therapy must be evaluated and adequate duration of therapy at a given dose assessed before dose increases or medication changes are undertaken.

A single antihypertensive agent should be used initially unless BP is over 200 mm Hg systolic or 120 mm Hg diastolic, in which case more than one medication should be started simultaneously. Care should be given not to start at too high a dose, especially in patients over 65 years of age. Patients with these high levels of blood pressure will respond to low doses and be brought out of the range in which target organ damage is a likely possibility. Frequent visits and rapid titration are much more appropriate than is aggressive therapy directed at treating blood pressure number rather than rate of decrease.

Although diuretics and beta blockers have been used predominantly in clinical trials demonstrating efficacy, there is adequate evidence that central alpha-2 agonists and peripheral sympathetic blockers when used together with diuretics also are effective in decreasing morbidity and mortality (earlier studies of efficacy used reserpine, guanethidine, and methyldopa). ACE inhibitors have been shown to be effective in decreasing mortality in patients with heart failure, and preventing LV remodeling and heart failure in patients with decreased LV function and segmental wall motion abnormalities attributed to myocardial ischemia and infarction. Both ACE inhibitors and nondihydropyridine calcium antagonists may have beneficial effects on maintaining renal function in diabetics and in those with chronic renal disease unassociated with renovascular disease. These findings are useful in determining selection of a first line agent.

ADHERENCE CONSIDERATIONS

There are several principles that will increase adherence : (1) limit dosage to once a day medication, if possible; (2) communicate regularly with the patient to determine side effects and ensure adherence; (3) check for orthostasis after initiation of medications, especially in elderly individuals. The use of nurses and other health professionals for followup, and reliance on one pharmacy to fill prescriptions help with adherence. It is most important for the physician to listen to the patient in regard to perceived side effects of medication, expense of drugs, and ancillary nontraditional formulations which the patient may consider either for elevated blood pressure or other health conditions. Seemingly refractory hypertension, i.e., blood pressures which remain above 140 mm Hg systolic or 90 mm Hg diastolic, is often the result of inadequate drug dosage or the choice of the wrong agents than patient noncompliance with prescribed dosage. If the patient is actually taking the proper doses of two or more properly selected antihypertensive agents and is still not at goal level of BP, secondary causes of hypertension should be looked for. Greater emphasis should be placed on weight loss and reduction of sodiun intake, and ambulatory blood pressure monitoring should be considered to look for "office resistance."

Concerns had been expressed about excessive lowering of blood pressure based upon so-called "J-curve" in which increased cardiovascular events develop with lowering of the diastolic pressure below 85 mm Hg. The Hypertension Optimal Treatment (HOT) Study clearly showed that there is no "J" curve in hypertension even in those without pre-existing ischemic heart disease.[16]

The elimination of antihypertensive agents after a period of adequate BP control has also been a subject of some debate. Slow, progressive reduction of therapy should be considered if (1) the patient has maintained BP at target levels for one year of more and (2) the patient has adhered to lifestyle modifications. Since at least 25-50% of patients demonstrate early increases in BP after drug cessation, frequent followup visits (perhaps semi-monthly) are recommended for the first 3-6 months after drug decrease or cessation.

HYPERTENSIVE EMERGENCIES

The situations in which blood pressure elevation leads to immediate or potential life threatening events over a period of hours or days are rare. Such emergencies or urgencies result from the direct effects of blood pressure elevation as well as superimposition of hypertension upon underlying disease. There is no specific blood pressure threshold for a hypertensive emergency. Preeclampsia of pregnancy may be associated with target organ damage at stage 1 or stage 2 hypertensive levels. In general, emergencies or urgencies are associated with systolic blood pressure levels above 180 mm Hg and/or diastolic blood pressure levels above 110 mm Hg with evidence for one or more of the following findings: (1) CNS, such as stroke, transient ischemic attack, or symptoms such as headache, blurring of vision, or decreased mentation; (2) exudates, hemorrhage or papilledema in the optic fundus; (3) major findings of arterial disease including aortic dissection, aneurysm or arterial obstruction; (4) cardiac abnormalities including ischemia or heart failure; (5) acute renal damage including rapidly increasing creatinine, marked proteinuria, or oliguria.

The concerns about interventions in these cases are (1) that targets for lowering BP vary with the underlying condition- in general, blood pressure decrease should be cautious in cerebrovascular events (completed stroke or TIA) but vigorous with aortic dissection and pre-eclampsia, and intermediate with other conditions; (2) with rapid interventions, blood pressure should be reduced by about 25% within minutes to several hours, with a general target of no less than 160/100 mmHg after 6-8 hours (except with aortic dissection and preeclampsia); (3) for emergencies, intravenous medications using infusions will allow accurate monitoring of antihypertensive effects; (4) early addition of oral agents should be done as soon as the patient can take oral medications; (5) efforts should be made to substitute definitive therapy for emergency medication as soon as practicable.

In our experience, there are several approaches which have been fraught with danger: (1) administration of sublingual nifedipine, which may produce precipitous, excessive decreases in blood pressure; (2) reliance on early intravenous drug combinations which complicate efforts to convert therapy to definitive oral medication.

Some caveats about specific hypertensive emergencies: (1) with evidence of stroke or transient ischemic events, determine as soon as possible whether a cerebrovascular hemorrhage has occurred. The use of fibrinolytic agents after stroke requires especially careful blood pressure monitoring, with use of intravenous antihypertensive agents should BP rise much above 180/110 mm Hg. (2) Aortic dissection should be diagnosed as rapidly as possibly by CT scan or transesophageal echocardiogram (in the case of thoracic dissection). (3) In the case of renal failure, it is prudent to exclude renovascular disease. Aortic dissection and acute myocardial infarction or unstable angina are the only hypertensive emergencies in which the rate of blood pressure rise in early systole as well as the absolute BP must be considered. Thus, not only should antihypertensive medications be administered by adjunctive agents which decrease the rate of LV contraction (beta-blockers) and avoidance of agents with reflex sympathetic effects (e.g. hydralazine, diazoxide). Drugs such as magnesium sulfate, methyldopa and hydralazine are excellent first line drugs in eclampsia but would not be considered as first line agents in other hypertensive emergencies.

In hypertensive emergencies, it is important to determine the circumstances surrounding the event as well as the clinical findings themselves. Special consideration includes (1) cocaine or amphetamine use, (2) delerium tremens in a patient developing hypertension following surgery, (3) use of cyclosporine as an immunosuppressive agent, (4) use of certain dietary substances such as cheeses and wines in patients on monoamine oxidase inhibitors (5) precipitous withdrawal of certain antihypertensive agents, especially clonidine (6) excessive sympathetic response (pheochromocytoma, postoperative after withdrawal from sympatholytic antihypertensive agents).

TREATMENT OF SECONDARY HYPERTENSION

In those few patients with identifiable causes of hypertension, specific interventions vary in their success. Coarctation of the aorta is relieved by surgical intervention but residual hypertension may be present in relation to the duration of hypertension pre-operatively. Primary aldosteronism is treated by surgery when an adenoma is present but by a spironolactone, amiloride or triamterene with sodium restriction if bilateral adrenal hyperplasia is present. In some cases, glucocorticoid-remediable hyperaldosteronism may be the etiology and glucocorticoids will successfully reduce blood pressure. In pheochromocytoma: phenoxybenzamine, a noncompetitive alpha-receptor blocker, or an alpha-1 blocker such as prazosin, should be used initially, and beta-blockers only after alpha blockade is induced, to prevent the paradoxic increases in blood pressure that occurs when beta blockers are used without alpha blockers. Surgery is almost invariably necessary.When malignant pheochromocytoma is present, or when tumors are unresectable, metyrosine, an agent which inhibits tyrosine hydrolase, may be useful to diminish catecholamine production. In renovascular hypertension, surgery or angioplasty is preferred and is more successful in lowering blood pressure in fibromuscular hyperplasia of young women than atherosclerotic renovascular disease in the elderly. ACE inhibitors and angiotensin receptor blockers are to be avoided with bilateral disease but may be especially effective with unilateral disease. In polycystic kidney disease, ACE inhibitors may slow the progression of the disease, though this has not been proven unequivocally. Dialysis and transplant are necessary in patients with end stage renal disease.

SPECIAL POPULATIONS

Racial and Ethnic Minorities

Although hypertension occurs in all ethnic groups, certain differences apply. For African Americans, hypertension is more prevalent and target organ damage more severe for given blood pressure than in other groups. Nonetheless, adequate declines in blood pressure and decreases in cardiovascular events can be accomplished with appropriate medication. This is especially important because of the higher stroke and heart disease mortality , and hypertension-related end-stage renal disease in African Americans. Diuretics especially are effective in blood pressure lowering[17]. Calcium antagonists and alpha-beta blockers (labetalol, carvedilol) are also especially effective.

Hispanic patients have a high prevalence of type II diabetes, and therefore efforts should be especially made to bring blood pressures down to target levels of below 130/85 mm Hg. Blood pressure levels in hypertension are the same as or lower than comparative levels in non-Hispanic whites.

East Asians are particularly responsive to antihypertensive therapy compared with whites, and my need lower doses than whites. Asian Indians are at high risk for cardiovascular disease and have a very high prevalence of insulin resistance and type II diabetes.

Women's Issues

Compared to men with similarly elevated blood pressures, especially in stage 1 hypertension, women have less target organ damage. Thus, in Stage 1 hypertension, lifestyle modification may therefore be pursued for periods of up to a year before antihypertensive drug therapy is started.

Oral contraceptive use may be associated with increased blood pressures. Development of hypertension under these circumstances is best treated by discontinuation of estrogen use, unless the risks of pregnancy are higher than the risks of hypertension, or other contraceptive use is impractical.

The development of pregnancy in hypertensive individuals on antihypertensive women requires discontinuation of beta-blockers in early pregnancy and ACE inhibitors and angiotensin receptor blockers throughout pregnancy [18]. Because of this, it is recommended that treatment using these agents be avoided in women in the childbearing period not on adequate contraception. In early pregnancy before the 20th week, methyldopa is an efficacious and safe agent. In hypertension developing after the 20th week, methyldopa and hydralazine are appropriate agents. Diuretics should not be initiated during pregnancy, but can be continued if they were part of the antepartum regimen in women with chronic hypertension.

In women receiving hormone replacement therapy, blood pressure may occasionally increase so that periodic evaluation is necessary. Oral estrogen is probably the main cause as with oral contraceptives. The effects of transdermal estrogens on blood pressure are not established. Progestins alone do not increase blood pressure.

Hypertension in the Elderly

In patients above the age of 60, systolic blood pressure becomes more important in predicting adverse cardiovascular events, and a substantial percentage of individuals (well over 50%) have either isolated systolic hypertension or both systolic and diastolic hypertension. Although essential (primary) hypertension is predominantly seen, renovascular hypertension associated with atherosclerosis must be considered in elderly patients with the onset of hypertension after age 55 or 60.

There is still some debate about whether elderly patients with stage I isolated systolic hypertension (systolic blood pressure between 140-159 mm Hg and diastolic blood pressure < 90 mm Hg) should be treated with antihypertensive agents [19]. Although these individuals are definitely at increased risk, controlled clinical trials of isolated systolic hypertension in the elderly have included only individuals with systolic pressures > 160 mm Hg, so that outcome efficacy of therapy at lower levels of systolic pressure is still unproven.

In the use of antihypertensive strategies in the elderly, low dosages of medication should be used initially, about 1/2 the usual dose as in younger individuals. Thiazide diuretics have clearly demonstrated efficacy in reducing mortality and morbidity in the elderly in controlled clinical trials. In the Systolic Hypertension in the Elderly Program (SHEP), the beta blocker atenolol was added if chlorthalidone alone did not reduce blood pressure to goal [19]. There is also recent evidence that a long acting dihydropyridine calcium antagonist (nitrendipine), with an ACE inhibitor added if needed to get blood pressure to goal level, decreased fatal and non-fatal stroke. On the other hand, drugs to be used cautiously are agents that produce significant postural changes or adversely affect cognitive function (peripheral adrenergic blockers, central alpha-2 agonists).

HYPERTENSIVE AGENTS IN COEXISTING DISEASE

A newly diagnosed hypertensive individual may have underlying conditions not necessarily associated with the blood pressure increase and in which clinical conditions are considered stable (i.e., no hypertensive emergency or urgency). Special conditions to consider in supporting a choice of initial antihypertensive agent include coronary artery disease, left ventricular failure, atrial dysrhythmias, peripheral arterial disease, and renal parenchymal disease.

Patients with stable angina, a past history of myocardial infarction, or other evidence for coronary artery disease should be given beta-blockers or long acting calcium antagonists preferentially. On the other hand, there is recent evidence from clinical observations and meta-analysis that short acting calcium antagonists, especially dihydropyridines, may be harmful, as well as agents which may produce reflex sympathetic response or sympathomimetic activity (hydralazine, beta blockers with intrinsic sympathomimetic activity). After a Q-wave infarction, ACE inhibitors, and beta blockers are recommended. After a non-Q wave infarction, diltiazem or verapamil should be considered for antihypertensive treatment because it may decrease non-fatal recurrent infarction when post-infarct LV systolic performance is normal (LV ejection fraction > 50%).

In patients with evidence of LV systolic dysfunction, with or without a past history of covert clinical LV failure, or with mild to moderate failure, an ACE inhibitor and diuretic are complementary antihypertensive agents. Angiotensin receptor blockers may also be beneficial. In severe chronic heart failure, the alpha-beta blocker carvedilol, with antihypertensive properies, also has beneficially affected prognosis. On the other hand, in the elderly with evidence of mild pulmonary edema associated with diastolic (but not systolic) LV dysfunction, beta blockers or nondihydropyridine calcium antagonists, especially verapamil, may be useful agents. Many of the latter include patients are elderly subjects with small left ventricles, in which systolic performance may actually be hyperdynamic and ejection fraction greater than normal.

With chronic atrial fibrillation and hypertension, long acting verapamil or diltiazem, or a long acting beta blocker (without intrinsic sympathomimetic activity) is an appropriate choice.

In peripheral arterial disease, there are no precepts except the obvious one of attempting to use arterial vasodilators and avoid beta-blockers, which are the only antihypertensive agents that initially increase peripheral vascular resistance.

In renal parenchymal disease, efforts are needed not only to lower the blood pressure, but also to slow renal disease progression. With mild to moderate disease, blood pressure should be lowered to 130/85 mm Hg. If proteinuria in excess of 1 gm/24 hours is present, more aggressive blood pressure lowering, to 125/75 mm Hg, should be implemented. ACE inhibitors, with diuretics, are the agents of choice with mild renal disease. ACE inhibitors should be used cautiously if creatinine is > 3 mg/dl unless dialysis is being undertaken. Thiazide diuretics can be used unless the glomerular filtration rate is < 30 ml/min, at which level loop diuretics are more effective antihypertensive agents, and are usually necessary to reduce blood volume and control blood pressure.

Diabetes mellitus presents another special case in which blood pressure should be lowered below the standard recommendation of 140/90 mm Hg to 130/85 mm Hg. ACE inhibitors, calcium antagonists (especially nondihydropyridines), alpha-1 blockers, and diuretics are all useful. ACE inhibitors are especially preferred with microalbuminuria or other evidence of diabetic nephropathy, especially those with type 1 diabetes. There is also some evidence that nondihydropyridine calcium antagonists may be protective as well.

Since hyperlipidemia is an important risk factor for coronary artery disease, there has been concern about using antihypertensive agents that adversely affect lipid profiles. For example, beta blockers (except those with intrinsic sympathomimetic activtiy) decrease HDL-cholesterol and increase triglycerides. Thiazide and loop diuretics (but not indapamide), increase LDL-cholesterol as well as having adverse effects on HDL-cholesterol and triglyceride levels, at least in the first several months of therapy and at high doses. On the other hand, alpha-1 blockers decrease LDL-cholesterol and raise HDL-cholesterol. However, there is no evidence that the use of agents with adverse lipid effects in order to lower blood pressure will increase cardiovascular risk. In some studies (TOMHS and others), the adverse change in lipid levels by diuretics and beta-blockers is not a long term effect. Finally, evidence from clinical trials following acute myocardial infarction indicates overwhelmingly that a beta-blocker decreases cardiovascular mortality and is mandated in that circumstance, if there are no contraindications. Antihypertensive drug effects associated with other drugs and conditions are listed in Table 8.

Table 8. Antihypertensive Drug Effects on Other Drugs and Conditions

Diuretics	Raise lithium levels
Beta blockers	Hepatic enzyme induction
	Mask insulin induced hypoglycemia
	Increase cocaine effects
	Potentiate clonidine withdrawal effects
ACE inhibitors	Raise lithium levels
	Raise potassium levels when used with potassium sparing diuretics
Calcium antagonists	Increase cyclosporin levels [not felodipine, isradipine, nifedipine]
Verapamil	Decrease lithium levels
Verapamil, diltiazem	Decrease digoxin, quinidine, theophylline, sulfonylureas
Central alpha-2 agonists	
Clonidine	Potentiate anesthetics
Methyldopa	Increase lithium levels

Modified from Table 11[2]

LOOKING TO THE FUTURE: EVOLVING STRATEGIES

The evidence that effective advances in awareness, treatment, and control of hypertension have reversed are based upon part 2 of the NHANES III survey and suggest the need to re-emphasize the importance of treating hypertension to goal levels.

There is added emphasis on the importance of target organ damage and other cardiovascular risk factors in considering drug interventions, and in bringing target blood pressures to still lower values than 140/90 mm Hg in diabetics and individuals with parenchymal renal disease.

Newer antihypertensive classes of agents include the angiotensin receptor blockers, which may provide a similar spectrum of action without the side effects of cough seen with ACE inhibitors.

The concept of the limited echocardiogram, if appropriate attention is placed on measurement technique, will allow more comprehensive diagnosis of LVH, a robust risk factor for cardiovascular mortality and morbidity, independent of covariate risk factors.

More attention to lifestyle modification in individuals with high normal blood pressure may prevent the development of hypertension.In this regard, population approaches using community programs and resources will assist in promoting prevention and increasing awareness of the risks and prevalence of hypertension.

Finally, increasing evidence for genetic factors that may facilitate the development of hypertension should serve to identify individuals at increased risk and focus preventive practices in a more efficient manner.

SUMMARY

Recent guidelines on the classification of blood pressure indicate the importance of recognizing high normal blood pressure as well as hypertensive levels as an indication for intervention. The presence of other cardiovascular risk factors or target organ damage even with slightly elevated blood pressure levels is a reason for initiating antihypertensive drug therapy. Ambulatory blood pressure monitoring provides a mean of establishing blood pressure variations which may determine whether elevated blood pressure levels in the office really reflect establish hypertension, and for optimizing the diurnal distribution of drug dosage.

Specific therapy may be determined not only on the basis of blood pressure but also by concomitant conditions such as left ventricular hypertrophy, coronary heart disease and heart failure. Lifestyle modifications such as limitation of sodium intake, limitation of alcohol intake, increased activity, and weight reduction are important adjuncts in controlling blood pressure. Keeping care inexpensive and simple is the key to successful patient compliance. In practical terms, this means once or twice a day drug dosage, and drug combinations in one pill if possible.

Efforts must be redoubled to reduce blood pressure to goal in as many hypertensives as possible.There is a large body of incontravertible evidence indicating the benefit of treatment. Yet, barely more than a quarter of hypertensive Americans are receiving enough therapy to take full advantage of these advances. For those over 65 years of age, less than 10% are at JNC VI goal. We must apply the many techniques available. The clear reduction which can be expected in stroke, heart failure, coronary heart disease, and renal failure, will be an apt reward for these efforts.

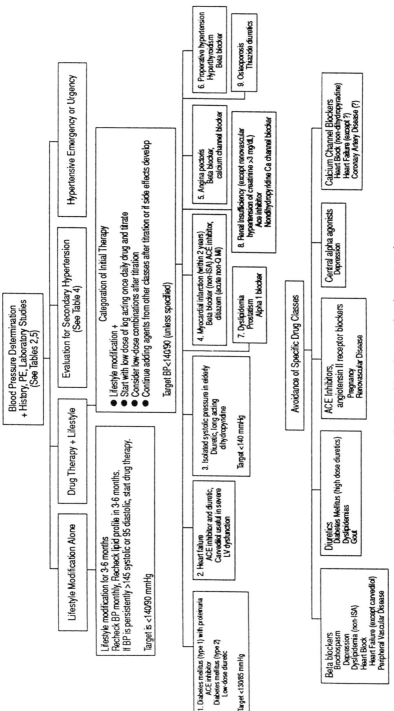

Figure 1: An algorithm for treating hypertension.

ACKNOWLEDGEMENT

The authors acknowledge the excellent secretarial assistance by Carmen Trujillo-Garcia.

References

1.   Guidelines for the treatment of mild hypertension. Memorandum from a WHO/ISH meeting. J Hypertens 1992;11:905-918.

2.   The sixth report of the Joint National Committee on Prevention, Detection, Evaluation, and Treatment of High Blood Pressure. Arch Int Med 1997; 157: 2412-2445.

3.   Pickering T, for an American Society of Hypertension ad hoc panel. Recommendations for the use of home (self) and ambulatory blood pressure monitoring. Am J Hypertens 1995; 9: 1-11.

4.   Koren MJ, Devereux RB, Casale PN, Savage DD, Laragh JH. Relation of left ventricular mass and geometry to morbidity and mortality in uncomplicated essential hypertension. Ann Int Med 1991;114:345-352.

5.   Black HR, Weltin G, Jaffe CC. The limited echocardiogram: a modification of standard echocardiography for use in routine evaluation of patients with systemic hypertension. Am J Cardiol 1991:67:1027-1030.

6.   Levy D, Garrison RJ, Savage DD et al. Prognostic implications of echocardiographically determined left ventricular mass in the Framingham Heart Study NEngl J Med 1990:322-1561-1566.

7.   Schmieder RE, Martus P, Klingbeil A. Reversal of left ventricular hypertrophy in essential hypertension: a meta-analysis of randomized double-blind studies. JAMA 1996;275: 1507-1513.

8.   Materson BJ, Reda DJ, Cushman WC, et al, for the Department of Veterans Affairs Cooperative Study Group on Antihypertensive Agents. Single-drug therapy for hypertension in men: a comparison of six antihypertensive agents with placebo. N Engl J Med 1993;328:914-921.

9.   Neaton JD, Grimm RH Jr, Prineas RJ, et al, for the Treatment of Mild Hypertension Study Research Group. treatment ofMild Hypertension Study: final results. JAMA 1993;270;713-724.

10. Liebson PR, Grandits GA, Dianzumba S, et al, for the Treatment of Mild Hypertension Study Research Group. Comparison of five antihypertensive monotherapies and placebo for change in left ventricular mass in patients receivibng nutritional- hygienic therapy inthe Treatment of Mild Hypertension Study (TOMHS). Circulation 1995;91:698-706.

11. Mahoney LT, Schieken RM, Clarke WE, Lauer RM. Left ventricular mass and exercise responses predict future blood pressure. The Muscatine Study. Hypertension 1988;12:206-213.

12. Devereux RB. Does increased blood pressure cause left ventricular hypertrophy and vice versa? Ann Int Med 1990;112:157-159.

13. Collins R, Peto R, Mac Mahon S, et al. Blood pressure, stroke, and coronary heart disease. Part 2: short-term reductions in blood pressure: overview of randomized drug trials in their epidemiological context. Lancet 1990;335:827-838.

14.   Black HR, Yi J-Y. A new classification scheme for hypertension based on relative and absolute risk with implications for treatment and reimbursement. Hypertension 1996;28: 719-724.

15.   Alderman, MH. Blood pressure management: individualized treatment based on absolute risk and the potential of benefit. Ann Int Med 1993;119:329-335.

16.   Hansson L, Zanchetti A, Carruthers SG, et al. Effects of intensive blood-pressure lowering and low-dose aspirin in patients with hypertension: Primary results of the Hypertension Optimal Treatment (HOT) randomised trial. Lancet 1998;351:1755-1763.

17.   Moser M. Can the cost of care be contained and quality of care maintained in the management of hypertension? Arch Int Med 1994;154:1665-1672.

18.   Sibai BM. Treatment of hypertension in pregnant women. N Engl J Med 1996;335: 257-265.

19.   Systolic Hypertension in the Elderly Program Cooperative Research Group. Implications of the Systolic Hypertension in the Elderly program. Hypertension 1993;21:335-343.

8

SELECTION OF BALLOON CATHETER THERAPY FOR PATIENTS WITH MITRAL AND AORTIC VALVE STENOSIS

Ted Feldman, MD
The University of Chicago Hospital, Chicago, IL

PERCUTANEOUS TRANSVENOUS MITRAL COMMISSUROTOMY

Percutaneous transvenous mitral commissurotomy (PTMC) was innovated by Inoue, performing the first procedure in 1982 using a unique balloon catheter system.[1] The balloon is designed to operate somewhat like a pulmonary artery flotation catheter and after it is introduced into the left atrium it can be "floated" into the left ventricle then used to split the fused mitral commissures completely. The availability of percutaneous methods for accomplishing mitral commissurotomy has allowed for broader patient selection than has been traditional for surgical methods.[2] The ease of percutaneous therapy, the relatively traumatic nature of the procedure, and the short hospital stay makes application of mitral commissurotomy to a broad segment of the population of patients with rheumatic mitral stenosis highly feasible. Randomized comparisons of PTMC with both open and closed surgical commissurotomy have demonstrated equivalent acute and long term results.[3] Thus, PTMC is the procedure of choice for the vast majority of patients with mitral stenosis.

Most patients with mitral stenosis present with the sine quo non of this disease, dyspnea on exertion. It is also common for patients with mitral stenosis to limit their activity rather than to report dyspnea with increasing activity. A careful history and physical and in addition to non-invasive testing is critical. Stress testing is helpful in the evaluation of patients whose symptoms are ambiguous or from whom history is difficult to elicit.[4] Patients who cannot perform on a treadmill may undergo dobutamine stress echocardiography to demonstrate alternations in the transmitral pressure gradient with exertion.[5] Treadmill exercise testing with expired gas analysis is another valuable method for quantification of exercise tolerance and is especially useful in serial testing in patients whose clinical picture is unclear.[6]

ECHOCARDIOGRAPHY:

Echocardiography is the mainstay of the non-invasive of mitral stenosis. The transthoracic echocardiogram provides an evaluation of all of the chamber sizes, associated valve lesions, and the mitral leaflet and subvalvular apparatus morphology. Doppler ultrasound provides a measure of the level of pulmonary hypertension and assessment of the severity of associated tricuspid and aortic valve lesions. Symptomatic patients with predominant mitral stenosis, mild mitral regurgitation or less, and mitral apparatus morphology that appears suitable are the ideal candidates for PTMC. The morphologic evaluation of the mitral valve and subvalvular apparatus morphology has been based conventionally on the echocardiographic score.[7] The scoring system evaluates leaflet thickening, subvalvular deformity, calcification, and leaflet mobility as the major features of valve deformity on a maximum of 4 scale. Thus, valves that are minimally deformed will have a score under 6, while those with severe deformity will have a score approaching 16. A variety of investigations have evaluated echocardiographic score as a means to predict acute and long term outcomes of balloon commissurotomy. The acute results of the procedure are similar or slightly less good in patients with echo scores greater than 8 compared to those with lower scores.[8] The long term results are less good in patients with scores greater than 8 and even less good in patients with scores of 12 or greater. These differences in outcome are related to the overall severity of the rheumatic disease process in these patients. It has not been demonstrated that mitral valve replacement offers better long term outcome in these patients with more severe valve disease and no direct comparison between PTMC and valve replacement surgery yet exists.[9]

Echo scores clearly define those patients that are ideal candidates for this procedure with scores 8 or less. Those with scores of 12 or greater clearly also have a less good result, although they may not fairly be compared with surgical commissurotomy. In fact, those with scores greater than 12 are often elderly patients who are poor candidates for surgery (or not candidates for surgery) and PTMC has a special role in this group. Patient selection is especially difficult for the group with scores of 9 - 12. These are often good candidates for surgical valve replacement and less than ideal for PTMC. Whether PTMC as a first strategy offers an advantage has not clearly been defined.

The symmetry of commissural fusion on short axis echo exam has also proven useful for predicting the acute results of PTMC.[10] In some patients commissural fusion is symmetric while in others it is highly asymmetric. Those with symmetric fusion (even if the valve is calcified) are more likely to have good results after balloon dilatation.[11] When the commissures are asymmetrically fused and especially when one commissure is densely fused and calcified while the other remains relatively open, the balloon will drift to the open side as it inflates without effecting a great dilating force on the fused side. It is, thus, difficult to open the fused commissure in these patients and the results of PTMC are not as often dramatic as they are in patients with symmetrical commissural fusion.

EVALUATION OF LEFT ATRIAL THROMBUS:

Echocardiography is most critical for evaluating patients for potential left atrial thrombus prior to PTMC.[12] Appendage thrombus is detected easily using transesophageal echocardiography. Prior to the widespread use of transesophageal echo exams, most patients were treated with Coumadin for 4 - 6 weeks prior to PTMC. The procedure was then performed with the recognition that embolic events would complicate between 1 and 4% of procedures. Since the use of pre-PTMC transesophageal echocardiography has become routine, stroke rarely complicates the procedure. Those without prior history of anticoagulation therapy, patients with atrial septal or free wall atrial thrombus, or those with large and mobile thrombi in the appendage should not undergo PTMC. They may be treated with oral anticoagulant therapy for 3 - 6 months and then a repeat transesophageal examination may be performed to see if the thrombus has resolved. This strategy is successful in a large proportion of the patients who have therapy deferred during anticoagulation therapy in this manner. In many cases the thrombus will appear improved but not completely resolved, with an echo dense appearance in the distal appendage consistent with old, organized clot. A great deal of judgment is required regarding the risk of embolic stroke in patients with mobile atrial thrombus since this is such a catastrophic complication and can be avoided by either additional anticoagulation or surgical commissurotomy.

Some patients have organized thrombus in the atrial appendage with a history of long term anticoagulation therapy. PTMC may be undertaken with relatively low risk of dislodgment of these organized thrombi.[13] Some operators have reported good clinical outcomes in very carefully selected patients with left atrial appendage thrombus. One of the unique elements of use of the Inoue balloon that must be considered in these cases is the potential to steer the balloon from the left atrium across the mitral valve using the stylette that is part of the Inoue balloon apparatus. Special care must be taken to avoid allowing the balloon tip to catch in the left atrial appendage. Frequently the tip of the balloon will drift into the left upper or left lower pulmonary veins and it is sometimes difficult to distinguish this from the atrial appendage fluoroscopically.

PROCEDURE RESULTS:

The clinical results of PTMC have been reported by many groups from all over the world.[14,15] There is uniformly a decline in the left atrial mean pressure and the transmitral pressure gradient and an increase in the cardiac output and mitral valve area. The mitral valve area typically increases from 1.0 cm² to 1.8 to 2.0 cm². The pulmonary artery pressure declines from 20 to 30% immediately after PTMC and often by an additional 50% or more after six months.[16] When a large decrease in pulmonary artery pressure occurs acutely during a procedure, patients often spontaneously comment on a sense of relief from their shortness of breath while still on the catheterization table. The long term results are similar to series reported for both closed and open surgical commissurotomy in the past.

PROCEDURE COMPLICATIONS:

The most important complication of balloon commissurotomy is an increase in the degree of mitral regurgitation. Fortunately, severe increases in mitral regurgitation are infrequent. In the North American Inoue Balloon Registry fewer than 3% of patients underwent valve replacement during the procedure hospitalization as a result of the PTMC procedure.[17] Catastrophic mitral regurgitation of a 4+ grade occurs in less than 3% and an increase in mitral regurgitation of 3 or 4 grades occurs in a total of 3.7% of patients. 1/3 of patients have an increase in mitral regurgitation of one grade. Altogether about 2/3 of patients have 1+ or less mitral regurgitation at the end of the procedure.

Decreases in mitral regurgitation have been described in a small number of patients. This is probably related to variations in ventriculographic technique and loading conditions but it is plausible that in some patients leaflet co-optation is improved by commissurotomy with a resultant decrease in mitral regurgitation. Some studies have found that the degree of mitral regurgitation seen immediately post procedure decreases a few months following balloon dilatation. A number of mechanisms may be involved in this long term resolution of mitral regurgitation. The valve annulus may be stretched acutely and then recoils over time with the diminution in the degree of regurgitation. It is also possible that the balloon traumatizes the papillary muscles in some cases, contributing transiently to post procedure mitral regurgitation.

It is our experience that mitral regurgitation is related either commissural tearing or to damage to the chordae tendineae.[18] The second mechanism, damage to the chordae, may be minimized or eliminated if care is taken to be sure that the balloon moves freely along the long axis of the ventricle between the valve and the apex after the mitral valve is crossed. The maneuver of probing towards the left ventricular apex with the partially inflated balloon insures free movement of the catheter. If the balloon shaft seems to kink or the tip of the balloon appears angulated or eccentric, the balloon may be withdrawn into the left atrium and the valve may be recrossed to gain a better orientation for balloon inflation.

A variety of other complications may occur. Ventricular perforation is almost unheard of with the Inoue balloon while it occurs consistently in 1 - 2% of patients treated using the double balloon technique. Complications related to transseptal puncture occur with a frequency of about 1% in most series. This may be operator related and appears to decrease as operators become more experienced with PTMC and transseptal technique.[19]

Stroke is a rare occurrence now that transesophageal echocardiographic screening is used widely. TIA or stroke episodes may occur when related to embolization from catheters or wires. It is important to distinguish a clinical picture simulating TIA that can occur as a consequence of sedative or local anesthetic use. This latter problem is especially common in patients over age 80 years.

Despite the large atrial septal punctures used to gain access for the balloons, atrial septal defect is not an important complication of this procedure. Shunt ratios of greater than 1.5:1 occur in only 3 - 5% of patients and many of these resolve within the first few months after the procedure. Atrial septal defect is likely to be persistent only in those patients with an incomplete valve opening who thus maintain a pressure gradient from the left atrium to the right atrium. Residual atrial septal defect is usually noted by colored Doppler but is detectable by oximetry in less than 12% and is clinically important in only 1 - 2% of patients. Some of these shunts that are noted early after PTMC are no longer present after a few months. The cases that require surgical closure of the atrial puncture site are most often those where inadequate valve dilatation has resulted in persistent left atrial hypertension, which maintains the shunt over time.

PATIENT SELECTION

A major element of successful PTMC procedures is good patient selection. The traditional criteria for commissurotomy candidates include a pliable mitral valve and little subvalvular disease. These patients have done well using both surgical and catheter methods. Long term follow-up on this group of patients has shown excellent results with about 70% remaining improved over a 5 - 7 year follow-up period using PTMC.

An AHA/ACC task force has recently proposed guidelines for therapy for patients with mitral stenosis. Asymptomatic patients with pulmonary hypertension at rest or with exercise, and most symptomatic patients should be considered for PTMC or valve replacement. The following three flow charts (Figure1-3) show a decision tree for selection of therapy in asymptomatic patients, those with Class I-II symptoms, and severely symptomatic patients with Class III-IV limitations. Therapy for patients with no symptoms or symptoms and moderate stenosis is predicated largely on the pulmonary artery pressure at rest or with exercise.

Figure 1. Asymptomatic Patients With Pulmonary Hypertension

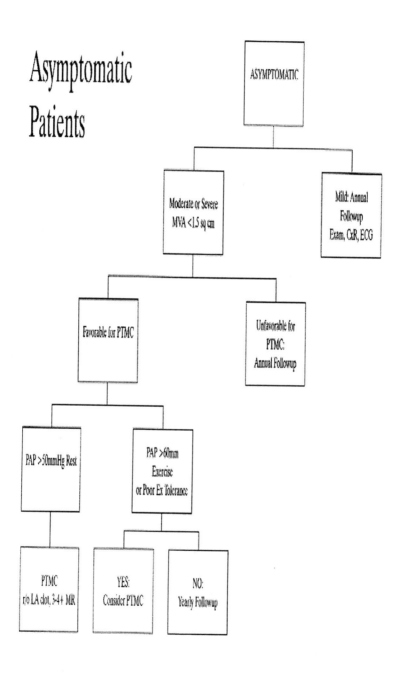

Figure 2. Symptomatic Patients - NYHA Class II

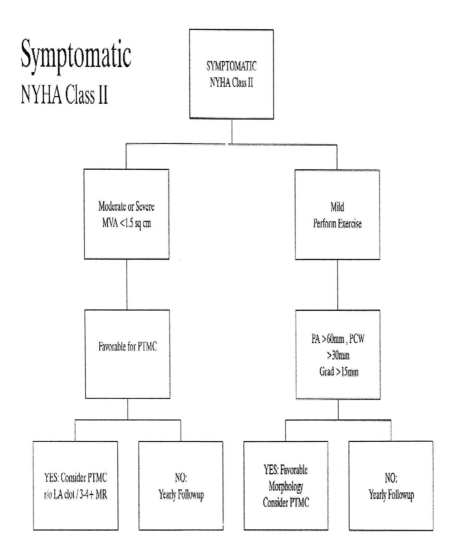

Figure 3. Symptomatic Patients – NYHA Class III-IV

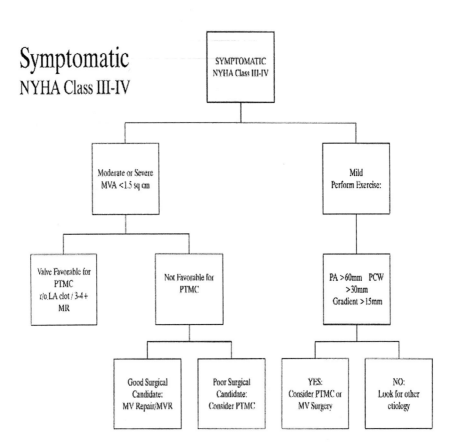

Symptomatic
NYHA Class III-IV

A major consideration for patient selection is the presence or absence of other valvular lesions. The decision to proceed with PTMC may be influenced in both directions. The patient with severe aortic insufficiency and severe mitral stenosis will likely need to undergo double valve replacement to have meaningful clinical improvement. On the other hand, a patient with moderate aortic insufficiency and severe mitral stenosis in whom the need for aortic valve replacement is not well defined may benefit from balloon dilatation of the mitral valve even when the mitral valve morphology is not ideal. The PTMC procedure will allow the patient a period of time to determine whether the aortic lesion will ultimately require valve replacement. Double valve replacement might be deferred until a point at which it is clearly indicated or likely to result in greater clinical improvement. Patients with associated coronary disease can undergo PTCA and PTMC at a same session procedure. If there are additional valvular lesions, waiting 6 - 12 months to determine the durability of the PTCA results may allow a simpler valve operation without the need for associated coronary artery bypass surgery.

Tricuspid regurgitation is the lesion that most commonly confounds the decision making process in patient selection for PTMC. It is often difficult to determine whether tricuspid regurgitation is primary or secondary with associated pulmonary hypertension. Since most patients have a significant decrease in their pulmonary artery pressure following PTMC, tricuspid regurgitation can be expected to improve in the majority even when there is rheumatic deformity of the tricuspid valve. In uncertain situations an observation period following balloon dilatation may be necessary to determine whether tricuspid annuloplasty will ultimately be important.

SPECIAL CONSIDERATIONS FOR PATIENT SELECTION:

A number of special patient populations are especially well suited for PTMC. Some elderly patients with extreme valve deformity and significant co-morbid associated illnesses may have palliation from PTMC with excellent short term results.[20] Patients who are dependent on intravenous vasopressor therapy and in the Intensive Care Unit are in this category. Short term palliation allows them to be discharged from the hospital and greatly expedites their medical management. Elderly patients who are Class IV at home may be given significant mobility and independence for periods ranging from ½ year to up to 4 years.

Pregnant patients are another group for whom PTMC is ideally suited.[21,22] Those who have signs of pulmonary congestion during pregnancy present at a point where therapy is critically needed. The Inoue procedure can be performed with only a few minutes of fluoroscopy time. With transthoracic echocardiographic monitoring of the procedure, right heart catheterization is not necessary, which helps minimize the fluoroscopy time. When right heart catheterization is performed from the femoral approach, special care must be taken to have the patient move onto the left side during passage of a catheter or wire through the inferior vena cava so that the uterus does not compress the movement of the catheter into the right atrium. PTMC results have been reported by many groups and pregnant patients.[21,22] The results are excellent, though concern remains regarding the long term effects of radiation on the child. If catastrophic mitral regurgitation does result from the procedure in pregnant patients, the results are obviously dire for both mother and fetus. The goal of the procedure is thus hemodynamic improvement, rather than a "perfect" result.

The procedure is best performed late in the fifth month and in the sixth month of the pregnancy. At this point organogenesis is largely complete and the risks of precipitating early labor are as low as they can be. Fluoroscopy time can usually be kept under ten minutes. Transesophageal echocardiographic assistance to minimize fluoroscopy time has not been helpful in our practice. The trauma of esophageal intubation in one case precipitated contractions which required intra-procedure magnesium therapy.

PTMC FOR VALVE REPLACEMENT CANDIDATES:

The use of PTMC in valve replacement candidates (with significant valve deformity) remains controversial. Commissurotomy has been used predominately in patients with pliable valves and the classical loud opening snap and the long term results are well established. Randomized and longitudinal comparisons of PTMC and surgical commissurotomy have both shown no differences in acute or long term outcome.[7-14]
PTMC has lower procedure mortality than valve surgery and has allowed the use of this procedure in patients who might otherwise undergo valve replacement surgery but the long term results of PTMC in these patients has not been compared with valve replacement in randomized trials. No randomized comparisons have been made between valve replacement surgery and balloon commissurotomy in patients with valves that are not well suited by traditional criteria for commissurotomy.

We have examined the results of PTMC in these otherwise typical mitral valve replacement patients. In the North American Inoue Registry we found three year event-free survival of 62% and a six year event free survival of 44% in this group.[2,24]
This is in contrast to a 70% five year event-free survival overall in the Registry and in prior reports of surgical commissurotomy. The use of PTMC must be considered in relation to the outcome of mitral valve replacement surgery [25]. Surgical mortality is usually between 3 and 8%. The incidence of thromboembolic and bleeding complications, infections, and reoperations range between 6 and 8% per patient per year after valve replacement. Patients who undergo valve replacement represent a sicker population than those who have surgical commissurotomy and direct comparisons between mitral valve surgery and mixed populations of PTMC patients

(including both ideal and non-ideal commissurotomy candidates) do not yield a reasonable picture of the outcomes in these two different groups.

Prior studies have compared patients with echocardiographic scores that are low compared to those that are higher.[26] The results of PTMC procedures are clearly less good in patients with echo scores greater than 8 compared to those with scores less than 8 as are the long term outcomes. This has led some to select patients for PTMC only when the echo scores are low. The patients with a higher echo score usually undergo mitral valve replacement rather than commissurotomy. Thus, comparing these surgical patients with commissurotomy patients rather than with mitral valve replacement outcomes is inappropriate.

No direct comparisons have been made between the outcome of mitral valve replacement and balloon commissurotomy in patients with similar clinical characteristics. Patients with greater degrees of valve deformity and higher pulmonary artery pressures with associated right heart failure represent a different spectrum than those in whom commissurotomy has traditionally been performed. A randomized trial would be the only way to definitively resolve this patient selection issue and none has been performed to date. Three to four year event-free survival of patients undergoing PTMC with poorly suited valves for commissurotomy are about 60% and the results of surgical series show an annual major event rate ranging 6 - 8% after the in-hospital surgical events occur. The comparison of patients with non-ideal valves for commissurotomy and historical controls from surgery thus suggest that the results from balloon dilatation may not differ substantially from surgical results using valve replacement in similar patients. After a five year period, substantial morbidity occurs in surgery patients because they represent a sicker population compared to those that have either balloon or surgical commissurotomy. A patient with significant mitral valve deformity who undergoes PTMC as initial therapy has a 60% chance of avoiding mitral valve replacement for at least a few years. The probability of mitral valve replacement in this group is thus 30 - 40%. If this patient undergoes mitral valve replacement as initial therapy, the probability of mitral valve replacement in the same time period is, of course, 100%.

MILD MITRAL STENOSIS:

Patients with mild mitral stenosis represent an additional special challenge.[27,28] Patients with a mitral valve area greater than 1.5 generally do not have symptoms, though some will have obvious classical symptoms of mitral stenosis. The decision to perform PTMC may be undertaken easily when symptoms are present. When these patients are very large in physical size, the valve area index may be smaller than the absolute valve area. This helps simplify decision making further. Patients with mild symptoms create a decision making dilemma. No data exists regarding the long term consequences of

PTMC in this group. Coexisting pulmonary hypertension at rest or with exercise is an indication for intervention. The acute results of the procedure in patients with mild mitral stenosis are often dramatic. Valve areas between 2.5 and 3.0 cm^2 are commonly achieved. Whether this has an impact on the natural history of the disease is speculative. Some of these patients will certainly develop mitral regurgitation if left untreated and converting them to treated commissurotomy patients may be greatly beneficial. On the other hand, the complications that occur from the procedure in these patients may offset these long term results to an unclear degree.

BIOPROSTHETIC VALVES:

Patients with bioprosthetic valves have undergone balloon dilatation.[29,30] Rare cases of successful procedures have been described. Pathologic studies have shown a tendency for fragmentation of the valve leaflets as a result of the balloon dilatation. This procedure cannot be recommended routinely for patients with prosthetic stenosis due to these pathologic findings. Since the mechanism of stenosis in bioprosthetic valves does not involve commissural fusion, PTMC will probably have limited durability in these cases. Tricuspid valve leaflet fragmentation and embolization may be less clinically important or catastrophic and balloon dilatation of stenotic bioprosthetic tricuspid valves may thus be safer to attempt as a palliative therapy in patients who have no other alternative. PTMC has been successfully performed in patients with prior mitral annuloplasty rings without any special modifications of technique.[31,32]

PRIOR SURGICAL COMMISSUROTOMY:

About 15% of patients having PTMC procedures have undergone surgical commissurotomy in the past. These patients are well suited for balloon dilatation and have excellent acute results. The longer term results of PTMC in these patients are not as good as for patients without prior commissurotomy.[33] This appears to be largely because these patients have had rheumatic heart disease for a much longer period of time and have associated greater levels of pulmonary hypertension and multi-valve lesions. In the North American Inoue Registry, prior commissurotomy emerged as the most predictive single variable for the need for surgical valve replacement late after PTMC. The utility of the procedure in these patients depends heavily on the goals of therapy for an individual patient.

COST:

The costs of catheter commissurotomy are obviously significantly less than surgical commissurotomy or valve replacement surgery in the United States. The material cost for balloon catheters is between $1,000 and $3,000 depending on the types of balloons and supplies used and the usual hospital stay is one night for the older patients and commonly completely outpatient for patients 50 years of age or younger. Typical cost for catheter commissurotomy on a one night stay basis is between $8,000 and $12,000 while surgical commissurotomy or valve replacement surgery ranges between $20,000 and $60,000.

Outside the United States cost considerations are significantly different. Disposable supplies may make up the greater part of the cost and closed surgical commissurotomy in some settings actually represent a less expensive alternative. This is particularly true in countries such as India.

The development of more reliably reusable catheters has helped cut costs in the third world. Multi-use of devices intended for single use is usual practice in many parts of the world. The Inoue balloon catheter is used 3-5x routinely while double balloons or multi-track balloons are used even more frequently. A reusable metal mitral commissurotomy modeled after the Tubbs dilator has just been developed and promises to help reduce costs in some parts of the world where this procedure is most needed.

AORTIC VALVULOPLASTY

Balloon aortic valvuloplasty created great excitement when it was initially introduced.[42-45] The procedure promised in its early development to be an alternative to surgical valve replacement. Balloon dilatation of the aortic valve yields an increase in aortic valve area, a fall in transvalve pressure gradient and an increase in cardiac output. This is accomplished percutaneously from a femoral puncture without need for surgical incision. There is immediate clinical improvement in the vast majority of patients, with substantially less morbidity than surgical valve replacement. It was quickly discovered, however, that the results of this procedure are not long lasting and, thus, not a reasonable alternative for patients who are good candidates for operative valve replacement.[45,46] The short durability of this procedure resulted in a rapid move away from the use of balloon aortic valvuloplasty even in cases where surgery was felt to be very high risk. Despite the lack of enthusiasm for this procedure today, a number of important clinical indications still remain for balloon aortic valvuloplasty.

RESULTS OF BALLOON AORTIC VALVULOPLASTY

Valve area increases between 60% and 100% in almost all patients. The transvalve pressure gradient declines by at least 50%. The valve area after dilatation ranges between 0.7 cm^2 and 1.1 cm^2. Even a small increase in valve area is associated with dramatic clinical improvement. If the valve area is larger than 0.5 cm^2 prior to valvuloplasty, post dilatation areas of 1.0 or more cm^2 are common. It should be appreciated that prosthetic aortic valve areas (both mechanical and porcine) have an area between 0.9 and 1.2 cm^2.[47] Small women have prosthetic areas at the smaller end of this range. These valve areas are all substantially less than the normal 2.5 to 4.0 cm^2 area and it is notable that the areas resultant from both valvuloplasty and valve replacement provide adequate hemodynamics. Prosthetic-patient mismatch syndromes are occasionally seen after surgery but in the valvuloplasty patient population, since the patients are so sick at the outset, very small increments in valve area are typically associated with significant clinical improvements.

The greatest limitation of this procedure is the recurrence of stenosis in virtually all patients.[48] Most patients will have anatomic and symptomatic restenosis somewhere between 6 months and 18 months after valvuloplasty though some remain clinically improved for as long as 2-5 years. Survival is clearly not improved by aortic valvuloplasty.

The mechanism of restenosis is related to the mechanism of the relief of stenosis. The valve is calcified and trileaflet in these patients, with thickening of the valve cusps and the absence of commissural fusion. The calcium deposits are nodular and densely encased in a fibrotic capsule on the superior surface of the valve leaflet. This fibrous encapsulation is responsible for the lack of embolization of calcific debris during balloon valvuloplasty. After valvuloplasty, multiple fractures occur in the calcific nodules which create hinge-like areas with improved leaflet mobility. The restenosis process involves the regrowth of fibrous tissue in these cracks or hinge points.[49] Ossification of these fissures may occur as well. The active process of restenosis follows a time course consistent with new scar tissue formation.

CURRENT INDICATIONS FOR AORTIC BALLOON VALVULOPLASTY:

There are currently six major clinical situations in which this procedure is useful (Table 1).

Table 1. Indications for Aortic Valvuloplasty

1. Cardiogenic shock
2. Bridge to surgery.
3. Pre-operative for non-cardiac surgery.
4. Vasopressor/ICU dependent with high surgical risk.
5. Diagnostic test in low gradient/low output setting.
6. Poor surgical risk/advanced age.
7. Congenital aortic stenosis.
8. Rheumatic aortic stenosis.

Patients who present with aortic stenosis and cardiogenic shock may have an immediate salutary hemodynamic response. Balloon dilatation can be used at the time of initial catheterization and decisions regarding later therapy can be made after the patient has been stabilized. Second, patients with severe left ventricular dysfunction in whom aortic valve replacement is planned may have the procedure as a "bridge" to surgery. As soon as left ventricular performance is improved they may then undergo surgery with less risk. The pre-renal azotemia that these patients commonly have may improve over a period of just a few days. Patients with aortic stenosis that is discovered during evaluation for major non-cardiac surgery may have valvuloplasty[4] pre-operatively. The non-cardiac operation can be performed without either the anticoagulation or delay engendered by valve replacement. This occurs most commonly in patients with malignancies that require operation. Fourth, patients who have been hospitalized for a protracted period and are not candidates for valve replacement surgery may undergo balloon valvuloplasty with very successful short term improvement. Patients who are on vasopressor therapy and cannot be weaned may often be switched to less intensive medical therapy. This will facilitate transfer out of the ICU and often discharge to home. Valvuloplasty can not be expected to improve their long term prognosis but may give them a improved quality of life either in or outside of the hospital. There are patients in whom valvuloplasty can be used as a diagnostic evaluation. When the valve area is between 0.7 and 0.9 cm^2 and the cardiac output and transvalvular pressure gradient are low, it is often difficult to evaluate the likelihood for a response to valve replacement. The severity of valve stenosis is also difficult to evaluate in this group. Poor ventricular function makes therapy difficult. Valve replacement can be performed as a first therapy and if patients have an improvement in left ventricular function, they survive. Unfortunately, those who do not have improvement in left ventricular performance have extremely high perioperative mortality. Balloon dilatation may, thus, be used to select those patients likely to have improvement in ventricular function and the greater benefit from later surgical valve replacement therapy. If the symptoms in left ventricular performance improve after balloon valvuloplasty, valve replacement can be performed with a high expectation for longer term success.

Most common are symptomatic patients with high surgical risks. The extremely elderly are the greatest single sub group in this category. Patients over age 80 and certainly those over age 90 have substantial risks for mortality and morbidity when they undergo aortic valve replacement. In addition to the mortality risk, stroke and protracted hospital courses are common. Another common high risk surgical patient group are those with extreme degrees of chronic lung disease in whom the risks of mechanical ventilation perioperatively are at the extremes. A significant number of these patients require a long recovery period in a chronic care facility. Aortic valvuloplasty is attractive in these patients. In our own practice, patients over age 90 are a major component of this group.

Excellent results have also been reported in younger patients with congenital aortic stenosis, and in patients with rheumatic stenosis.[50,51] This latter group is under appreciated as a population who can have excellent results from valvuloplasty. Acute results have been less good in patients with bicuspid aortic stenosis. The evaluation of balloon dilatation for stenotic bioprosthetic valves using in vitro testing has been very poor. Prosthetic tissue may be very friable and often it is not calcified. The potential for leaflet perforation, evulsion, and embolization is significant.

COMPLICATIONS OF AORTIC VALVULOPLASTY:

The major complications of balloon aortic valvuloplasty are ventricular perforation from the catheter or guide wire and femoral arterial complications related to the large sheath size. Cardiac tamponade from catheter perforation has been reported in 1% of cases. Vascular surgery for femoral arterial complications may be necessary in as many as 5% of patients. Significant hematomas occur in 10 - 20% of patients and transfusion rates are as high as 20%. Critically ill patients with multi organ system failure do not recover predictably and will often have a complicated post-procedure course, if they recover. With increasing experience, arterial complications may be expected to decrease.

Bundle branch block may occur as the balloon contacts the ventricular septum. Patients with pre-existing bundle branch block may develop complete heart block due to balloon compression of the calcific atrioventricular plate with impingement on the conducting system. Temporary pacemaker use may be necessary in some cases. In rare patients, permanent pacemaker implantation is necessary after the procedure. Severe aortic regurgitation is rare. In fact, we have had no experiences with severe aortic insufficiency in our entire experience with this procedure over the last decade and do not routinely perform aortography or even echocardiography post procedure to evaluate aortic valve insufficiency. It is a clinical concern only when the aortic diastolic pressure drops significantly or there are obvious clinical sequelae during the procedure. Leaflet avulsion may occur, usually with 23 mm diameter balloons or a 20 mm balloon in a small patient. The major contraindication posed by pre-valvuloplasty aortic insufficiency is that when regurgitation is the major lesion, balloon dilatation will not result in hemodynamic improvement. A progressive low cardiac output state may occur after valvuloplasty, which may be fatal. This may result from prolonged or repeated balloon inflations and left ventricular outflow obstruction with resultant depression of cardiac output.

As outflow tract obstruction is acutely worsened by the balloon, chamber dilatation occurs and ventricular pressure generation decreases. Coronary artery perfusion pressure may drop and create problems in patients with coronary artery disease. Ventricular tachycardia during balloon inflations may also contribute to left ventricular depression. A rest period between inflations of several minutes may be necessary to avoid this problem. The aortic pressure should rebound to at least baseline during these breaks. If the valve has been opened adequately, the aortic pressure will rise above its baseline level due to better transmission of left ventricular pressure across the outflow tract. It is of course necessary to wait for resolution of ischemic ECG changes and any symptoms that might occur in between balloon inflations.

References

1   Inoue K, Owaki T, Nakamura T, Kitamura F, Miyamoto N: Clinical application of transvenous
     mitral commissuromtomy by a new balloon cathter. J Thorac Cardiovasc Surg 87:394-402, 1984.

2   Ellis LB, Singh JV, Morales DD, Harken DE. Fifteen to twenty year study of one thousand patients
     undergoing closed mitral valvuloplasty. Circulation 1973;48:357-64.

3   Reyes VP, Raju BS, Wynee J, Stephenson LW, Raju R, Fromm BS, Rajagopal P, Mehta P, Singh
     S, Rao DP, Satyanarayana PV, Turi ZG. Percutaneous balloon valvuloplasty compared with open
     surgical commissurotomy for mitral stenosis. New Engl Med. 1994;331:961-7.

4   McKay CR, Kawanishi DT, Kotlewski A, Parise K, Odom-Maryon T, Gonzalez A.
     Hemodynamics 3 months after double-balloon, catheter balloon valvuloplasty treatment of patients
     with symptomatic mitral stenosis. Circulation. 1998;77:1013-21.

5   Marzo KP, Herrmann HC, Mancini DM. Effect of balloon mitral valvuloplasty on exercise
     capacity, ventilation and skeletal muscle oxygenation. J A, Coll Cardiol. 1993;21(4):856-65.

6   Wilkins GT, Weyman AE, Abascal VM, Block PC, Palacios IF. Percutaneous balloon dilitation of
     the mitral valve: an analysis of echocardiographyic variables related to outcome and the mechanism
     of dilataion. Br Heart J. 1988;60:299-308.

7   Feldman T, Carroll JD, Isner JM, Chisholm RJ, Holmes DR, Massumi A, Pichard AD, Herrmann
     HC, Stertzer SH, O'Neill WW, Dorros G, Sundram P, Bashore TM, Ramaswamy K, Jones LS,
     Inoue K. Effect of valve deformity on results and mitral regurgitation after Inoue balloon
     commissurotomy. Circulation. 1992;85:180-7.

8   Post JR, Feldman T, Isner J, Herrmann HC. Inoue balloon mitral valvotomy in patientswith severe
     valvular and a subvalvular deformity. J Am Coll Cardiol. 1995;25:1129-36.

9   Feldman T, Herrmann HC, Carroll JD, Ramaswamy K, Mobis JM, Harrison JK, Pichard AD,
     Holmes DR, Rothbaum DA, Dorros G, Bailey SR, Feldman R, Margolis JR, Ramee SR. Balloon
     valvotomy for non-ideal commissurotomy candidates. J Am Coll Cardiol. 1995;25:90A.

10   Fatkin D, Roy P, Morgan JJ, Feneley MP. Percutaneous balloon mitral valvotomy with the Inoue single-
     balloon catheter: commissural morphology as a determinant of outcome. J A Coll Cardiol. 1993;21:390-7.

11   Levin TN, Feldman T, Bednarz J, Carroll JD, Lang RM. Transesophageal echocardiographic evaluation of
     mitral valve morphology to predict outcome after balloon mitral valvotomy. Am J Cardiol. 1994;73:707-10.

12   Tessier P, Mercier LA, Burelle D, Bonan R. Results of percutaneous mitral commissurotomy in patients with a left
     atrial appendage thrombus detectedby trransesophageal echocardiography. J Am Soc Echo. 1994;17:394-9.

13   Chen WJ, Chen MF, Liau CS, Wu CC, Lee YT. Safety of percutaneous transvenous balloon mitral commissurotomy
     in patients with mitral stenosis and thrombus in the left atrial appendage. Am J Cardiol. 1992;70:117-9.

14   Feldman T. Hemodynamic results, clinical outcome, and complications of Inoue balloon mitral
     valvotomy. Cathet Cardiovasc Diagn. Suppl 2:2-7, 1994.

15   Trevino AJ, Ibarra M, Garcia A, Uribe A, de la Fuente F, Bonfil MA, Feldman T. Immediate
     and long-term results of balloon mitral commissurotomy for rheumatic mitral stenosis: comparison
     between Inoue and double-balloon techniques. Am Heart J. 1996;131:530-6.

16   Ribeiro PA, al Zaibag M, Abdullah M. Pulmonary artery pressure and pulmonary vascular
     resistance before and after mitral balloon valvotomy in 100 patients with severe mitral valve
     stenosis. Am Heart J. 1993;125:1110-4.

17   Feldman T, Carroll JD, Herrmann HC, Holmes DR, Bashore TM, Isner JM, Dorros G, Tobis JM. Effect of balloon size and stepwise inflation technique on the acute results of Inoue mitral commissurotomy. Cathet Cardiovasc Diagn. 1993;28:199-205.

18   Herrmann HC, Lima JA, Feldman T, Chisholm R, Isner J, O'Neill W, Ramaswamy K. Mechanisms and outcome of severe mitral regurgitation after Inoue balloon valvuloplasty. J Am Coll Cardiol. 1993;22:783

19   Anonymous. Complications and mortality of percutaneous balloon mitral commissurotomy. A report from the National Heart, Lung, and Blood Institute Balloon Valvuloplasty Registry. Circulation. 1992;85:2014-24.

20   Tuzcu EM, Block PC, Griffin BP, Newell JB, Palacios IF. Immediate and long-term outcome of percutaneous mitral valvotomy in patients 65 years and older. Circulation. 1992;85:963-71.

21.   Iung B, Cormier B, Elias J, Michael PL, Nallet O, Porte JM, Sananes S, Uzan S, Vahanian A, Acar J. Usefulness of percutaneous balloon commissurotomy for mitral stenosis during pregnancy. Am J Cardiol. 1994;73:398-400.

22.   Stephen SJ. Changing patterns of mitral stenosis in childhood and pregnancy in Sri Lanka. J Am Coll Cardiol. 1992;19:1276-84.

23.   Feldman T, Herrmann HC, Rothbaum DA, Bashore TM, Ramee SR, Carroll JD, Dorros G, Pichard AD, Isner JM, Feldman RC, Bailey SR, Holmes DR, O'Neill WW, Massumi A, Robis JM, Kawanishi DR. Late outcome after percutaneous mitral commissurotomy: six year results of the N. American Inoue balloon registry. J Am Coll Cardiol. 1997;29:226A.

24.   Feldman T, Herrman HC, Carroll JD, Ramaswamy K, Tobis JM, Harrison JK, Pichard AD, Holmes DR, Rothbaum DA, Dorros G, Bailey SR, Feldman R, Margolis JR, Ramee SR. Balloon valvotomy for non-ideal commissurotomy candidates. J Am Coll Cardiol. 1995;25:90A.

25   Hammermeister KE, Sethi GK, Henderson WG, Oprian C, Kim T, Rahimtoola S. A comparison of outcomes in men 11 years after heart-valve replacement with a mechanical valve or bioprosthesis. Veterans affairs cooperative study on valvular heart disease. New Engl J Med. 1993;328:1289-96.

26   Feldman T, Carroll JD. Valve deformity and balloon mechanics in percutaneous transvenous mitral commissurotomy. Am Heart J. 1991;121:1628-33.

27   Pan M, Medina A, Suarez de Lezo J, Romero M, Hernandez E, Segura J, Melian F, Pavlovic D, Jimenez F, Vivancos R. et al. Balloon valvuloplasty for mild mitral stenosis. Cathet Cardiovasc Diagn. 1991;24:1-5.

28   Herrmann HC, Feldman T, Isner JM, Bashore T, Holmes DR Jr, Rothbaum DA, Bailey SR, Dorros G. Comparison of results of percutaneous balloon valvuloplasty in patients with mild and moderate mitral stenosis to those with severe mitral stenosis. The North American Inoue Balloon Investigators. Am J Cardiol. 1993;71:1300-3.

29   Spellberg RD, Mayeda GS, Flores JH. Balloon valvuloplasty of a stenosed mitral bioprosthesis. Am Heart J. 1991;122:1785-7.

30   Lin PJ, Chang JP, Chu JJ, Chang CH, Hung JS. Balloon valvuloplasty is contraindicated in stenotic mitral bioprostheses. Am Heart J. 1994,127:724-6.

31   Feldman T, Levin T, Kabour A: Percutaneous transvenous mitral commissurotomy following carpentier ring annuloplasty. J Invasive Cardiol. 1997,9:184-7.

32   Jang IK, Block PC, Newell JB, Tuzcu EM, Palacios IF. Percutaneous mitral balloon valvotomy for recurrent mitral stenosis after surgical commissurotomy. Am J Cardiol. 1995;75:601-5.

33   Herrman HC, Ramaswamy K, Isner JM, Feldman TE, Carroll JD, Pichard AD, Bashore TM, Dorros G,, Massumi GA, Sundram P. et al. Factors influencing immediate results, complications, and short-term follow-up status after Inoue balloon mitral valvotomy: a North American multi center study. Am Heart J. 1992,124:160-6.

34   Feldman T. Innovations in transseptal catheterization and balloon mitral commissurotomy. Cathet Cardiovasc Diagn. 1995;36:188.

35   Inoue K. Percutaneous transvenous mitral commissurotomy using the Inoue balloon. Eur Heart J. 1991;12:Suppl B:99-108.

36   Feldman T, Herrmann HC, Inoue K. Technique of percutaneous tansvenous mitral commissurotomy using the balloon catheter. Cathet Cardiovasc Diagn. 1994;Suppl 2:26-34.

37   Inoue K, Feldman T. Percutaneous transvenous mitral commissurotomy using the Inoue balloon catheter. Cathet Cardiovasc Diagn. 1993;28:119-25.

38   Berland J, Rocha P, Choussat A, Lefebvre T, Fernandez F, Rath P. Balloon mitral valvotomy by using the Twin-AT catheter: immediate results and complications in 110 patients. Cathet Cardiovasc Diagn. 1993;28:126-33.

39   Stefanadis C, Kouroukliz C, Stratos C, Piotsavos C, Tentolouris C, Toutouzas P. Percutaneous balloon mitral valvuloplasty by retrograde left atrial catheterization. Am J Cardiol. 1990;65:650-4

40   Park SJ, Kim JJ, Park SW, Song JK, Do YC, Lee SJ. Immediate and one-year results of percutaneous mitral balloon valvuloplasty using Inoue and double-balloon techniques. Am J Cardiol. 1993;71:938-43

41   Levin TN, Feldman T, Carroll JD. Effect of atrial septal occlusion on mitral area after Inoue balloon valvotomy. Cathet Cardiovasc Diagn. 1994;33:308-14.

42   Letac B, Cribier A, Koning R, Lefebvre E. Aortic stenosis in elderly patients aged 80 or older. Treatment by percutaneous balloon valvuloplasty in a series of 92 cases. Circulation. 1989,80:1514-20.

43   Safian RD, Berman Ad, Diver DJ, McKay LL, Come PC, Riley MF, Warren SE, Cunningham MJ, Wyman RM, Weinstein JS, et al. Balloon aortic valvuloplasty in 170 consecutive patients. N Engl J Med. 1988,319:125-30.

44   Percutaneous balloon aortic valvuloplasty. Acute and 30-day follow-up results in 674 patients from the NHLBI Balloon Valvuloplasty Registry. Circulation. 1991,84:2383-97.

45   Otto CM, Mickel MC, Kennedy JW, Alderman EL, Bashore TM, Block PC, Brinker JA, Diver D, Ferguson J, Holmes DR Jr., et al: Three year outcome after balloon aortic valvuloplasty. Insights into prognosis of valvular aortic stenosis. Circulation. 1994,89:642-50.

46   Bernrard Y, Etievent J, Mourand JL, Anguenot T, Schiele F, Guseibat M, Bassand JP: Long-term results of percutaneous aortic valvuloplasty compared with aortic valve replacement in patients more than 75 years old. J Am Coll Cardiol. 1992,20:796-801.

47   Khuri SF, Folland ED, Sethi GK et al, and the participants in the VA Cooperative Study on Valvular Heart Disease: Six month postoperative hemodynamics of the Hancock heterograft and the Bjork-Shiley prosthesis: Results of a Veterans Administration cooperative prospective randomized trial.. J A, Coll Cardiol 1998;12:8.

48   Feldman T, Galgov S, Carroll JD. Restenosis following successful balloon valvuloplasty:bone formation in aortic valve leaflets. Cathet Cardiovasc Diag 1993, 29:1-7.

49   Hayes SN, Holmes DR Jr, Nishimura RA, Reeder GS. Palliative percutaneous aortic balloon valvuloplasty before noncardiac operations and invasive diagnostic procedures. Mayo Clinic Proceedings. 1989;64:753-7.

50   Sandhu SK, Lloyd TR, Crowley DC, Beekman RH. Effectiveness of balloon valvuloplasty in the young adult with congential aortic stenosis. Cathet Cardiovasc Diagn. 1995;36:122-127.

51   Ueda K, Tamai H, Yung-Sheng H, Ono S, Kosuga K, Tanaka S, Matsui S, Minami M, Nakamura T, Motohara S, Uehata H. Eight-year outcome of rheumatic aortic stenosis after percutaneous balloon aortic valvuloplasty. Circulation 1996, 94:369.

9

CONGESTIVE HEART FAILURE CLINICS AND OTHER STRATEGIES FOR COST EFFECTIVE MANAGEMENT

Marc A. Silver, MD
Christ Hospital Heart Failure Institute, Oak Lawn, IL

HEART FAILURE--A MODEL FOR SUCCESS

Heart failure is epidemic in the United States (1). Fueled by our successes in preventing short-term mortality in acute coronary artery syndromes as well as the aging of our population, the overall impact has been an annual escalation in the number of patients developing the overt syndrome of heart failure. With our understanding that the overtly symptomatic patient with heart failure is one who has had long standing derangement of structure, function, neurohormones and metabolism, it is not surprising that heart failure is both difficult to treat and often resistant to that treatment. Likewise, because of its chronicity and recurring nature, heart failure is also a national economic burden both in terms of expenses for patients, families, institutions and payers as well an emotional burden for those who have and treat this syndrome (2).

Out of this situation, however, have arisen a variety of innovative and effective approaches that can impact favorably resource utilization for heart failure at all ends of the spectrum. In this chapter, I will review, in brief, some of these approaches, their rationale and, where available, some of the outcome measurements supporting their use.

The Heart Failure Admission

Perhaps one of the most difficult areas in which to discuss resource utilization is that of the heart failure patient who is admitted to the hospital. For over 1.2 million primary heart failure admissions each year nearly twenty three billion dollars are spent in providing this care. It would seem that advances could be made in delimiting these admissions and / or in curtailing their cost. Several problems underlie this difficult situation. The first factor is that the majority of patients admitted to the hospital today for decompensated heart failure have a very advanced form of heart failure. For example in a study performed by Stevenson et al (3) demonstrated that the majority of the patients admitted are in New York Heart Association functional class 4, have evidence of marked activation of the sympathetic nervous system, have significant pulmonary arterial hypertension and have a low cardiac index. Additionally, adding to the difficulty advanced age and multiple co-morbidities. We have all witnessed the heart failure admission become easily transformed into an exceedingly long hospital stay as the focus shifts from treating the heart failure towards evaluation of the renal insufficiency or diabetes mellitus. There is little in the way of guidelines for the heart failure admission (4); however, the goals of the heart failure admission can be summarized in Table I. below.

Table I. Goals for the Heart Failure Admission

Establish cause for the admission/decompensation
Symptom Relief
Complete Diuresis
Attenuate/ Prevent End-Organ Damage
Enhance Oral Pharmacologic Regimen
Decrease or Attenuate Readmission

Even before considering the goals for the heart failure admission it is worthwhile to recall that once a patients proceeds from either having no symptoms or mild symptoms into the land of advanced symptoms requiring hospital admission, almost certainly that patients life will be foreshortened and certainly changed. Therefore, it is worth a very careful look at where the patient stands on the heart failure timeline. As is expressed in the algorithm found at the end of this chapter, no matter at which point the patient "enters" the heart failure spectrum a useful strategy involves a more chronic disease management approach

Regarding the establishment of the cause for the admission, it is useful to think of the admission as an opportunity to better understand what the particular cause in the individual patient that upset the precarious balance within most patients with advanced heart failure live. For some patients investigation will also include diagnostics that discloses the etiology of the patient's heart failure. This, in fact, is an important initial step since determining that the patient has active myocardial ischemia, for example, allows focus on the required steps to treat the underlying problem with the ultimate goal being prevention of further decline in left ventricular function and attenuation of the symptoms of heart failure.

There is, in fact, controversy about the ideal way to provide symptom relief for most patients admitted for heart failure. Lowering an elevated left ventricular filling pressure which may be the hallmark of a decompensated patient with either systolic or diastolic dysfunction is one of the goals. This can be achieved by using alone or in combination diuretics, vasodilators or inotropic agents. There are potential benefits and pitfalls to each approach; but perhaps the point to be made is early administration of some therapy. Reassessment within a short time frame is necessary to decide if the path chosen has been effective and if not to move ahead with another strategy. Several clinical trials are underway to specifically address the outcome of heart failure patients treated during acute decompensation in a variety of ways including early use of inotropic agents, use of naturetic peptides and even the diagnostic use of a pulmonary artery catheter. Results of these trials will hopefully give us more objective data upon which to plan a strategy for hospitalized patients.

Related to symptom relief is the goal of complete diuresis. Readmission rates for the heart failure patient are enormously high and often related to an incomplete diuresis in the initial admission. This lead rapidly to diuretic resistance as well as poor gastrointestinal absorption and metabolism of other heart failure medications which lead to further decompensation and subsequent readmission. Again, no clear guideline exists for determining a "dry" state but at a minimum there should be some assessment made on the basis of clinical exam (lung crackles, jugular venous pressure, hepatomegaly, skin turgor) as well as laboratory assessment.

A major goal of the heart failure admission is the recognition that the patient is now in a high-risk category; that is high risk for subsequent readmission. Therefore every attempt should be made to identify the targets for intervention to lower the risk for that patient. Identification of the cause and type of heart failure are important first steps. Often attention focuses on the actual treatment of the volume overload or the orthopnea that little attention is focused on the underlying etiology. Identification of an etiology such as myocardial ischemic, is critical in directing the patients evaluation and perhaps subsequent course. Similarly, echocardiographic determination of either impaired or intact left ventricular systolic function also may vary the diagnostic and / or therapeutic path.

Other common factors such as dietary abuses or medication non-compliance impact on the admission and subsequent readmission. Early identification by careful questioning by medical and nursing staff as well as by social workers and other staff members can often provide clues that might ordinarily be missed in the routine medical evaluation.

Considerable attention has been given to the importance of attaining adequate doses of oral medications particularly angiotensin converting enzyme inhibitors. There is increasing support for target dose at and beyond those used in clinical trials with evidence supporting decreased readmission rates for those patients attaining the higher target doses. At the end of the heart failure admission usually several forces are working to limit the hospital length of stay including the patients own perception of improved functional status. Nevertheless, ensuring an adequate, well tolerated and well-understood oral regimen may go a long way towards compensating for an additional hospital day.

Finally, one of the commonly overlooked goals of the admission is the initiation or expansion of heart failure education for the patient and the family. While the acute or sub-acute setting is not an ideal place to initiate chronic patient education, it may be an ideal opportunity to get a patient interested in further education follow-up. This education-based approach has been shown to be cost effective in reducing hospital readmission even in elderly patients with heart failure (2,5,6).

The Emergency Department

In most hospitals the emergency department is a large if not the predominant source for heart failure admissions. Here again, faced with the acutely decompensated patient goals are critical in determining the most effective way to evaluate and treat the patient. In many ways, despite the acuity level in the Emergency Department, many of the same principles in the chapter algorithm apply such as an understanding of the left ventricular function and prognostic profile and use of symptom relieving as well as survival promoting therapies. Perhaps most important is to not let either the patient of the physician get lost in the acuity. Perhaps one of the key goals for the Emergency Department is in assuring the initiation of the chronic disease management that these patients will require. Keeping the patient on a seamless path is crucial.

Whatever algorithm is used to exclude myocardial ischemia for the arriving heart failure patient, several quick steps including oxygen delivery and intravenous diuretics can initiate rapid patient improvement. Additional use of vasodilator therapy and perhaps even inotropic therapy for the appropriate patient can be effective. The ability to utilize an observational area for the heart failure patient has been shown to be a useful and cost-effective strategy. If patients use a single hospital or hospital system, then early identification of the patient who has previously had heart failure either using a paper or electronic record can also expedite treatment. The ability to have the patient seen and followed within a 24 hour period, perhaps in the physicians office or a heart failure clinic (see below) make decision to discharge the improved patient easier from the Emergency Department.

In the Emergency Department or once actually admitted to the hospital, then, there are several key principals to enhance the efficacy and decrease resource utilization as listed in Table II.

Table II. General Approaches in the Hospital Emergency Department and In-Patient Units

Early identification of a heart failure patient
Knowledge of left ventricular function
Knowledge of etiology
Knowledge of precipitating factors
Rapid delivery of safe, inexpensive therapy (oxygen, diuretics, nitrates)
Frequent evaluation of the efficacy of therapy--escalate as needed
Avoid repeated diagnostics. Always ask: • "Will knowing this result change my treatment?" • "Do I want to know the result now when the patient is decompensated or latter when well compensated?"
Have a plan to achieve best oral medical therapy. If this will not be attained in the hospital assure an early follow-up visit in order to proceed with the plan.

The Heart Failure Clinic

Because of the need for chronic education and care of heart failure patients as well as the gap that exists between acute hospital based care and physician office care specialized centers have been developed generically called heart failure centers or clinics.

Often, the motivation for the development of the heart failure clinic has been the attention to the frequency of hospitalization and subsequent re-hospitalization for many patients with heart failure. The heart failure clinic, then, is often an outgrowth of an institutional task force related to the health care costs of caring for patients with a chronic disease. As far as a target for heart failure clinic activities goes, this, too, if often seemingly straightforward. Frequently, when deficits in patient understanding or education (2) are identified or even inadequate utilization of standard medical therapy (7) and then these approaches are targeted. On rarer occasions, the development of a heart failure clinic is a prospective approach to offering a comprehensive continuum of care for a targeted disease or population. Regardless of the approach initiating the development the structure and function of the clinic is similar in either circumstance. It has been my experience that a nurse has usually been selected as the initial team member to investigate or initiate the development of the heart failure clinic; on occasion the initial facilitator is a physician.

An extremely wide variety of approaches have been utilized throughout the United States. This is a reflection of the varied needs and resources available to individual institutions and practices. Therefore, the term "heart failure clinic" means different things to different people. The spectrum of activities that may be offered in a heart failure clinic or program are listed in Table III.

Utilization of a protocolized approach often makes proper up-titration of drugs, like beta blockers, easier and enhances the ability to attain target doses. Perhaps because of the difficulty of educating patients who are frequently elderly with associated cognitive deficits, or who are ill during a short-stay hospital admission, education remains one of the critical services a heart failure clinic can offer most patients. (5)

Location of the clinic is variable and can be adjacent to the hospital where patients may come on an elective basis to receive education, dietary instruction, exercise and supervision. Similarly they can be in physician offices or wherever resources are adequate to meet the needs of the patients. Hospital based clinics allow the staff to utilize hospital personnel such as therapists, rehabilitation nurses, social workers and dietitians

Table III. Services Offered in Heart Failure Clinics

Education for Patients and Families
Education for Primary Care Physicians and Cardiologists
Nurse Telemanagement
Telephone Triage
Critical Pathway (Hospital) and Guideline Development
Out-Patient Inotropes and Intravenous Diuretics
Beta blocker and ACEI titration programs
Rehabilitation and Exercise Training
Heart Transplantation Evaluation
Clinical Research

without having to have these individuals dedicated to the clinic. Clinics usually are outgrowths of an area of expertise and interest that already exists within the institution such as cardiac or pulmonary rehabilitation, a cardiac support group or a physicians office. Ideally, there should also be a space reserved for patient education conferences and lectures as well as private patient-family conferences. Access to a library of heart failure related materials and Internet access is also extremely useful.

Identifying which patients should be enrolled in the heart failure clinic is usually obvious at first. Those at the highest risk of recurrent admission or those in need of advanced service are the patients to target. Later as the process proceeds many other ways of targeting patients exist such as looking at common drug combinations or use of services or diagnostics. Still another, perhaps more proactive way, is to look at patients at risk for heart failure as is discussed below (see screening the asymptomatic patient).

Outcomes with Heart Failure Clinics

There is increasing experience using a heart failure clinic model and both case control and randomized trials demonstrate the efficacy of this approach. One of the initial studies to look prospectively at such an approach was conducted by Rich et. al (6). Although the patients in this study were identified within the hospital setting much of the specialized treatment of the patients in the study group were carefully coordinated by heart failure nurses who insured telephone or direct contact via home care nurses or directly with home visits or calls by the heart failure nurses. Using this approach there was not only improved survival in the patients initially being discharged alive but also a 56% reduction in subsequent readmission to the hospital. Multiple readmissions were also prevented and although not significant in this population readmission for non-heart failure related causes was also reduced.

Not only have improved symptoms, quality of life, decreased hospitalization and improved exercise tolerance been attributed to effective management in heart failure clinics (6,8,9) but a reduction in cost in caring for heart failure patients has also been described (6, 10-12).

West et al. from Stanford recently described their experience with home based comprehensive disease management for 51 patients with symptomatic heart failure. (12) Based on a system applied to risk factor modification for coronary artery disease (13) they employed a physician supervised but nurse run program that implemented guideline driven goals and clinical monitoring all done via telephone contact. Through this approach the investigators demonstrated decreased dietary sodium intake (38%), enhanced oral medication dosing as well as improved functional status and exercise tolerance. With the heart failure program they also were able to reduce general out-patient visits, emergency room visits and hospital admissions.

Screening for the Asymptomatic Patient

We know that the clinical syndrome of heart failure is preceded by months and usually years of molecular and structural changes that set the stage for appearance of overt heart failure. Often, this is heralded by early, transient symptoms and more commonly by markers for the disease such as impaired exercise and elevated levels of neurohormones. Additionally we are aware of certain high-risk populations for the development of heart failure including patients who have had a myocardial infarction, diabetics and hypertensives. It seems prudent then, to consider some form of screening at least for patients with risk of heart failure. This is not so far-fetched as one might imagine. Considering all the evidence that lipid lowering drugs prevent primary and secondary myocardial infarction, certainly, prevention of additional myocardial damage by use of pharmacotherapy can be seen as a reasonable outcome of a heart failure screening program that includes evaluation of a patients lipids.

The Future of Heart Failure Clinics

One of the problems that we face is the disconnect that exists between the understanding of the value of the heart failure clinic and its ability to be reimbursed for services rendered. For example, despite evidence demonstrated above (12) in most cases hospital fees would have been reimbursed by most payers had the patient been hospitalized, yet there is little in the way of reimbursement coding for most heart failure services. Increasingly reimbursement may be obtained for extended nursing visits or for the home care visits but there is more difficulty in obtaining reimbursement for the required frequent telephone contact. That is why, thus far, it has been at-risk managed care organizations, who see the economic benefit of utilizing specialized heart failure services. With a larger span of capitated reimbursement, perhaps utilization of heart failure clinics will also spread. Also, anticipated might be a merging of borders of some of the common overlapping chronic disease processes such as diabetes, renal insufficiency and heart failure. There are many common educational and medical threads amongst these disease processes and since these are such common co-morbidities for the heart failure patient, the heart failure clinic might well expand its borders to become a broader chronic disease management clinic.

Finally, nowhere more than among chronic disease states are patients expressing interest in and utilizing complimentary and alternative medical approaches. Because of the generally lower tech-higher touch approach of the heart failure clinic, this might be the logical setting to scientifically explore the value and potential benefit of some of these complimentary approaches.

SUMMARY

Because of the growing number of patients with symptomatic heart failure and the economic impact heart failure has on society, we have witnessed an expansion of programs aimed at attenuating their disease. One of the outgrowths of this effort has been the development of the heart failure clinic. These variably structured and focused clinic usually employ a multidisciplinary approach including patient and family education, drug titration and initiation, telemangement, data collection and research. There is evidence that a variety of these approaches are successful in attenuating disease severity and utilization of expensive in-patient resources. Growth and refinement of the heart failure clinic will continue for years to come.

An Algorithm for effective heart failure management: A continuum of care

Regardless where along the heart failure continuum the patient is encountered, several key elements (a-f) are critical to patient care, improved outcomes and effective resource utilization. This approach, at either end of the disease spectrum is shown below and discussed in the text.

Key Features:
- Must be able to incorporate the patient at any point along the continuum
- Flow should be seamless

Advanced, Symptomatic (Admission)

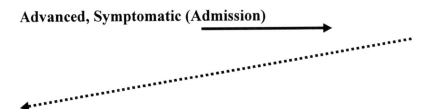

Objectify LV function and prognostic profile:
  a) Use symptom relieving / survival promoting medications
  b) Begin chronic disease management with emphasis on recurring and consistent education
  c) Target outcome measures
  d) Employ a focused variety of techniques for disease management
  e) Reevaluate progress / review options
  f) Consider investigational approaches

Consider complimentary / alternative approaches

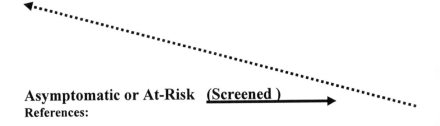

Asymptomatic or At-Risk (Screened)
References:

References:

1. O'Connell JB, Bristow MR. The economic impact of heart failure in the United States; time for a different approach. Journal of Heart Lung Transplant, 1994; 13: S107-S112.

2. Silver MA. Patient knowledge of fundamentals in chronic heart failure. Congestive Heart Failure. 1996;2(2):11-13.

3. Stevenson WG, Stevenson LW, Middlekauff HR, et al. Improving survival for patients with advanced heart failure: study of 737 consecutive patients. J Am Coll Cardiol 1995;26:1417-1423.

4. Konstam M, Dracup K, Baker D, et al. Heart Failure: Evaluation and Care of Patients with Left Ventricular Systolic Dysfunction. Clinical Practice Guideline No. 11. AHCPR Publication No. 94-0612. Rockville, MD: Agency for Health Care Policy and Research, Public Health Service, U.S. Department of Health and Human Services. June 1994.

5. Silver MA. Success with Heart Failure. Help and hope for the millions with congestive heart failure. Second Edition. New York: Plenum Press, 1998

6. Rich MW, Beckham V, Wittenberg C, Leven CI, Freedland KE, Carney RM. A multidisciplinary intervention to prevent the readmission of elderly patients with congestive heart failure. N Engl J Med 1995;333:1190-1195.

7. McDermott, MM, Lee P, Mehta S, Gheorghiade M. Patterns of angiotensin-converting enzyme inhibitor prescriptions, educational interventions, and outcomes among hospitalized patients with heart failure. Clin Cardiol 1998;21:261-268.

8. Smith LE, Fabbri SA, Pai R, Ferry D, Heywood JT. Symptomatic improvement and reduced hospitalization for patents attending a cardiomyopathy clinic. Clin Cardiol 1997;20:949-954.

9. Hanumanthu S, Butler J, Chomsky D, Davis S, Wilson JR. Effect of a heart failure program on hospitalization frequency and exercise tolerance. Circulation 1997;96:2842-2848.

10. Chapman DB, Torpy J. Development of a heart failure center: a medical center and cardiology practice join forces to improve care and reduce costs. Am J Man Care 1997;3:431-437.

11. Fonarow GC, Stevenson LW, Walden JA, et al. Impact of a comprehensive heart failure management program on hospital readmission and functional status of patients with advanced heart failure. J Am Coll Cardiol 1997;30:725-732.

12.   West JA, Miller NH, Parker KM, et al.   A comprehensive
       management system for heart failure improves clinical outcomes
       and reduces medical resource utilization.   Am J Cardiol
       1997;79:58-63.

13.   DeBusk RF, Miller NH, Superko R, et al. A case management system
       coronary risk factor modification following acute myocardial infarction.
       Ann Intern Med 1994;120:721-729.

10

Resource Utilization in Atrial Fibrillation

Sudhir Wahi MD, FCCP
Allan L Klein MD, FRCP(C), FACC
Department of Cardiology, Cleveland Clinic Foundation, Cleveland, OH

INTRODUCTION

Atrial fibrillation is a commonly encountered rhythm disturbance characterized by an irregular and often rapid pulse rate. Mechanically, the rapid and irregular depolarization of the atria causes an alteration in the length of individual cardiac cycles resulting in irregular filling of the left ventricle during diastole and a varying pulse volume. The characteristic findings of atrial fibrillation on a surface electrocardiogram include an irregularly irregular ventricular response associated with a loss of discrete individual P-waves and/or the presence of irregular fibrillatory waves. Atrial fibrillation is usually well tolerated by most patients, but can occasionally cause hemodynamic instability particularly at rapid ventricular response rates.

Prevalence and Incidence of Atrial Fibrillation

Atrial fibrillation is the most common sustained arrhythmia seen in clinical practice, with an estimated incidence of over 2 million cases in the United States [1]. The prevalence of atrial fibrillation in the general population is approximately 0.4% [1, 2]. It is primarily a disease of the elderly population, with more than 50% of patients being ≥ 75 years of age [1]. The prevalence and incidence of atrial fibrillation increases with advancing age (Figure 1), affecting 0.2% of the population 25-34 years old, 2-5% older than 60 years old, and 10% older than 80 years old [1-5]. Atrial fibrillation though rarely life threatening itself, is responsible for far greater hospitalization days than any other arrhythmia [6] (Figure 2). This essentially includes admission for the investigation and management of the rhythm disturbance, hemodynamic instability or worsening congestive cardiac failure. Additional hospital admission days for complications of atrial fibrillation such as strokes and heart failure and are more difficult to account for accurately. The association with thromboembolic disease and stroke is one of the most important sequelae of atrial fibrillation. A 4-to-6-fold increase (15-fold with a history of rheumatic heart disease) makes atrial fibrillation one of the most potent risk factors for stroke in the elderly and the most common cause of embolic stroke. [2, 7-10].

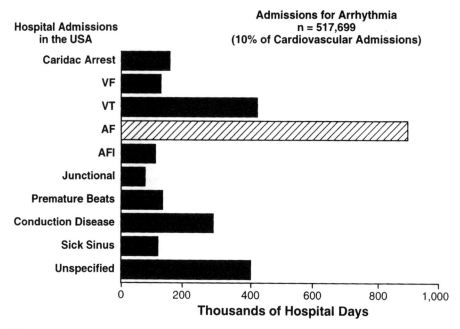

Fig 1:   Estimated Atrial Fibrillation Prevalence in the United States Population. (With permission from *Scientific American Medicine* [147]).

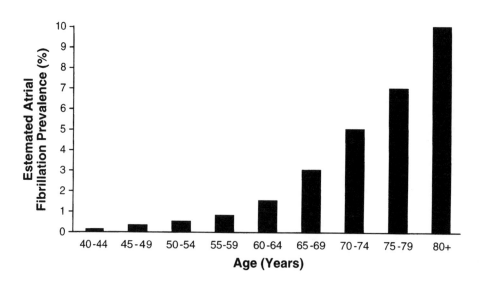

Fig 2:   Number of hospital admission days in the United States for arrhythmias. (With permission from *Am J Cardiol* [148]).

Hypertension and coronary artery disease are the commonest cardio-vascular conditions associated with atrial fibrillation [11]. Besides these conditions, rheumatic mitral valve disease, mitral annular calcification and mitral valve prolapse and numerous medical conditions including pericarditis, pulmonary embolism, chronic lung disease, thyrotoxicosis and metabolic abnormalities predispose to the development of atrial fibrillation. Data from the Framingham study shows that age, valvular heart disease, congestive heart failure, diabetes mellitus and hypertension are independent risk factors for the development of atrial fibrillation [3].

Development of atrial fibrillation is an important public health problem, with a significant bearing on the health care resources in the managed care era. Atrial fibrillation is associated with a two-fold increase in total and cardiovascular mortality [2], and a 5 fold increase in the risk of embolic stroke in the absence of adequate anti-coagulation [9]. With the rather high prevalence rate in the ≥ 75 years age group, atrial fibrillation is easily the most potent risk factors for cardiogenic stroke in the elderly. In the 50 to 59 year age group, the estimated risk of stroke from atrial fibrillation is 1.5%, but rises disproportionately to almost 30% in the 80 to 89 age population [9, 10].

Occurrence of atrial fibrillation in the absence of any pre-existing conditions or structural cardio-vascular problems is known as lone or primary atrial fibrillation [5, 12, 13]. The reported frequency of lone atrial fibrillation is approximately 10%, and mostly these patients are less than 65 years of age. [5, 12, 13]. Lone atrial fibrillation is not associated with an increased risk of stroke in the under 60 years age group [12], but the risk increases in those older than 60 years [13].

Besides the risk of embolic stroke, atrial fibrillation may have other hemodynamic consequences. Atrial fibrillation is characterized by the rapid electrical activation, with multiple waves of depolarization [14-16]. This is associated with an inappropriately rapid heart rate, loss of effective atrial mechanical function and results in a decrease in cardiac output. There is a loss of normal atrio-ventricular synchrony and an irregular ventricular response. Varying R-R interval on the electrocardiogram and varying effective diastolic filling periods lead to widely varying stroke volumes and a reduction in the cardiac output, [17]. Prolonged uncontrolled atrial fibrillation with irregular and rapid ventricular response can lead to a deterioration of left ventricular function and a tachycardia induced cardiomyopathy [18].[19].

Pathophysiology and Electrophysiology:

The commonly accepted hypothesis regarding the electrophysiologic mechanisms for the development of atrial fibrillation was first described by Moe and co-workers [14-16]. According to their multiple wavelet hypothesis, atrial fibrillation develops due to multiple intra-atrial reentrant circuits that are continuously wandering and changing. These have been documented in animal models and humans [20-22]. The perpetuation or termination of atrial fibrillation depends upon the average number of wavelets present. [20, 23-25]. An average of 3-6 intra-atrial reentrant circuits are required for perpetuation of atrial fibrillation [20, 23]. It has been demonstrated in an animal model that persistent atrial fibrillation may develop after repeated induction of atrial fibrillation [26]. Duration of the atrial fibrillation is an important criteria in determining the initial success to cardiovert and thereafter maintain the patient in normal sinus rhythm [27]. Chronic atrial fibrillation also results in histological changes in the atria including atrophy, fibrosis and enlargement [28, 29] and the restoration of effective mechanical function of the atrial after cardioversion is delayed dependent on the duration of atrial fibrillation [30].

In atrial fibrillation, there is a loss of normal atrio-ventricular synchrony and an irregular ventricular response. Changing R-R interval on the electrocardiogram and varying effective diastolic filling periods lead to widely varying stroke volumes and a reduction in the cardiac output [17]. Prolonged uncontrolled atrial fibrillation with irregular and rapid ventricular response can lead to a dilatation of the left ventricle with global deterioration of left ventricular function and a tachycardia induced cardiomyopathy [18],[19]. This may be partially or completely reversible following adequate rate control [19, 31]. Electrical remodeling of the atrium has also been shown to be significantly attenuated by reducing the influx of the intracellular calcium accumulation using calcium channel antagonists [32].

Clinical Manifestations:
Occasionally patients with atrial fibrillation may be asymptomatic. Most patients complain of various symptoms, which are largely related to the loss of atrio-ventricular synchrony, uncontrolled ventricular rate, underlying cardiac condition and associated medical problems.

Symptoms may range from palpitations due to the irregular rapid heart rate to angina due to ischemia precipitated by the decreased diastolic ventricular and coronary filling. Decrease in cardiac output from the loss of atrial contractility can lead to or worsen congestive heart failure and even cause pulmonary edema. Fatigue and dyspnea on exertion are the other frequently reported symptoms, which may again be related to the reduction in cardiac output or rapid ventricular rate (Figure-3). Thrombo-embolism and stroke may be the first clinical presentation of the patient in atrial fibrillation.

Management strategies and Resource Utilization:

The goals of therapy in patients with atrial fibrillation include maintaining hemodynamic stability, reducing the risk of thromboembolism and to prevent or reverse the tachycardia induced cardiomyopathy and an overall effort to reduce the morbidity and mortality. (Table I).

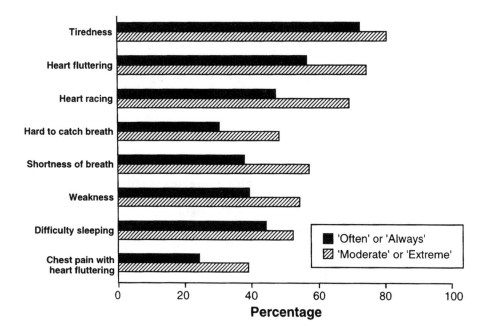

Fig 3:   Symptoms of atrial fibrillation among a population of patients about to undergo radiofrequency ablation of the atrioventricular (AV) node and pacemaker implantation. (Modified with permission from *Am J Cardiol* [148]).

Table 1.   TARGETS OF THERAPY FOR ATRIAL FIBRILLATION

TARGETS OF THERAPY	GOALS OF THERAPY

Symptoms from palpitations
   Irregular heart beats
   Rapid ventricular rates
	Maintenance of sinus rhythm
	Control of AV nodal conduction

Impaired hemodynamics
   Loss of AV synchrony
   Rapid ventricular rates
	Maintenance of sinus rhythm
	Control of AV nodal conduction

Risk of thromboembolism	Reduction in risk of systemic embolism/stroke

Tachycardia-induced cardiomyopathy
   Ventricular cardiomyopathy
   Atrial cardiomyopathy
	Control of ventricular rate, AV nodal conduction
	Maintenance of sinus rhythm

Increase in mortality	Improvement in survival

Obtained with permission from Mina Chung, M.D.

Management:

A careful history and physical examination, followed by an E.C.G and laboratory studies to investigate thyroid dysfunction or electrolyte imbalance are important to tailor therapy for any individual patient. A transthoracic echocardiogram for the assessment of left atrial size, ventricular function and valvular function is indicated for all patients. A functional stress test and / or cardiac catheterization may be required for an individual patient and can be planned after the non-invasive assessment of patients with atrial fibrillation.

The medical management of atrial fibrillation has been discussed extensively in some recently published reviews [33-35]. A detailed discussion of the individual therapeutic options available is beyond the scope of this text. As eluded to earlier, the main efforts in these patients is the control of the ventricular rate, as well as achievement and maintenance of sinus rhythm. Along with these measures adequate anticoagulation is very important to reduce the risks of thromboembolism and stroke.

Control of ventricular rate

This can be achieved by use of pharmacological agents that slow the atrio-ventricular nodal conduction, namely, digoxin, beta-blockers and calcium channel blockers. All these agents have been well examined clinically [36-46]. Non-pharmacological measures for ventricular rate control include complete atrio-ventricular nodal (or His bundle) ablation with implantation of a permanent rate-responsive [47-50]. The procedure is mostly limited to patients whose symptoms are difficult to control and are due to rapid ventricular rates. The disadvantages of the procedure include the dependence on a permanent pacemaker, a possible small risk of late sudden death [51, 52].

Restoration of Sinus Rhythm

Electrical cardioversion is the most effective method of conversion to sinus rhythm especially in the hemodynamically unstable patient [53]. The need and duration of anticoagulation before cardioversion is discussed in the next section (see below). High-energy *internal cardioversion* (200-360 J) has also been used successfully for refractory cases [54, 55]. The pharmacological agent, procainamide, can also be used for cardioversion in an elective patient [56, 57]. Ibutilide is another intravenous agent that has been approved as a drug for the conversion of atrial flutter and fibrillation [58].

Maintenance of sinus rhythm

This requires use of an antiarrhythmic agent, particularly in patients with frequent or resistant atrial fibrillation, underlying cardiovascular disease, or enlarged atria. Class IA (quinidine, procainamide, disopyramide), IC (flecainide, propafenone), IA/B/C (moricizine), III (sotalol, amiodarone) are the pharmacological antiarrhythmic agents available [59-71]. Class IA / IC agents can cause QT interval prolongation and are associated with a high incidence of proarrhythmia, including torsade de pointes. These agents should be used cautiously in patients with underlying coronary heart disease [72, 73].

Resource Utilization:

In the era of cost containment and managed care, allocation of resources has to be optimized carefully to keep the health care management costs in check without compromising patient safety. In spite of being the most frequently encountered rhythm disorder and being responsible for greater hospitalization than all forms of ventricular arrhythmias together, no uniformly accepted approach for management is available. Guidelines are available for various therapeutic measures like anti-coagulation, rate control and cardioversion but therapy needs to be customized to an individual patient.

At the heart of the management debate for atrial fibrillation patients the main issues are the risks and benefits of achieving and maintaining normal sinus rhythm versus adequate ventricular rate control in majority of atrial fibrillation patients [74]

Rate vs. Rhythm control

In recent years the approach to the management of atrial fibrillation is changing significantly. In the era of managed care, risks and benefits of any management strategy need to be well supported clinically. With the newer treatment options and better understanding of the mechanisms and consequences of the arrhythmia, a more aggressive approach to try and convert to normal sinus rhythm is being advocated by most groups. The earlier this is done, better are the chances of success in being able to convert and maintain sinus rhythm [27]. Simultaneously, decreasing the adverse effects on the myocardial function due to the AV dyssynchrony and rapid ventricular rate.

Atrial fibrillation usually does not cause an acute hemodynamic compromise, but similar to other chronic diseases like hypertension, hypercholesterolemia and diabetes mellitus produces a more insidious but significant structural and functional detriment. There are numerous reasons to attempt to cardiovert atrial fibrillation to sinus rhythm (Table II). Atrial fibrillation accounts for more days of hospitalization than all ventricular arrhythmias combined (Figure-2) In a study by Baily et al. atrial fibrillation alone accounted for nearly 900 thousand hospital admission days [6]. Patients with atrial fibrillation spend an estimated average of 5 days in hospital at a cost of $4800, which represents a total cost of $1 billion dollars annually [35]. The admissions may be necessary due to exacerbation of congestive heart failure, stroke or investigation and treatment of the rhythm disturbance. All of these significantly increase the health care costs involved in the management of these patients.

Table II: Reasons for restoring Sinus Rhythm in Patients with Atrial Fibrillation.

* Appropriate / physiological rate control
* Regularization of heart rhythm
* Restoration of atrial contribution to cardiac output
* Improvement in hemodynamics
* Maintenance of normal electrophysiology
* Prevention of left atrial dilation
* Prevention of left ventricular dysfunction
* Relief of symptoms (dyspnea, fatigue, chest pain, palpitations, etc.); improved quality of life
* Reduce thrombo-embolic complications

In the presence of pre-existing diastolic dysfunction or restrictive filling of the left ventricle, loss of the atrial contribution to the left ventricular filling due to atrial fibrillation coupled with an abbreviated diastolic filling time due to a rapid ventricular rate leads to a reduced stroke volume and can precipitate congestive cardiac failure. This situation automatically translates into higher health care expenses acutely and on a long term. This provides another reason favoring rhythm rather than rate control in these patients.

Converting back to sinus rhythm has adequately been shown to improve the exercise capacity and maximal oxygen consumption. [75-80]. This has been observed regardless of the underlying cardiac disease [78]. In some patients this may not be demonstrable immediately and can parallel the improvement in atrial mechanical function. This increase in exercise capacity has a significant impact on the "quality of life". As discussed earlier, maintaining sinus rhythm has a beneficial effect on the left ventricular function and avoids the development and progression of a ventricular cardiomyopathy due to a rapid ventricular rate and varying cardiac cycle length.

Having elaborated on the advantages of restoring sinus rhythm, the fact is that in nearly 75% patients without maintenance antiarrhythmic therapy, atrial fibrillation will recur. Duration of atrial fibrillation preceding the cardioversion [81, 82], left atrial diameter [83], left ventricular function [84] functional class and underlying etiology [82] have a bearing on the likelihood of recurrence of atrial fibrillation. These factors may help to identify patients with atrial fibrillation to gain the maximum benefit from adopting a more energetic approach to restore sinus rhythm.

Ventricular proarrhythmias, including torsade de pointes, are recognized complications of antiarrhythmic therapy, and were reviewed recently in patients with atrial fibrillation [85]. Data from the Stroke Prevention in Afib.(SPAF-1) trial [86] concluded that antiarrhythmic therapy significantly increases the risk of cardiac mortality in patients with a history of congestive cardiac failure. In the light of this finding, it is imperative to initiate therapy with one of the anti-arrhythmic agents after admission in-hospital for all patients with underlying heart disease and congestive cardiac failure. With nearly 86% patients with persistent and more than half of those paroxysmal atrial fibrillation having structural heart disease, it will certainly increase the cost of management of these patients at the initiation of therapy and then needing regular surveillance and monitoring to adjust drug dosage.

Management decisions in patients who develop recurrent sustained atrial fibrillation are unresolved at present, more so for patients who are able to tolerate the arrhythmia with minimal or no symptoms. Should these patients be subjected to a repeat cardioversion, electrical or pharmacological, or is it acceptable to let them maintain atrial fibrillation. The Atrial Fibrillation Follow-up Investigation of Rhythm Management (AFFIRM) [87] (Figure-4) - a large randomized multi-center clinical trial sponsored by the National Institute of Health is currently underway. It has been designed to address this concern and test the hypothesis that in patients with atrial fibrillation, total mortality with primary therapy intended to maintain sinus rhythm is equal to that with primary therapy intended to control heart rate. The study is intended to recruit over 5000 patients at completion. It will also address the issues whether bleeding, secondary to anti-coagulation, is commoner in the patients maintained on rate control. It will also examine whether arrhythmia related mortality is higher in the group in sinus rhythm, and that stroke and thrombo-embolism occur more often in the heart rate control patients.

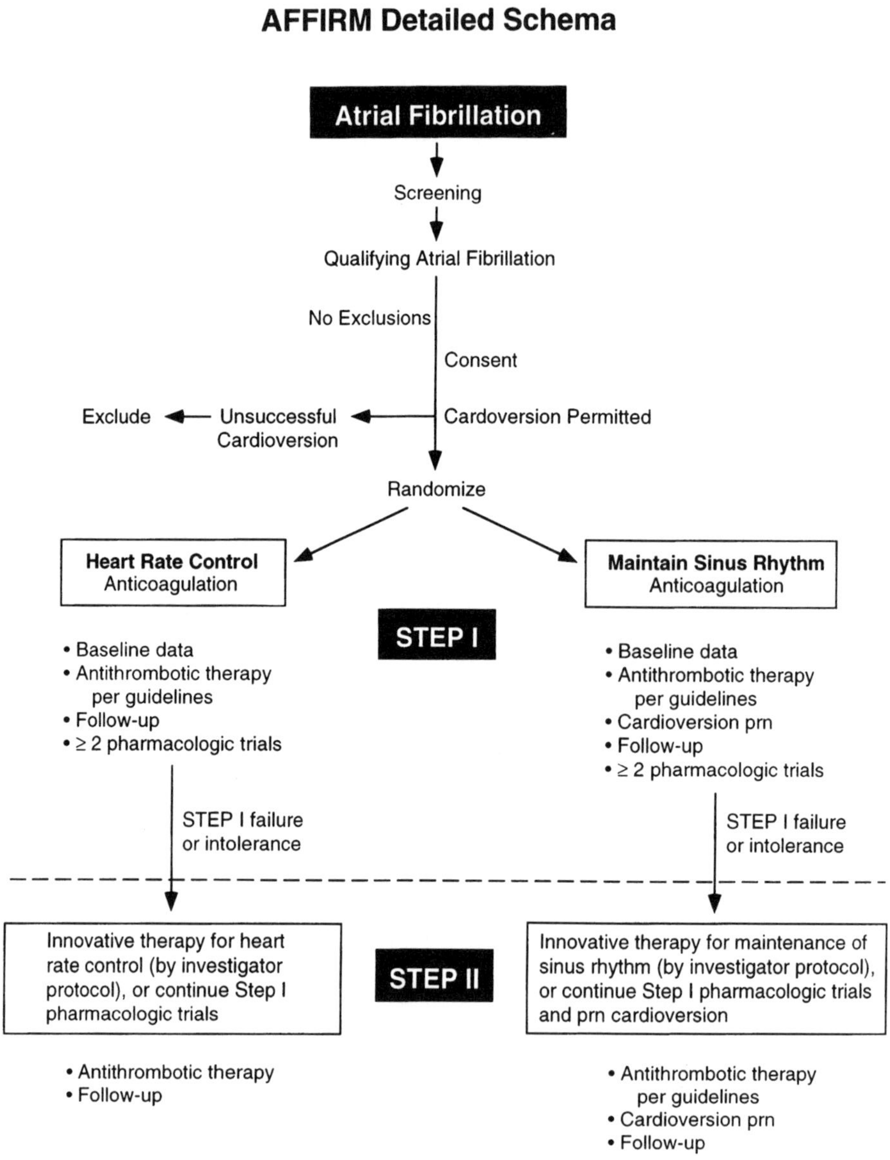

AFFIRM Detailed Schema

Fig 4: An outline of the AFFIRM Study. Anticoagulation in the group randomized to attempted maintenance of sinus rhythm is at the discretion of the investigators. "Innovative therapy" for heart rate control includes atrioventricular nodal ablation or modification. Innovative therapy for maintenance of sinus rhythm includes the maze operation or atrial pacing. (From The AFFIRM investigators, with permission[87]).

Stroke and Atrial Fibrillation

Impaired atrial mechanical function in patients with atrial fibrillation leads to stasis of blood in the left atrium and left atrial appendage. This is often recognized as spontaneous echo contrast [88] on transthoracic or transesophageal echocardiography, and is regarded as a precursor for the development of a thrombus in the left atrium or atrial appendage [88, 89]. Nearly 45% of all embolic strokes in are due to atrial fibrillation [90].

Rationale and Approach to Anti-coagulation

Atrial fibrillation is an important risk factor for ischemic stroke, especially in the older population.[9] In persons with normal sinus rhythm, the risk of stroke increases from 4.5/1000 person years in their 60s, to 9/1000 person years in their 70s and 14.3/1000 person years in their 80s. Development of atrial fibrillation increases this risk 5 fold across these age groups. In practice, atrial fibrillation accounts for nearly 14% of all strokes above the age of 60 years or 75,000 strokes per year in the United States [9, 91].

In the 1980s, the five randomized trials were done to assess the benefit of anticoagulation in reducing the risk of strokes in patients with atrial fibrillation. They showed a relative reduction of risk ranging from 52% to 86%. All trials were stopped prematurely due to the marked benefit from warfarin (Table III). More importantly more than 25% of the strokes in the warfarin treated group occurred in patients not taking their prescribed medications. Another interesting observation from these trials was that the lowest anticoagulation target was as effective as the higher intensities. Pooled data from these 5 trials revealed a 68% relative risk reduction [92].

Aspirin was thought to be an alternate agent for patients unable to take warfarin. However data from several studies [93-95] comparing varying doses of aspirin to warfarin and placebo, failed to show any significant reduction in the rate of strokes. Pooled data from the 5 primary prevention trials (Table IV) shows warfarin therapy has clear benefit and significant reduction in the risk of strokes in all age groups except patients under 65 years of age. In these relatively younger patients, with no other risk factors the risk for stroke was 1% in the control group and did not change with anticoagulation.

The concerns about bleeding complications, as an argument for not initiating anticoagulation in patients with atrial fibrillation is not substantiated. The increase of major intracranial hemorrhage in the 5 randomized trials was 0.2% per year. Rate of a bleeding complication requiring transfusion or hospitalization was 1.8% per year. New results from clinical practice [96-98] confirm these findings and the intensity of anticoagulation is mainly responsible for the bleeding risk. The risk of intracranial hemorrhage increases sharply if the prothrombin time ratio (PTR) is > 2 (INR>4) (Figure-5). [98] Likewise the lowest effective INR for the benefit of reducing the stroke risk is 2.0, below which the risk escalated sharply [99] (Figure-6).

Table III: Randomized Trials of Anticoagulation for Atrial Fibrillation

	AFASAK	BAATAF	SPAF	CAFA	SPINAF	EAFT
Anticoagulation target	INR 2.8-4.2	PTR 1.2-1 5	PTR 1.3-1.8	INR 2-3	PTR 1.2-1.5	INR 2.5-4
Subjects, n	335	212	210	187	260	225
Emboli, n	4	2	6	5	4	20
Annual rate	1.6%	0.41%	2.3%	2.5%	0.88%	3.9%
Control subjects, n	336	208	211	191	265	214
Emboli, n	21	13	18	11	19	50
Annual rate	5.5%	3.0%	7.4%	5.2%	4.3%	12.3%
Preventive efficacy	71%	86%	69%	52%	79%	66%
95% CI	3-90%	51-96%	27-85%	(-36)-87%	52-90%	43-80%

Abbreviated titles of trials: AFASAK = Atrial Fibrillation, Aspirin, Anticoagulation Study; BAATAF = Boston Area Anticoagulation Trial for Atrial Fibrillation; CAFA = Canadian Atrial Fibrillation Anticoagulation Study; EAFT = the secondary prevention European AF Trial; SPAF = Stroke Prevention in Atrial Fibrillation; SPINAF = Veterans Affairs Stroke Prevention in Nonrheumatic Atrial Fibrillation Study.

INR = international normalized ratio; PTR = prothrombin time ratio; CI = confidence interval Preventive efficacy is the relative risk reduction calculated as (1-RR) x 100, where RR is the annual rate in the anticoagulation group divided by the annual rate in the control group.
Adapted with permission from Ann Epidemiol.[146]

Table IV: Pooled Analysis of First Five Afib Trial: Efficacy of Warfarin by Risk Category [&]

Risk Category	Control		Warfarin	
	# Strokes	Rate (95%CI)	# Strokes	Rate (95% CI)
Age< 65 years:				
No Risk factor	3	1.0% (0.3-3.1)	3	1.0% (0.3-3.0)
f 1 risk factor	16	4.9% (0.3-8.1)	6	1.7% (0.8-3.9)
Age 65-75 years:				
No Risk factor	16	4.3% (2.7-7.1)	4	1.1% (0.4-2.8)
f 1 risk factor	27	5.7% (3.9-8.3)	7	1.7% (0.9-3.4)
Age > 75 years:				
No Risk factor	6	3.5% (1.6-7.7)	3	1.7% (0.5-5.2)
f 1 risk factor	13	8.1% (4.7-13.9)	2	1.2% (0.3-5.0)

[&] The first 5 trials are AFASAK, BAATAF,CAFA, SPAF, and SPINAF (listed in footnote to TableIII). Risk factors are history of hypertension, diabetes, or prior stroke or transient ischemic attack. Rate is annual rate; CI is confidence interval.

Adapted with permission from Arch Intern Med.[92]

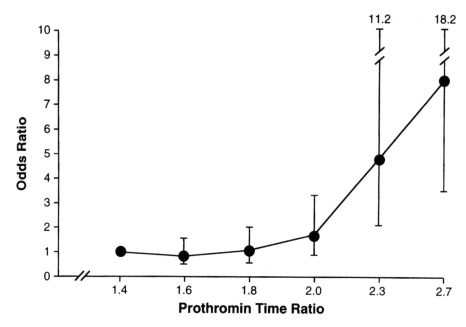

Fig 5:   The odds ratio of intracranial hemorrhage among patients receiving warfarin as a function of
the prothrombin time ratio of 1.0 –1.5. 95% confidence limits are indicated. (Reprinted with
permission from *Ann Intern Med.* [98]).

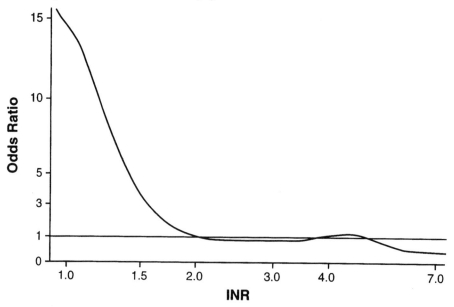

Fig 6:   The odds ratio for ischemic stroke among patients with atrial fibrillation receiving warfarin as
a function of the international normalized ratio (INR). (The reference category is INR of 2.0.
Reprinted with permission from *N Engl J Med*[145]).

Risk modification with anticoagulation therapy is the most efficient example of cost to benefit ratio seen with any medical intervention. [100, 101] The benefit achieved is immediate, with a significant reduction in the risk of stroke in all age groups tested. The prescriptions for anticoagulation have increased dramatically since the results of the primary prevention trials appeared. However only a third of all atrial fibrillation patients are receiving anticoagulation treatment.

The recommendation should be that all patients with atrial fibrillation especially over the age of 65 years to receive warfarin unless contraindicated. Good monitoring and data management to keep the INR between 2 – 3. Surveillance and care of these patients to be undertaken by personal specifically dedicated for the anticoagulation clinics in all health maintenance organizations (HMOs).

Role of Echocardiography

Transthoracic Echocardiography

Enhanced resolution of the two dimensional echocardiographic images due to the technical improvements in the ultrasound equipment make the transthoracic echocardiogram an attractive and versatile tool for the initial screening of patients with atrial fibrillation.
Transthoracic echocardiography allows a non-invasive and accurate measurement of left atrial size and function [102, 103]. Left atrial enlargement is seen in nearly 77% patients with atrial fibrillation compared to only 27% in patients with normal sinus rhythm [104]. The presence of left atrial enlargement decreases the likelihood of maintaining sinus rhythm long-term [105, 106]. Doppler echocardiography is useful in the assessment left atrial function.

Left atrial appendage is a small pouch present anterior to the left atrium and is a common site for the development of the left atrial thrombus in these patients with atrial fibrillation. Left atrial appendage can be screened in less than 20% patients when using transthoracic imaging alone [107, 108]. Visualization of the left atrial appendage is significantly better with the transesophageal approach.

Transthoracic echocardiography has the convenience of easy accessibility and performance, however has a comparatively lower sensitivity estimated at only 39% to 63% [107-110] but a high specificity [111-113] for the detection of thrombi in the left atrial appendage and left atrium.

Transesophageal Echocardiography

Development of the flexible transesophageal echocardiography (TEE) probe has improved the capability to visualize the more posterior structures of the heart, which are poorly visualized by transthoracic echocardiography. Higher frequency transducers (5MHz – 7MHz) with TEE compared to lower frequency transducers (2 MHz – 2.5MHz) used in transthoracic echocardiography significantly improves the structural resolution. The exclusion of a pre-existing thrombus in the left atrium or appendage, precludes the need for prolonged anticoagulation prior to cardioversion. The feasibility of the TEE guided cardioversion has been assessed by different groups [114-118]. There has been sufficient experience gained with this procedure clinically, and it can be performed safely with minimal complication [119]. The issue of safety in the performance of TEE has been well established even in hospitalized and critically ill patients [120]. The improved image resolution with TEE has the advantage of a significantly higher sensitivity and specificity of 95% – 99% for the detection of thrombi [113, 118, 121, 122] (Figure – 7).

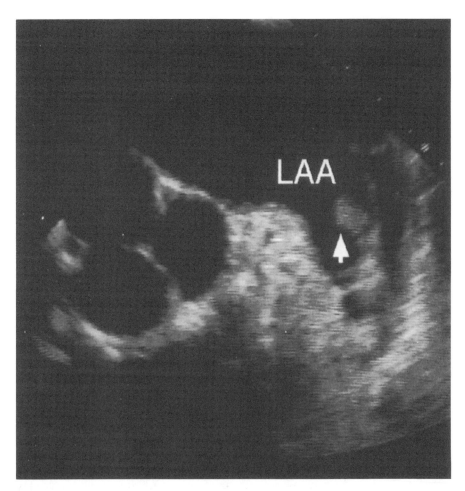

Fig 7:   Left atrial appendage visualized on TEE demonstrating a large clot in the appendage. (With permission from *Ann Intern Med* [137].

In a recent report the Stroke Prevention in Atrial Fibrillation III (SPAF III) investigators examined the association between the previously identified independent clinical risk factors for stroke in patients with atrial fibrillation with the transesophageal echocardiographic features correlating with the risk.[123]. Presence of left atrial appendage thrombi, dense spontaneous echo contrast, impaired mechanical function of the left atrial appendage and complex aortic plaque are related to the risk stratification for stroke in these patients. The left atrial and appendage mechanical function rather than size were more reliable markers of risk, and these can be better assessed by TEE.

Transesophageal echocardiography guided cardioversion

Electrical cardioversion is a standard procedure to convert atrial fibrillation to normal sinus rhythm. This is associated with a 0.6% – 5.6% risk of thrombo-embolism [124]. The risk is significantly greater for patients not on anticoagulation therapy [125]. In some studies [126-128] the risk of thromboembolism was not correlated with the presence or absence of anticoagulation. It is traditionally believed that thromboembolism is related to the dislodgment of an existing thrombus in the left atrium and left atrial appendage [128]. The temporal relationship of successful cardioversion shows that most events occur few hours to few weeks after cardioversion. This may be related to the lag between the return of the electrical and mechanical activity of the atria. Grimm et al. [129, 130] recently reported that there might be stunning of the left atrial appendage post cardioversion. This highlights the need for adequate anticoagulation at the time of the cardioversion and up to 4 weeks later. [131] Long term anticoagulation will be needed for patients with an underlying structural cardiac disorder, cardiomyopathy, mitral valve disease or a previous history of embolism.

Manning et al. performed TEE in 94 patients with atrial fibrillation hospitalized for cardioversion. They reported atrial thrombi in 12 (13%) patients, in whom cardioversion was deferred and were given long term anticoagulation therapy. They had a 95% success rate in cardioversion, with no embolic complications in patients undergoing TEE guided early cardioversion if atrial thrombi could be excluded [115].

In a follow-up larger series with a similar patient population, Manning et.al. [118] found atrial thrombi in 34 (15%) of 230 atrial fibrillation patients hospitalized for cardioversion. Once again they reported no embolic events in their patients in whom the TEE was negative for a thrombus. Three patients with atrial thrombi in whom the cardioversion was deferred died suddenly, which according to them was most likely secondary to a systemic embolism.

In another study using TEE, Black et.al. [116] identified atrial thrombi in 5 (12%) of the 40 patients screened. In their series patients without thrombi underwent cardioversion without short-term anticoagulation. They reported cerebral embolism in one patient 24 hours following a successful cardioversion. A repeat transesophageal echocardiogram done 4 day later revealed a new left atrial thrombus not seen on the precardioversion study In a series of 66 patients with non-valvular atrial fibrillation, Fatkin reported embolic events in 4 patients shortly after restoration of normal sinus rhythm following cardioversion. None of these patients were therapeutically anticoagulated. The findings from these non-randomized studies suggest, there is an approximately 10 –15% prevalence of atrial thrombi in atrial fibrillation. Although TEE identifies the left atrial thrombi accurately, anticoagulation is still necessary post–cardioversion to prevent thrombus formation and embolization during the period of atrial stunning [130-134].

Presently, patients undergoing electrical cardioversion are conventionally treated with anti-coagulation for three weeks before and four weeks after cardioversion to decrease the risk of thrombo-embolism. TEE with short term anticoagulation is being proposed as a novel strategy to guide anticoagulation management in patients undergoing electrical cardioversion. This approach has several advantages over the conventional approach of 7 weeks of anticoagulation. First, TEE would be able to detect left atrial appendage thrombi that increase the risk of embolic stroke after cardioversion. Thus screening the patients for thrombi with TEE before cardioversion may reduce the incidence of embolic events resulting from cardioversion by deferring cardioversion. Second, in the majority of patients without left atrial appendage thrombi, earlier cardioversion will shorten the period of anticoagulation and lower the risk of bleeding complications. The cost savings of preventing an embolic stroke and of decreasing bleeding complications and allowing earlier cardioversion in patients without thrombi may more than offset the cost of the TEE guided strategy. Finally, earlier cardioversion is believed to increase the likelihood of successful return to and maintenance of sinus rhythm.

To assess the proposed advantages of the TEE guided cardioversion, the ACUTE (Assessment of Cardioversion Using Transesophageal Echocardiography) pilot study, a randomized multicenter clinical trial was performed [135]. The study involved 126 atrial fibrillation patients scheduled for cardioversion, who were randomized to either TEE guided cardioversion or conventional therapy. The patients in the TEE guided group were therapeutically anti-coagulated during and for 4 weeks post-cardioversion according to the study protocol [7]. Atrial thrombi were reported in 13% of patients randomized to the TEE guided group, in whom the cardioversion was then deferred and full anticoagulation administered. No embolism was reported in the 38 patients with a negative TEE, who had early cardioversion. One patient in the conventional therapy group had peripheral embolism. The authors reported a considerably shorter time to cardioversion in the TEE group, 0.6 weeks compared to 4.8 weeks in the conventional therapy group (p<0.01). The bleeding complications were documented to be higher in the conventional therapy group. This randomized pilot trial supports the previous studies, that TEE guided cardioversion is feasible and safe, however the study was not powered to detect differences in clinical outcomes between the two TEE guided and conventional approach.

Whether this TEE guided strategy with shorter-term anticoagulation is clinically safer, more efficacious and more cost-effective than the conventional anticoagulation approach is being tested in a large international randomized multi-center trial the "Assessment of Cardioversion Using Transesophageal Echocardiography (ACUTE)". The study design of the ACUTE trial expected to enroll nearly 3000 patients, was published recently [136]. Similar to the pilot study, patients will be randomized to the conventional or TEE guided arm for cardioversion. The patients in the conventional arm will be anticoagulated for 3 weeks prior and 4 weeks after the cardioversion. The patients undergoing TEE guided cardioversion will be anticoagulated before the TEE and cardioversion and for 3 weeks following it (Figure 8). The primary endpoints include ischemic stroke, transient ischemic episodes, and systemic embolization for 8 weeks after enrollment, and secondary endpoints including major and minor bleeding, all cause mortality, success of cardioversion and cost effectiveness. The study has randomized 1115 patients in 70 centers worldwide until November 1998.

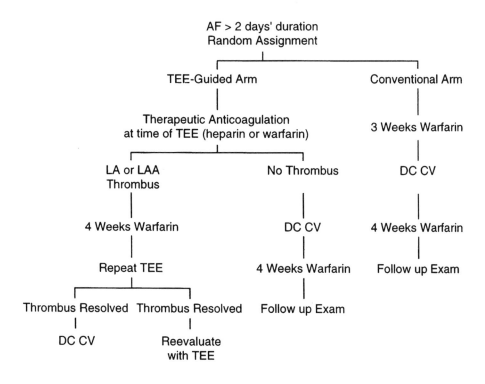

Fig 8:   Diagram of the ACUTE Protocol (With permission from the ACUTE investigators [136]).

Controversy of TEE guided vs. conventional anticoagulation approach :

Currently, both the conventional anticoagulation approach and the TEE are being employed in clinical practice as the standard of care, although neither one has been validated in a comprehensive comparative study with adequate sample size. Since the report by Manning et al [115] , and the ACUTE pilot study [137] describing the safety and feasibility of the TEE guided approach, many cardiologists have begun to employ this approach as their standard of care. The main reasons for the rapid acceptance of the TEE guided approach within the medical community, despite the lack of controlled clinical trials, seems to relate to its perceived safety, the convenience of the procedure for the patient and physician, and the fact that it enables cardioversion earlier without a prolonged waiting period. At our own institution, which is a leader in this field, the TEE guided approach has been increasingly in an average of 14.7% of the 3329 electrical cardioversions since 1991. Within the United States it is estimated that this approach is being used in 20% to 30% of all cardioversions. In the recently published management guidelines for atrial fibrillation by the American Heart Association and the American College of Cardiology [138], endorsed the conventional approach and the TEE guided approach was suggested as an alternative approach. Similarly, guidelines for the clinical application of echocardiography stated that large multicenter trials are needed to address this issue [139]. Prystowsky has highlighted the limitations of the TEE guided approach, including missing thrombi by the TEE, cost of repeated TEE if thrombi are present, and the experience of TEE operators in the community.

The findings from the ACUTE pilot study clearly support the cost effectiveness of the TEE guided the approach to restore normal sinus rhythm early [140]. Using the cost effectiveness model analysis, they found the TEE-guided anticoagulation management strategy to be cost effective primarily due to the lowered risk of embolic stroke. They reported a 27% cost reduction by the TEE guided early cardioversion in comparison to the conventional approach of anticoagulation and delayed cardioversion, and projected cost savings of $51700 for every 100 patients treated. In another model Seto et al. also found the TEE guided approach to be the least costly per quality-adjusted life year amongst the three different management strategies tested [141]. This issue will be convincingly resolved with the completion of the large ongoing randomized prospective multi-center ACUTE trial. The results of this study will have a significant impact on society given the vast numbers of patients with atrial fibrillation undergoing electrical cardioversion (> 100,000) and the costs associated with strokes and stroke aftercare, with more than 2000 strokes and approximately $64000 per stroke, nearly $128 million dollars [100, 135, 142, 143].

Summary:

With some exceptions, at least an attempt should be made to try and restore sinus rhythm in all patients with atrial fibrillation. Especially in patients where the arrhythmia is of a recent onset. Patients with a longstanding history of atrial fibrillation have a low likelihood of maintaining sinus rhythm on the long term. In patients with significant underlying structural heart disease it may be more difficult to restore normal sinus rhythm. Incidentally these patients symptomatically stand to gain most by maintaining sinus rhythm.

The overall success of maintaining normal sinus rhythm offers the real possibility of lowering management costs incurred from frequent hospitalization and complications of anticoagulation or the arrhythmia itself. The ACUTE pilot study demonstrates the clear benefits of lowered costs, complications and possibly improved long term success in maintaining sinus rhythm by accepting the transesophageal guided early cardioversion approach.

The cost benefit analysis of the various approaches to the management of patients with atrial fibrillation is constantly changing as more is understood about the arrhythmia and newer pharmacological and non-drug approaches to the management are evolved. A number of ongoing trials like the large National Heart Lung and Blood Institute in the United States, funded multi-center trial, Atrial Fibrillation Follow-up Investigation of Rhythm Management (AFFIRM), the Rate Control vs. Electrical cardioversion (RACE) trial in the Netherlands, the Prognosis In Atrial Fibrillation (PIAF) study in Germany and the International multi-center study Assessment of Cardioversion Utilizing Transesophageal Echocardiography (ACUTE) would enable us to get a better handle on the most effective strategy in the management of atrial fibrillation.

References:

1. Feinberg, W.M., J.L. Blackshear, A. Laupacis, R. Kronmal, and R.G. Hart, Prevalence, age distribution, and gender of patients with atrial fibrillation. Analysis and implications. Arch Intern Med, 1995. **155**(5): p. 469-73.

2. Kannel, W.B., R.D. Abbott, D.D. Savage, and P.M. McNamara, Coronary heart disease and atrial fibrillation: the Framingham Study. Am Heart J, 1983. **106**(2): p. 389-96.

3. Kannel, W.B., R.D. Abbott, D.D. Savage, and P.M. McNamara, Epidemiologic features of chronic atrial fibrillation: the Framingham study. N Engl J Med, 1982. **306**(17): p. 1018-22.

4. Cairns, J.A. and S.J. Connolly, Nonrheumatic atrial fibrillation. Risk of stroke and role of antithrombotic therapy. Circulation, 1991. **84**(2): p. 469-81.

5. Furberg, C.D., B.M. Psaty, T.A. Manolio, J.M. Gardin, V.E. Smith, and P.M. Rautaharju, Prevalence of atrial fibrillation in elderly subjects (the Cardiovascular Health Study). Am J Cardiol, 1994. **74**(3): p. 236-41.

6. Baily, D., M.H. Lehmann, D.N. Schumacher, R.T. Steinman, and M.D. Meissner, Hospitalization for arrhythmias in the United States: importance of atrial fibrillation.(Abstr.). J Am Coll Cardiol, 1992. **19**: p. 41A.

7. Laupacis, A., G. Albers, J. Dalen, M. Dunn, W. Feinberg, and A. Jacobson, Antithrombotic therapy in atrial fibrillation. Chest, 1995. **108**: p. 352S-359S.

8. Wolf, P.A., T.R. Dawber, H.J. Thomas, and W.B. Kannel, Epidemiologic assessment of chronic atrial fibrillation and risk of stroke: the Framingham study. Neurology, 1978. **28**(10): p. 973-7.

9. Wolf, P.A., R.D. Abbott, and W.B. Kannel, Atrial fibrillation: a major contributor to stroke in the elderly. The Framingham Study. Arch Intern Med, 1987. **147**(9): p. 1561-4.

10. Wolf, P.A., R.D. Abbott, and W.B. Kannel, Atrial fibrillation as an independent risk factor for stroke: the Framingham Study. Stroke, 1991. **22**(8): p. 983-8.

11. Davidson, E., I. Weinberger, Z. Rotenberg, J. Fuchs, and J. Agmon, Atrial fibrillation. Cause and time of onset. Arch Intern Med, 1989. **149**(2): p. 457-9.

12. Kopecky, S.L., B.J. Gersh, M.D. McGoon, J.P. Whisnant, D.R. Holmes, Jr., D.M. Ilstrup, and R.L. Frye, The natural history of lone atrial fibrillation. A population-based study over three decades. N Engl J Med, 1987. **317**(11): p. 669-74.

13. Brand, F.N., R.D. Abbott, W.B. Kannel, and P.A. Wolf, Characteristics and prognosis of lone atrial fibrillation. 30-year follow-up in the Framingham Study. Jama, 1985. **254**(24): p. 3449-53.

14. Moe, G., On the multiple wavelet hypothesis of atrial fibrillation. Arch Int Pharmacodyn Ther., 1962. **140**: p. 83 - 88.

15. Moe, G. and J. Abildskov, Atrial fibrillation as a self sustaining arrhythmia independent of focal discharge. Am Heart J, 1959. **58**: p. 59 - 70.

16. Moe, G., W. Rheinboldt, and J. Abildskov, A computer model of atrial fibrillation. Am Heart J, 1964. **67**: p. 200 - 220.

17. Naito, M., D. David, E.L. Michelson, M. Schaffenburg, and L.S. Dreifus, The hemodynamic consequences of cardiac arrhythmias: evaluation of the relative roles of abnormal atrioventricular sequencing, irregularity of ventricular rhythm and atrial fibrillation in a canine model. Am Heart J, 1983. **106**(2): p. 284-91.

18. Packer, D.L., G.H. Bardy, S.J. Worley, M.S. Smith, F.R. Cobb, R.E. Coleman, J.J. Gallagher, and L.D. German, Tachycardia-induced cardiomyopathy: a reversible form of left ventricular dysfunction. Am J Cardiol, 1986. **57**(8): p. 563-70.

19. Grogan, M., H.C. Smith, B.J. Gersh, and D.L. Wood, Left ventricular dysfunction due to atrial fibrillation in patients initially believed to have idiopathic dilated cardiomyopathy. Am J Cardiol, 1992. **69**(19): p. 1570-3.

20. Allessie, M.A., P. Rensma, J. Brugada, J. Smeets, O. Penn, and C. Kirchhof, Pathophysiology of atrial fibrillation., in In Zipes D, Jalife J, eds. Cardiac Electrophysiology from Cell to Bedside. 1990, Saunders W.B.: Philadelphia. p. 548 - 59.

21. Cox, J.L., T.E. Canavan, R.B. Schuessler, M.E. Cain, B.D. Lindsay, C. Stone, P.K. Smith, P.B. Corr, and J.P. Boineau, The surgical treatment of atrial fibrillation. II. Intraoperative electrophysiologic mapping and description of the electrophysiologic basis of atrial flutter and atrial fibrillation. J Thorac Cardiovasc Surg, 1991. **101**(3): p. 406-26.

22. Konings, K.T., C.J. Kirchhof, J.R. Smeets, H.J. Wellens, O.C. Penn, andM.A. Allessie, High-density mapping of electrically induced atrial fibrillation in humans.Circulation, 1994. **89**(4): p. 1665-80.

23. Allessie, M.A., K. Konings, C.J. Kirchhof, and M. Wijffels, Electrophysiologic mechanisms of perpetuation of atrial fibrillation. Am J Cardiol, 1996. **77**(3): p. 10A-23A.

24. Wang, Z., P. Page, and S. Nattel, Mechanism of flecainide's antiarrhythmic action in experimental atrial fibrillation. Circ Res, 1992. **71**(2): p. 271-87.

25. Wang, J., G.W. Bourne, Z. Wang, C. Villemaire, M. Talajic, and S. Nattel, Comparative mechanisms of antiarrhythmic drug action in experimental atrial fibrillation. Importance of use-dependent effects on refractoriness. Circulation, 1993. **88**(3): p. 1030-44.

26. Wijffels, M.C., C.J. Kirchhof, R. Dorland, and M.A. Allessie, Atrial fibrillation begets atrial fibrillation. A study in awake chronically instrumented goats. Circulation, 1995. **92**(7): p. 1954-68.

27. Daoud, E.G., F. Bogun, R. Goyal, M. Harvey, K.C. Man, S.A. Strickberger, and F. Morady, Effect of atrial fibrillation on atrial refractoriness in humans. Circulation, 1996. **94**(7): p. 1600-6.

28. Paraskevaidis, I.A., D.T. Kremastinos, E.P. Matsakas, G.A. Tsetsos, G.N. Theodorakis, and P.K. Toutouzas, Transesophageal detection of early systolic reverse pulmonary venous flow in atrial fibrillation. Am J Cardiol, 1994. **73**(5): p. 392-6.

29. Manning, W.J., D.E. Leeman, P.J. Gotch, and P.C. Come, Pulsed Doppler evaluation of atrial mechanical function after electrical cardioversion of atrial fibrillation. J Am Coll Cardiol, 1989. **13**(3): p. 617-23.

30. Manning, W.J., D.I. Silverman, S.E. Katz, M.F. Riley, P.C. Come, R.M. Doherty, J.T. Munson, and P.S. Douglas, Impaired left atrial mechanical function after cardioversion: relation to the duration of atrial fibrillation. J Am Coll Cardiol, 1994. **23**(7): p. 1535-40.

31. Rodriguez, L.M., J.L. Smeets, B. Xie, C. de Chillou, E. Cheriex, F.Pieters, J. Metzger, K. den Dulk, and H.J. Wellens, Improvement in left ventricular function by ablation of atrioventricular nodal conduction in selected patients with lone atrial fibrillation. Am J Cardiol, 1993. **72**(15): p. 1137-41.

32. Tieleman, R.G., C. De Langen, I.C. Van Gelder, P.J. de Kam, J. Grandjean, K.J. Bel, M.C. Wijffels, M.A. Allessie, and H.J. Crijns, Verapamil reduces tachycardia-induced electrical remodeling of the atria [see comments]. Circulation, 1997. **95**(7): p. 1945-53.

33. Pritchett, E.L., Management of atrial fibrillation [see comments]. N Engl J Med, 1992. **326**(19): p. 1264-71.

34. Blackshear, J.L., S.L. Kopecky, S.C. Litin, R.E. Safford, and S.C. Hammill, Management of atrial fibrillation in adults: prevention of thromboembolism and symptomatic treatment. Mayo Clin Proc, 1996. **71**(2): p. 150-60.

35. Nattel, S., Newer developments in the management of atrial fibrillation. Am Heart J, 1995. **130**(5): p. 1094-106.

36. Hoffman, B.F., The pharmacology of cardiac glycosides. In: Rosen MR, Hoffman BF,eds. Cardiac therapy. The Hague: Martinus Nijhoff Publishers, 1983: p. 387 - 412.

37. Rawles, J.M., M.J. Metcalfe, and K. Jennings, Time of occurrence, duration, and ventricular rate of paroxysmal atrial fibrillation: the effect of digoxin [see comments]. Br Heart J, 1990. **63**(4): p. 225-7.

38. Anderson, J.L., E.M. Gilbert, B.L. Alpert, R.W. Henthorn, A.L. Waldo, A.K. Bhandari, R.W. Hawkinson, and E.L. Pritchett, Prevention of symptomatic recurrences of paroxysmal atrial fibrillation in patients initially tolerating antiarrhythmic therapy. A multicenter,double-blind, crossover study of flecainide and placebo with transtelephonic monitoring. Flecainide Supraventricular Tachycardia Study Group. Circulation, 1989. **80**(6): p. 1557-70.

39. Goldman, S., P. Probst, A. Selzer, and K. Cohn, Inefficacy of "therapeutic" serum levels of digoxin in controlling the ventricular rate in atrial fibrillation. Am JCardiol, 1975. **35**(5): p. 651-5.

40. David, D., E.D. Segni, H.O. Klein, and E. Kaplinsky, Inefficacy of digitalis in the control of heart rate in patients with chronic atrial fibrillation: beneficial effect of an added beta adrenergic blocking agent. Am J Cardiol, 1979. **44**(7): p. 1378-82.

41. DiBianco, R., J. Morganroth, J.A. Freitag, J.A. Ronan, Jr., K.M. Lindgren, D.J. Donohue, L.J. Larca, K.D. Chadda, and A.Y. Olukotun, Effects of nadolol on the spontaneous and exercise-

provoked heart rate of patients with chronic atrial fibrillation receiving stable dosages of digoxin. Am Heart J, 1984. **108**(4 Pt 2): p. 1121-7.

42.   Lang, R., H.O. Klein, E. Di Segni, J. Gefen, P. Sareli, C. Libhaber, D. David, E. Weiss, J. Guerrero, and E. Kaplinsky, Verapamil improves exercise capacity in chronic atrial fibrillation: double-blind crossover study. Am Heart J, 1983. **105**(5): p. 820-5.

43.   Hwang, M.H., J. Danoviz, I. Pacold, N. Rad, H.S. Loeb, and R.M. Gunnar, Double-blind crossover randomized trial of intravenously administered verapamil. Its use for atrial fibrillation and flutter following open heart surgery. Arch Intern Med, 1984. **144**(3): p. 491-4.

44.   Waxman, H.L., R.J. Myerburg, R. Appel, and R.J. Sung, Verapamil for control of ventricular rate in paroxysmal supraventricular tachycardia and atrial fibrillation or flutter: a double-blind randomized cross-over study. Ann Intern Med, 1981. **94**(1): p. 1-6.

45.   Atwood, J.E., J.N. Myers, M.J. Sullivan, S.M. Forbes, W.F. Pewen, and V.F. Froelicher, Diltiazem and exercise performance in patients with chronic atrial fibrillation. Chest, 1988. **93**(1): p. 20-5.

46.   Roth, A., E. Harrison, G. Mitani, J. Cohen, S.H. Rahimtoola, and U. Elkayam, Efficacy and safety of medium- and high-dose diltiazem alone and in combination with digoxin for control of heart rate at rest and during exercise in patients with chronic atrial fibrillation. Circulation, 1986. **73**(2): p. 316-24.

47.   Langberg, J.J., M. Chin, D.J. Schamp, M.A. Lee, J. Goldberger, D.N. Pederson, M. Oeff, M.D. Lesh, J.C. Griffin, and M.M. Scheinman, Ablation of the atrioventricular junction with radiofrequency energy using a new electrode catheter. Am J Cardiol, 1991. **67**(2): p. 142-7.

48.   Jackman, W.M., X.Z. Wang, K.J. Friday, D.M. Fitzgerald, C. Roman, K. Moulton, P.D. Margolis, A.J. Bowman, K.H. Kuck, G.V. Naccarelli, and et al., Catheter ablation of atrioventricular junction using radiofrequency current in 17 patients. Comparison of standard and large-tip catheter electrodes. Circulation, 1991. **83**(5): p. 1562-76.

49.   Yeung-Lai-Wah, J.A., J.F. Alison, L. Lonergan, R. Mohama, R. Leather, and C.R. Kerr, High success rate of atrioventricular node ablation with radiofrequency energy [see comments]. J Am Coll Cardiol, 1991. **18**(7): p. 1753-8.

50.   Trohman, R.G., T.W. Simmons, S.L. Moore, M.S. Firstenberg, D. Williams, and J.D. Maloney, Catheter ablation of the atrioventricular junction using radiofrequency energy and a bilateral cardiac approach. Am J Cardiol, 1992. **70**(18): p. 1438-43.

51.   Rosenquvist, M., M.A. Lee, L. Moulinier, M.J. Springer, J.A. Abbott, J. Wu, J.J. Langberg, J.C. Griffin, and M.M. Scheinman, Long-term follow-up of patients after transcatheter direct current ablation of the atrioventricular junction. J Am Coll Cardiol, 1990. **16**(6): p. 1467-74.

52.   Olgin, J.E. and M.M. Scheinman, Comparison of high energy direct current and radiofrequency catheter ablation of the atrioventricular junction [see comments]. J Am Coll Cardiol, 1993. **21**(3): p. 557-64.

53.   Lown, B., M.G. Perlroth, and S. Kaidbey, "Cardioversion" of atrial fibrillation. A report on the treatment of 65 episodes in 50 patients. N Eng J Med, 1963. **269**: p. 325 - 331.

54.   Levy, S., P. Lacombe, R. Cointe, and P. Bru, High energy transcatheter cardioversion of chronic atrial fibrillation. J Am Coll Cardiol, 1988. **12**(2): p. 514-8.

55.   Kumagai, K., Y. Yamanouchi, T. Hiroki, and K. Arakawa, Effects of transcatheter cardioversion on chronic lone atrial fibrillation. Pacing Clin Electrophysiol, 1991. **14**(11 Pt 1): p. 1571-5.

56.   Fenster, P.E., K.A. Comess, R. Marsh, C. Katzenberg, and W.D. Hager, Conversion of atrial fibrillation to sinus rhythm by acute intravenous procainamide infusion. Am Heart J, 1983. **106**(3): p. 501-4.

57.   Madrid, A.H., C. Moro, E. Marin-Huerta, J.L. Mestre, L. Novo, and A. Costa, Comparison of flecainide and procainamide in cardioversion of atrial fibrillation. Eur Heart J, 1993. **14**(8): p. 1127-31.

58.   Ellenbogen, K.A., B.S. Stambler, M.A. Wood, P.T. Sager, R.C. Wesley, Jr., M.C. Meissner, R.G. Zoble, L.K. Wakefield, K.T. Perry, and J.T. Vanderlugt, Efficacy of intravenous ibutilide for rapid termination of atrial fibrillation and atrial flutter: a dose-response study [published erratum appears in J Am Coll Cardiol 1996 Oct;28(4):1082]. J Am Coll Cardiol, 1996. **28**(1): p. 130-6.

59.   Byrne-Quinn, E. and A. Wing, Maintenance of sinus rhythm after DC reversion of atrial fibrillation: a double-blind controlled trial of long-acting quinidinebisulphate. British Heart Journal, 1970. **32**: p. 370-76.

60. Hjelms, E., Procainamide conversion of acute atrial fibrillation after open-heart surgery compared with digoxin treatment. Scand J Thorac Cardiovasc Surg, 1992. **26**(3): p. 193-6.

61. Laub, G.W., L. Janeira, S. Muralidharan, J.B. Riebman, C. Chen, M. Neary, J. Fernandez, M.S. Adkins, and L.B. McGrath, Prophylactic procainamide for prevention of atrial fibrillation after coronary artery bypass grafting: a prospective, double-blind, randomized, placebo-controlled pilot study. Crit Care Med, 1993. **21**(10): p. 1474-8.

62. Karlson, B.W., I. Torstensson, C. Abjorn, S.O. Jansson, and L.E. Peterson, Disopyramide in the maintenance of sinus rhythm after electroconversion of atrial fibrillation. A placebo-controlled one-year follow-up study. Eur Heart J, 1988. **9**(3): p. 284-90.

63. Clementy, J., M.N. Dulhoste, C. Laiter, I. Denjoy, and P. Dos Santos, Flecainide acetate in the prevention of paroxysmal atrial fibrillation: a nine-month follow-up of more than 500 patients. Am J Cardiol, 1992. **70**(5): p. 44A-49A.

64. Pietersen, A.H. and H. Hellemann, Usefulness of flecainide for prevention of paroxysmal atrial fibrillation and flutter. Danish-Norwegian Flecainide Multicenter Study Group. Am J Cardiol, 1991. **67**(8): p. 713-7.

65. Van Gelder, I.C., H.J. Crijns, W.H. Van Gilst, L.M. Van Wijk, H.P. Hamer, and K.I. Lie, Efficacy and safety of flecainide acetate in the maintenance of sinus rhythm after electrical cardioversion of chronic atrial fibrillation or atrial flutter. Am J Cardiol, 1989. **64**(19): p. 1317-21.

66. Connolly, S.J. and D.L. Hoffert, Usefulness of propafenone for recurrent paroxysmal atrial fibrillation. Am J Cardiol, 1989. **63**(12): p. 817-9.

67. Kyles, A.E., C.J. Murdock, J.A. Yeung-Lai-Wah, S. Vorderbrugge, and C.R. Kerr, Long term efficacy of propafenone for prevention of atrial fibrillation. Can J Cardiol, 1991. **7**(9): p. 407-9.

68. Pritchett, E.L., E.A. McCarthy, and W.E. Wilkinson, Propafenone treatment of symptomatic paroxysmal supraventricular arrhythmias. A randomized, placebo-controlled, crossover trial in patients tolerating oral therapy. Ann Intern Med, 1991. **114**(7): p. 539-44.

69. Weiner, P., R. Ganam, R. Ganem, F. Zidan, and M. Rabner, Clinical course of recent-onset atrial fibrillation treated with oral propafenone. Chest, 1994. **105**(4): p. 1013-6.

70. Suttorp, M.J., J.H. Kingma, E.R. Jessurun, A.H.L. Lie, N.M. van Hemel, and K.I. Lie, The value of class IC antiarrhythmic drugs for acute conversion of paroxysmal atrial fibrillation or flutter to sinus rhythm. J Am Coll Cardiol, 1990. **16**(7): p. 1722-7.

71. Clyne, C.A., N.A.d. Estes, and P.J. Wang, Moricizine. N Engl J Med, 1992. **327**(4): p. 255-60.

72. Echt, D.S., P.R. Liebson, L.B. Mitchell, R.W. Peters, D. Obias-Manno, A.H. Barker, D. Arensberg, A. Baker, L. Friedman, H.L. Greene, and et al., Mortality and morbidity in patients receiving encainide, flecainide, or placebo. The Cardiac Arrhythmia Suppression Trial [see comments]. N Engl J Med, 1991. **324**(12): p. 781-8.

73. Effect of the antiarrhythmic agent moricizine on survival after myocardial infarction. The Cardiac Arrhythmia Suppression Trial II Investigators. N Engl J Med, 1992. **327**(4): p. 227-33.

74. Sopher, S.M. and A.J. Camm, Atrial fibrillation: maintenance of sinus rhythm versus rate control. Am J Cardiol, 1996. **77**(3): p. 24A-37A.

75. Atwood, J.E., J. Myers, M. Sullivan, S. Forbes, S. Sandhu, P. Callaham, and V. Froelicher, The effect of cardioversion on maximal exercise capacity in patients with chronic atrial fibrillation. Am Heart J, 1989. **118**(5 Pt 1): p. 913-8.

76. Ueshima, K., J. Myers, C.K. Morris, J.E. Atwood, T. Kawaguchi, and V.F. Froelicher, The effect of cardioversion on exercise capacity in patients with atrial fibrillation. Am Heart J, 1993. **126**(4): p. 1021-4.

77. Gosselink, A.T., H.J. Crijns, M.P. van den Berg, S.A. van den Broek, H. Hillege, M.L. Landsman, and K.I. Lie, Functional capacity before and after cardioversion of atrial fibrillation: a controlled study. Br Heart J, 1994. **72**(2): p. 161-6.

78. Gosselink, A.T., E.B. Bijlsma, M.L. Landsman, H.J. Crijns, and K.I. Lie, Long-term effect of cardioversion on peak oxygen consumption in chronic atrial fibrillation. A 2-year follow-up. Eur Heart J, 1994. **15**(10): p. 1368-72.

79.   Lipkin, D.P., M. Frenneaux, R. Stewart, J. Joshi, T. Lowe, and W.J. McKenna, Delayed improvement in exercise capacity after cardioversion of atrial fibrillation to sinus rhythm. Br Heart J, 1988. **59**(5): p. 572-7.

80.   Lundstrom, T. and O. Karlsson, Improved ventilatory response to exercise after cardioversion of chronic atrial fibrillation to sinus rhythm. Chest, 1992. **102**(4): p. 1017-22.

81.   Waris, E., K.E. Kreus, and J. Salokannel, Factors influencing persistence of sinus rhythm after DC shock treatment of atrial fibrillation. Acta Med Scand, 1971. **189**(3): p. 161-6.

82.   Morris, J.J.J., R.H. Peter, and H.D. McIntosh, Electrical cardioversion of atrial fibrillation: immediate and long term results and selection of patients. Ann Intern Med, 1966.**65**: p. 216 - 231.

83.   Dethy, M., C. Chassat, D. Roy, and L.A. Mercier, Doppler echocardiographic predictors of recurrence of atrial fibrillation after cardioversion. Am J Cardiol, 1988. **62**(10 Pt 1): p. 723-6.

84.   Flugelman, M.Y., Y. Hasin, N. Katznelson, M. Kriwisky, A. Shefer, and M.S. Gotsman, Restoration and maintenance of sinus rhythm after mitral valve surgery for mitral stenosis. Am J Cardiol, 1984. **54**(6): p. 617-9.

85.   Prystowsky, E.N., Proarrhythmia during drug treatment of supraventricular tachycardia: paradoxical risk of sinus rhythm for sudden death. Am J Cardiol, 1996. **78**(8A): p. 35-41.

86.   Flaker, G.C., J.L. Blackshear, R. McBride, R.A. Kronmal, J.L. Halperin, and R.G. Hart, Antiarrhythmic drug therapy and cardiac mortality in atrial fibrillation.The Stroke Prevention in Atrial Fibrillation Investigators. J Am Coll Cardiol, 1992. **20**(3): p. 527-32.

87.   Atrial fibrillation follow-up investigation of rhythm management -- the AFFIRM study design. The Planning and Steering Committees of the AFFIRM study for the NHLBI AFFIRM investigators. Am J Cardiol, 1997. **79**(9): p. 1198-202.

88.   Black, I.W., A.P. Hopkins, L.C. Lee, and W.F. Walsh, Left atrial spontaneous echo contrast: a clinical and echocardiographic analysis. J Am Coll Cardiol, 1991. **18**(2): p. 398-404.

89.   Daniel, W.G., U. Nellessen, E. Schroder, B. Nonnast-Daniel, P. Bednarski, P. Nikutta, and P.R. Lichtlen, Left atrial spontaneous echo contrast in mitral valve disease: an indicator for an increased thromboembolic risk. J Am Coll Cardiol, 1988. **11**(6): p. 1204-11.

90.   Rittoo, D., G.R. Sutherland, P. Currie, I.R. Starkey, and T.R. Shaw, A prospective study of left atrial spontaneous echo contrast and thrombus in 100 consecutive patients referred for balloon dilation of the mitral valve. J Am Soc Echocardiogr, 1994. **7**(5): p. 516-27.

91.   Stroke Prevention in Atrial Fibrillation Study. Final results [see comments]. Circulation, 1991. **84**(2): p. 527-39.

92.   Risk factors for stroke and efficacy of antithrombotic therapy in atrial fibrillation. Analysis of pooled data from five randomized controlled trials [published erratum appears in Arch Intern Med 1994 Oct 10;154(19):2254]. Arch Intern Med, 1994. **154**(13): p. 1449-57.

93.   Petersen, P., G. Boysen, J. Godtfredsen, E.D. Andersen, and B. Andersen, Placebo-controlled, randomized trial of warfarin and aspirin for prevention of thromboembolic complications in chronic atrial fibrillation. The Copenhagen AFASAK study. Lancet, 1989. **1**(8631): p. 175-9.

94.   Secondary prevention in non-rheumatic atrial fibrillation after transient ischemic attack or minor stroke. EAFT (European Atrial Fibrillation Trial) Study Group [see comments].Lancet, 1993. **342**(8882): p. 1255-62.

95.   Investigators, T.S.P.i.A.F., A differential effect of aspirin on prevention of stroke in atrial fibrillation. J Stroke Cerebrovasc Dis, 1993. **3**: p. 181 - 188.

96.   Fihn, S.D., M. McDonell, D. Martin, J. Henikoff, D. Vermes, D. Kent, and R.H. White, Risk factors for complications of chronic anticoagulation. A multicenter study. Warfarin Optimized Outpatient Follow-up Study Group [see comments]. Ann Intern Med, 1993.**118**(7): p. 511-20.

97.   Cannegieter, S.C., F.R. Rosendaal, A.R. Wintzen, F.J. van derMeer, J.P. Vandenbroucke, and E. Briet, Optimal oral anticoagulant therapy in patients with mechanical heart valves [see comments]. N Engl J Med, 1995. **333**(1): p. 11-7.

98.   Hylek, E.M. and D.E. Singer, Risk factors for intracranial hemorrhage in outpatients taking warfarin. Ann Intern Med, 1994. **120**(11): p. 897-902.

99.   McCrory, D.C., D.B. Matchar, G. Samsa, L.L. Sanders, and E.L. Pritchett, Physician attitudes about anticoagulation for nonvalvular atrial fibrillation in the elderly. Arch Intern Med, 1995. **155**(3): p. 277-81.

100.   Gustafsson, C., K. Asplund, M. Britton, B. Norrving, B. Olsson, and L.A. Marke, Cost effectiveness of primary stroke prevention in atrial fibrillation: Swedish national perspective [see comments]. Bmj, 1992. **305**(6867): p. 1457-60.

101.   Gage, B.F., A.B. Cardinalli, G.W. Albers, and D.K. Owens, Cost-effectiveness of warfarin and aspirin for prophylaxis of stroke in patients with nonvalvular atrial fibrillation [see comments]. Jama, 1995. **274**(23): p. 1839-45.

102.   Hirata, T., S.B. Wolfe, R.L. Popp, C.H. Helmen, and H. Feigenbaum, Estimation of left atrial size using ultrasound. Am Heart J, 1969. **78**(1): p. 43-52.

103.   al, T.e., Dimensions and volumes of the left atrium and ventricle determined by single beam echocardiography. Br Heart J, 1972. **36**: p. 737-742.

104.   Aronow, W.S., C. Ahn, and I. Kronzon, Echocardiographic findings associated with atrial fibrillation in 1,699 patients aged > 60 years. Am J Cardiol, 1995. **76**(16): p. 1191-2.

105.   Hoglund, C. and G. Rosenhamer, Echocardiographic left atrial dimension as a predictor of maintaining sinus rhythm after conversion of atrial fibrillation. Acta Medica Scandinavica, 1985. **217**(4): p. 411-5.

106.   Dittrich, H.C., J.S. Erickson, T. Schneiderman, A.R. Blacky, T. Savides, and P.H. Nicod, Echocardiographic and clinical predictors for outcome of elective cardioversion of atrial fibrillation. American Journal of Cardiology, 1989. **63**(3): p. 193-7.

107.   Herzog, C.A., D. Bass, M. Kane, and R. Asinger, Two-dimensional echocardiographic imaging of left atrial appendage thrombi. Journal of the American College of Cardiology, 1984. **3**(5): p. 1340-4.

108.   Aschenberg, W., M. Schluter, P. Kremer, E. Schroder, V. Siglow, and W. Bleifeld, Transesophageal two-dimensional echocardiography for the detection of left atrial appendage thrombus. J Am Coll Cardiol, 1986. **7**(1): p. 163-6.

109.   DePace, N.L., R.L. Soulen, M.N. Kotler, and G.S. Mintz, Two dimensional echocardiographic detection of intraatrial masses. Am J Cardiol, 1981. **48**(5): p. 954-60.

110.   Schweizer, P., P. Bardos, R. Erbel, J. Meyer, W. Merx, B.J. Messmer, and S.Effert, Detection of left atrial thrombi by echocardiography. Br Heart J, 1981. **45**(2): p. 148-56.

111.   Pearson, A.C., A.J. Labovitz, S. Tatineni, and C.R. Gomez, Superiority of transesophageal echocardiography in detecting cardiac source of embolism in patients with cerebral ischemia of uncertain etiology. J Am Coll Cardiol, 1991. **17**(1): p. 66-72.

112.   Mugge, A., W.G. Daniel, A. Haverich, and P.R. Lichtlen, Diagnosis of noninfective cardiac mass lesions by two-dimensional echocardiography. Comparison of the transthoracic and transesophageal approaches. Circulation, 1991. **83**(1): p. 70-8.

113.   Mugge, A. and H.W.G.D. Kuhn, The role of transesophageal echocardiography in detection of left atrial thrombi. Echocardiography, 1993. **10**: p. 405 - 417.

114.   Stoddard, M.F., P.R. Dawkins, C.R. Prince, and R.A. Longaker, Transesophageal echocardiographic guidance of cardioversion in patients with atrial fibrillation. American Heart Journal, 1995. **129**(6): p. 1204-15.

115.   Manning, W.J., D.I. Silverman, S.P. Gordon, H.M. Krumholz, and P.S. Douglas, Cardioversion from atrial fibrillation without prolonged anticoagulation with use of transesophageal echocardiography to exclude the presence of atrial thrombi [see comments]. N Engl J Med, 1993. **328**(11): p. 750-5.

116.   Black, I.W., A.P. Hopkins, L.C. Lee, and W.F. Walsh, Evaluation of transesophageal echocardiography before cardioversion of atrial fibrillation and flutter innonanticoagulated patients. American Heart Journal, 1993. **126**(2): p. 375-81.

117.   Orsinelli, D.A. and A.C. Pearson, Usefulness of transesophageal echocardiography to screen for left atrial thrombus before elective cardioversion for atrial fibrillation. American Journal of Cardiology, 1993. **72**(17): p. 1337-9.

118.   Manning, W.J., D.I. Silverman, C.S. Keighley, P. Oettgen, and P.S. Douglas, Transesophageal echocardiographically facilitated early cardioversion from atrial fibrillation using short-term anticoagulation: final results of a prospective 4.5-year study [see comments]. J Am Coll Cardiol, 1995. **25**(6): p. 1354-61.

119.   Daniel, W.G., R. Erbel, W. Kasper, C.A. Visser, R. Engberding, G.R. Sutherland, E. Grube, P. Hanrath, B. Maisch, K. Dennig, and et al., Safety of transesophageal echocardiography.A multicenter survey of 10,419 examinations. Circulation, 1991. **83**(3): p. 817-21.

120. Pearson, A.C., R. Castello, and A.J. Labovitz, Safety and utility of transesophageal echocardiography in the critically ill patient. Am Heart J, 1990. **119**(5): p. 1083-9.
121. Mugge, A., H. Kuhn, P. Nikutta, J. Grote, J.A. Lopez, and W.G. Daniel, Assessment of left atrial appendage function by biplane transesophageal echocardiography in patients with nonrheumatic atrial fibrillation: identification of a subgroup of patients at increased embolic risk [see comments]. J Am Coll Cardiol, 1994. **23**(3): p. 599-607.
122. Manning, W.J., R.M. Weintraub, C.A. Waksmonski, J.M. Haering, P.S. Rooney, A.D. Maslow, R.G. Johnson, and P.S. Douglas, Accuracy of transesophageal echocardiography for identifying left atrial thrombi. A prospective, intraoperative study [see comments]. Ann Intern Med, 1995. **123**(11): p. 817-22.
123. Zabalgoitia, M., J.L. Halperin, L.A. Pearce, J.L. Blackshear, R.W. Asinger, and R.G. Hart, Transesophageal echocardiographic correlates of clinical risk of thromboembolism in nonvalvular atrial fibrillation. Stroke Prevention in Atrial Fibrillation III Investigators. J Am Coll Cardiol, 1998. **31**(7): p. 1622-6.
124. Black, I.W. and W.J. Stewart, The role of echocardiography in the evaluation of cardiac source of emboli; left atrial spontaneous echo contrast. Echocardiography, 1993. **10**: p. 429 - 439.
125. Bjerkelund, C.J. and O.M. Orning, The efficacy of anticoagulant therapy in preventing embolism related to D.C. electrical conversion of atrial fibrillation. Am J Cardiol, 1969. **23**(2): p. 208-16.
126. Rokseth, R. and D. Storstein, Quinidine therapy of chronic atrial fibrillation: The occurrance and mechanism of syncope. Arch Intern Med, 1963. **111**: p. 184 - 189.
127. Renekov, L. and L. McDonald, Complications in 220 patients with cardiac dysarrhythmias treated by phased direct current shock and indications for electroversion. Br Heart J, 1967 **29**: p. 926 - 936.
128. Goldman, M.J., The management of chronic atrial fibrillation. Prog Cardiovasc Dis, 1960. **2**: p. 465 - 479.
129. Grimm, R.A., D.Y. Leung, I.W. Black, W.J. Stewart, J.D. Thomas, and A.L. Klein, Left atrial appendage "stunning" after spontaneous conversion of atrial fibrillation demonstrated by transesophageal Doppler echocardiography. Am Heart J, 1995. **130**(1): p. 174-6.
130. Fatkin, D., D.L. Kuchar, C.W. Thorburn, and M.P. Feneley, Transesophageal echocardiography before and during direct current cardioversion of atrial fibrillation: evidence for "atrial stunning" as a mechanism of thromboembolic complications. J Am Coll Cardiol, 1994. **23**(2): p. 307-16.
131. Moreyra, E., R.S. Finkelhor, and R.D. Cebul, Limitations of transesophageal echocardiography in the risk assessment of patients before nonanticoagulated cardioversion from atrial fibrillation and flutter: an analysis of pooled trials. Am Heart J, 1995. **129**(1): p. 71-5.
132. Ewy, G.A., Optimal technique for electrical cardioversion of atrial fibrillation [editorial; comment] [see comments]. Circulation, 1992. **86**(5): p. 1645-7.
133. Salka, S., K. Saeian, and K.B. Sagar, Cerebral thromboembolization after cardioversion of atrial fibrillation in patients without transesophageal echocardiographic findings of left atrial thrombus. American Heart Journal, 1993. **126**: p. 722-724.
134. Black, I.W., D. Fatkin, K.B. Sagar, B.K. Khandheria, D.Y. Leung, J.M. Galloway, M.P. Feneley, W.F. Walsh, R.A. Grimm, C. Stollberger, and a.l. et, Exclusion of atrial thrombus by transesophageal echocardiography does not preclude embolism after cardioversion of atrial fibrillation. A multicenter study. Circulation, 1994. **89**(6): p. 2509-13.
135. Klein, A.L., R.A. Grimm, B. I.W., and e. al, Cost effectiveness of TEE-guided cardioversion with anticoagulation compared to conventional therapy in patients with atrial fibrillation (abstr). J Am Coll Cardiol, 1994: p. 128A.
136. Design of a clinical trial for the assessment of cardioversion using transesophageal echocardiography (The ACUTE Multicenter Study). Steering and Publications Committees of the ACUTE Study. Am J Cardiol, 1998. **81**(7): p. 877-83.
137. Klein, A.L., R.A. Grimm, I.W. Black, D.Y. Leung, M.K. Chung, S.E. Vaughn, R.D. Murray, D.P. Miller, and K.L. Arheart, Cardioversion guided by transesophageal echocardiography: the ACUTE Pilot Study. A randomized, controlled trial. Assessment of Cardioversion Using Transesophageal Echocardiography [see comments]. Ann of Intern Med, 1997. **126**(3): p. 200-9.

138. Prystowsky, E.N., D.W. Benson, V. Fuster, R.G. Hart, G.N. Kay, R.J. Myerberg, G.V. Naccarelli, and D.G. Wyse, Management of patients with atrial fibrillation: A statement for healthcare professionals from the subcommittee on electrocardiography and electrophysiology, American Heart Association. Circulation, 1996. **93**: p. 1262-1277.

139. Cheitlin, M.D., J.S. Alpert, W.F. Armstrong, and e. al., ACC/AHA guidelines for the clinical application of echocardiography: executive summary. A report of the American College of Cardiology/American Heart Association Task Force on Practice Guidelines (Committee on Clinical Application of Echocardiography). J Am Coll Cardiol, 1997. **29**: p. 862-79.

140. Rubin, D.N., R. Grimm, K. Arheart, S. Vaughn, and A.L. Klein, Cost Effectiveness of transesophageal echocardiography guided cardioversion with short-term anticoagulation compared to conventional therapy in patients with atrial fibrillation: The Assessment of Cardioversion Utilizing Transesophageal Echocardiography (ACUTE) Pilot Study. Unpublished data, 1997.

141. Seto, T.B., D.A. Taira, J. Tsevat, and W.J. Manning, Cost-effectiveness of transesophageal echocardiographic-guided cardioversion: a decision analytic model for patients admitted to the hospital with atrial fibrillation. J Am Coll Cardiol, 1997. **29**(1): p. 122-30.

142. Thorngren, M. and B. Westling, Utilization of health care resources after stroke. A population-based study of 258 hospitalized cases followed during the first year. Acta Neurologica Scandinavica, 1991. **84**: p. 303-10.

143. Shriver, M.E. and L.D. Prockop, The economic approach to the stroke work-up. Current Opinion in Neurology & Neurosurgery, 1993. **6**: p. 74-7.

144. Jenkins, L.S., K. Ellenbogen, N. Kay, M. Giudici, N. Jensen, R. Martin, and R. Bubein, Quality of life in patients with symptomatic atrial fibrillation. (Abstr.). Circulation, 1995. **92(suppl I)**: p. 490.

145. Hylek, E.M., S.J. Skates, M.A. Sheehan, and D.E. Singer, An analysis of the lowest effective intensity of prophylactic anticoagulation for patients withnonrheumatic atrial fibrillation [see comments]. N Engl J Med, 1996. **335**(8): p. 540-6.

146. Singer, D., Overview of the randomized trials to prevent stroke in atrial fibrillation. Ann Epidemiol, 1993. **3**: p. 563-567.

147. Chung, M. and Klein, A.L. Atrial fibrillation in: Scientific American medicine. New York: Scientific American, 1997, Chapter 1, Section IV, p.1-12.

148. Waktare, J.E.P. and Camm A.J, Acute treatment of atrial fibrillation: why and when to maintain sinus rhythm. Am J Cardiol, 1998. 81(5A): p.4C-15C.

11

CONGESTIVE HEART FAILURE

Durand E. Burns, MD
Minneapolis Heart Institute, Minneapolis MN
Maryl R. Johnson, MD
Northwestern University Medical School, Chicago IL

INTRODUCTION

The syndrome of congestive heart failure (CHF), defined as the inability of the heart to provide cardiac output commensurate to the metabolic needs of the body without calling on maladaptive compensatory mechanisms, affects more Americans and is responsible for more hospital admissions than any other medical condition. While the incidence of most forms of heart disease has declined over recent years, the incidence of heart failure is increasing, with more than 400,000 new cases of heart failure diagnosed in 1988, and nearly 700,000 new cases in 1992. It is estimated that with aging of the American population, the current prevalence of the condition (by some estimates approximately 5 million American people) will nearly double by the year 2030. "Heart failure and shock" is the highest volume diagnosis related group (DRG) in patients over the age of 65 years, and accounted for 841,285 hospital discharges in 1994. Current demographic and clinical trends contributing to the increasing prevalence of heart failure include an increased incidence of CHF with increased age, improvements in managing other heart disorders such as acute myocardial infarction, hypertension, and life-threatening arrhythmias, and prolongation of life in CHF patients with appropriate use of angiotensin converting enzyme (ACE) inhibitors and beta-blockers. The scope of the economic burden of CHF was outlined in a 1994 summary published by the Agency For Health Care Policy and Research stating that the total direct cost of heart failure treatment in the United States exceeded $10 billion per year, with a large majority of the cost being in hospital and nursing home days. Thus, resource utilization in CHF has become a prime focus in the current era of cost containment in provision of medical care, and strategies aimed at reducing acute hospital admissions and lengthy hospital stays for treatment of exacerbations of CHF will contribute greatly to reduction of resource utilization in this condition.

This chapter, after briefly outlining the pathophysiology of left ventricular systolic dysfunction and current therapy, will address tactics aimed at improvement in resource utilization for congestive heart failure, with the goal being prevention of acute crises necessitating hospitalization and the development of a cycle of dependency on acute care services. Broader application of such tactics could markedly reduce expenditures devoted to CHF care and at the same time improve the care patients receive.

PATHOPHYSIOLOGY OF CONGESTIVE HEART FAILURE

Figure 1 illustrates the pathophysiology of the heart failure state. Myocardial damage from any cause, or myocardial depression resulting from metabolic or pharmacologic factors, can produce myocardial dysfunction. The failing heart pumps a reduced cardiac output, and with this an elevation in ventricular filling pressure occurs in an attempt to maintain cardiac output via the Starling law. Additional compensatory mechanisms come into play, including stimulation of the sympathetic nervous system, vasopressin secretion, and stimulation of the renin/angiotensin/aldosterone system. In concert, these lead to sodium and water retention and venoconstriction, resulting in an increase in preload, as well as an increase in systemic vascular resistance, resulting in an increase in afterload. The increases in preload and afterload, although initially compensatory, exacerbate the heart failure syndrome, as elevated preload increases congestion and elevated afterload impedes cardiac output, particularly for the compromised ventricle.

Figure 1. The Pathophysiology of CHF

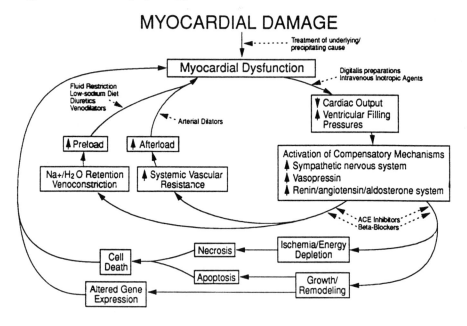

A diagrammatic representation of the pathophysiology of the congestive heart failure syndrome including sites of action of common treatment modalities. (Adapted from Johnson MR: Congestive heart failure: Diuretics, digitalis, and vasodilator therapy, in Parrillo JE (ed): Current Therapy in Critical Care Medicine, ed. 3. Philadelphia, Mosby, 1997, pp 109-115.)

MANIFESTATIONS OF THE HEART FAILURE SYNDROME

The symptoms and signs with which the patient with heart failure presents (Table 1) are related to both the low cardiac output and the elevated ventricular filling pressures which are part of the heart failure state. Low cardiac output produces the symptoms of weakness and fatigue and signs of pallor, mottling, and an ashen appearance. Increased filling pressure on the left side of the heart results in symptoms of pulmonary congestion (dyspnea, cough, paroxysmal nocturnal dyspnea, and orthopnea), with concomitant signs of tachycardia, an enlarged and displaced point of maximal impulse, a third and perhaps a fourth heart sound, a mitral regurgitation murmur, rales, and often physical examination evidence of a pleural effusion. Similarly, elevated preload in the right heart results in symptoms (anorexia, nausea, vomiting, abdominal pain, edema) and signs (right-sided S_3, tricuspid regurgitation, jugular venous distension, hepatomegaly, hepatic tenderness, ascites, edema) of systemic congestion. Increased preload on the left or right side of the circulation can produce significant weight gain.

Table 1. Manifestations of the heart failure syndrome

Abnormality	Symptoms	Signs
Low cardiac output	Weakness	Pallor
	Fatigue	Mottling
		Ashen appearance
		Cool extremities
		Diaphoresis
Increased LV*	Dyspnea	Tachycardia
filling pressure	Cough	Enlarged/displaced PMI
	Paroxysmal nocturnal dyspnea	S_3 with or without S_4
	Orthopnea	Murmur of mitral regurgitation
		Rales
		Decreased breath sounds at bases
Increased RV	Anorexia	Tachycardia
filling pressure	Nausea	Right-sided S_3
	Vomiting	Murmur of tricuspid regurgitation
	Abdominal pain	Elevated JVP
	Edema	Hepatomegaly
		Hepatic tenderness
		Ascites
		Edema

*LV = left ventricular; PMI = point of maximal impulse; RV = right ventricular; JVP = jugular venous pressure. *(Modified from Johnson MR: Congestive heart failure: Diuretics, digitalis, and vasodilator therapy, in Parrillo JE (ed): Current Therapy in Critical Care Medicine, ed 3. Philadelphia, Mosby, 1997, pp 109-115.)*

OVERVIEW OF THE TREATMENT OF CONGESTIVE HEART FAILURE

General treatment goals in congestive heart failure are to control symptoms, improve exercise tolerance and quality of life, prolong life, and reduce the number of hospitalizations and emergency room visits. In the current context of resource utilization particular emphasis is to be placed on prevention of costly acute hospitalization and intensive inpatient care.

Therapeutic modalities used in the treatment of heart failure can be reviewed in light of the pathophysiologic mechanisms of the development of the heart failure syndrome, as outlined in the previous section (see Figure 1). The initial goal is to improve the pumping function of the heart, thereby treating the heart failure syndrome at its onset. With this in mind, establishing a specific cause of the heart failure is important as treating the underlying etiology of the myocardial dysfunction provides the best opportunity for improving cardiac function, or at least slowing the progression of myocardial dysfunction.

The only oral agents currently available to improve ventricular function are the weakly inotropic digitalis glycosides. Intravenous inotropic agents (beta-agonists such as dobutamine and phosphodiesterase inhibitors such as milrinone and amrinone) may be of benefit in the acute care setting, as well as in selected outpatients as a component of chronic medical therapy.

Reduction of the workload of the heart, to provide a better balance between cardiac capacity and the metabolic demands of the body, can be accomplished by the use of systemic arterial vasodilators (ACE inhibitors, angiotensin receptor antagonists and direct-acting agents such as hydralazine), and in some cases by assisting the circulation with an intraaortic balloon pump or ventricular assist device. In some patients hospitalized with heart failure refractory to even the most aggressive medical treatment, decreasing the work of breathing by mechanical ventilation may be beneficial.

Control of sodium and water retention is necessary to decrease congestive symptoms. This is accomplished by placing the patient on a low salt (two gram sodium) diet, restricting fluid intake (generally 1000 to 1500 ml per day on an acute care basis, realizing that chronically a goal of 1500 to 1800 ml per day may be more realistic), and using loop diuretics, either alone or in synergistic combination with thiazides and/or potassium sparing agents. In severely affected patients who do not respond to these tactics, removal of fluid by hemodialysis, peritoneal dialysis, or continuous arteriovenous hemofiltration can be considered. In selected patients with pleural effusions or ascites, acute symptomatic relief can be achieved by thoracentesis or paracentesis. However, these modalities provide only temporary benefit since the fluid reaccumulates rapidly.

Mention must be made of drugs which may worsen heart failure or interfere with the efficacy or increase the toxicity of proven modalities of heart failure treatment. Medications such as first generation calcium channel antagonists, many antiarrhythmics, and nonsteroidal antiinflammatory agents should, if possible, be removed from the regimen of patients being treated for heart failure. Hypertension, angina and cardiac dysrhythmias can usually be controlled with agents which are at least neutral, and possibly beneficial, with regard to their effect on morbidity and mortality in patients with congestive heart failure.

COST-EFFECTIVE RESOURCE UTILIZATION IN THE EVALUATION AND MANAGEMENT OF CONGESTIVE HEART FAILURE

Several guidelines have been published regarding the evaluation and management of patients with systolic left ventricular dysfunction.[1-4] What follows represents a working synthesis of these guidelines and our practical experience in evaluating and caring for patients with heart failure due to systolic left ventricular dysfunction in the context of a specialized practice devoted to the comprehensive care of patients with heart failure.

The first step in the care of a patient who presents with CHF is to define the presence and severity of systolic dysfunction. This can be done by radionuclide angiography or echocardiography, with each study having its relative merits. Radionuclide angiography provides a more quantitative assessment of left ventricular, and particularly right ventricular, function, whereas echocardiography, especially when combined with Doppler data, provides additional information concerning valvular morphology and function and cardiac chamber size.

It is also important to define the underlying etiology of the heart failure, if possible, for only if a specific etiology can be defined and treated will the myocardial dysfunction generally be reversed. The most common cause of left ventricular dysfunction is coronary artery disease, and therefore every patient should have studies performed to determine if coronary disease is the etiology of left ventricular dysfunction. In patients with significant risk factors for coronary artery disease, or in whom the history or electrocardiogram suggests myocardial ischemia and/or infarction, the most cost-effective way to proceed is to go directly to coronary angiography. In those patients in whom the potential for coronary disease is lower, performing a stress nuclear or echocardiographic study and proceeding to coronary angiography only in patients with a study suggestive of myocardial ischemia is more prudent. In patients with coronary artery disease and evidence of ischemic but viable myocardium, revascularization by percutaneous transluminal coronary angioplasty, coronary stenting, or coronary artery bypass grafting should be undertaken. Only in this manner can hibernating myocardium be recruited and additional myocardial damage related to ischemia be prevented. Patients with significant hypertension should be aggressively treated and patients with valvular heart disease considered for reparative or replacement surgery prior to the time when ventricular dysfunction becomes so advanced that recovery of myocardial function is not possible. Those patients who have potential toxic (i.e., alcohol), metabolic (i.e., uremic) or nutritional (i.e., thiamine deficiency) causes of left ventricular dysfunction should be specifically counseled/treated. The fact that hypo- or hyperthyroidism can result in myocardial dysfunction should be considered and ruled out, particularly if patients have a history of atrial fibrillation or flutter, have evidence suggestive of thyroid disease, or are over age 65. A commonly forgotten contributor to heart failure is tachycardia. For those patients who have atrial arrhythmias with a rapid ventricular response, aggressive therapy is indicated, for conversion to normal sinus rhythm, or even slowing the ventricular response to the atrial arrhythmia, can significantly improve left ventricular function.

When no specific underlying etiology for the heart failure syndrome can be defined or ventricular dysfunction persists after specific therapy, aggressive medical management of heart failure becomes paramount. Digoxin, one of the oldest medications in the CHF armamentarium, is a weak positive inotropic agent. It is inexpensive and although it has been a mainstay in CHF treatment for years, only recently has it been studied in a controlled manner with regard to its impact on mortality and rates of hospitalization. In the Digitalis Investigation Group (DIG) study,[5] almost 7000 patients with a reduced left ventricular ejection fraction who were taking an ACE inhibitor and a diuretic were randomized to receive digoxin or placebo. After more than three years of follow-up, the digoxin-treated group had fewer overall hospitalizations. Hospitalizations for exacerbation of heart failure were reduced by approximately 28%, but an increased number of hospitalizations for suspected digitalis toxicity in the digoxin group partially offset this reduction. There was no significant difference in mortality between the two groups. Withdrawal of digoxin had previously been shown to result in increased hospitalization for heart failure,[6,7] and a cost analysis of these data has estimated that digoxin use would result in a large reduction in overall costs.[8] We generally prescribe digoxin therapy in patients with symptomatic left ventricular dysfunction, particularly those with ejection fractions of <30%, in an attempt to improve symptoms and decrease hospitalizations.

Angiotensin converting enzyme (ACE) inhibitors have clearly been shown to improve symptoms and reduce mortality and rates of hospitalization in patients with CHF.[9,10] Indeed, in patients with asymptomatic LV dysfunction, ACE inhibitors prevent the development of symptomatic heart failure.[11] A cost analysis of the SOLVD data suggested that treatment with ACE inhibitors had a favorable impact over four years of follow-up, reducing mortality at a savings of almost $720 per patient.[12] It must be emphasized that these results were achieved with doses of ACE inhibitors substantially higher than is the case in many physicians' practices (enalapril 10-20 mg b.i.d., captopril 25-50 mg t.i.d.), and many heart failure specialists feel that even higher doses may offer additional symptomatic benefits. For patients who are intolerant of ACE inhibitors, direct vasodilators (hydralazine and nitrates in combination) or angiotensin II receptor antagonists may provide similar benefits in terms of symptoms and exercise tolerance. The effects of these agents on mortality are less impressive or unknown and their effects on hospitalization rates have not been carefully studied.

In any heart failure practice, a major indication for hospital admission is volume overload. Adherence to a low sodium diet and fluid restriction, as previously discussed, decreases the tendency for volume overload, however, patients most often also require diuretic therapy to prevent and/or treat volume overload. We have found a stepwise approach to volume overload, as is used by most heart failure practices, to be beneficial. In patients who begin to retain volume, whether defined by a sudden weight gain or by symptoms or signs of volume overload, initiating or increasing the dose of an oral diuretic is generally the first step. If a patient becomes refractory to high doses of one of the loop diuretics, it may be beneficial to change to another loop diuretic. In addition, adding low dose metolazone (2.5 mg) can be beneficial, however, this should be done cautiously, and with close monitoring of fluid and electrolyte balance, because extensive diuresis can on occasion occur with only a single dose of this diuretic in combination with a loop diuretic. We also frequently give intravenous diuretics in the outpatient setting (either in the clinic or through the use of home health nurses) to those patients who have significant volume overload and are on a near optimized oral diuretic regimen. This may be enough to get the patient "over the hump", as diuresis may allow better forward cardiac output, due to reduced mitral and/or tricuspid regurgitation, as well as better absorption of oral medications due to the presence of less gut wall edema. If these maneuvers fail, the patient will most likely require inpatient therapy including such things as renal dose (two mcg/kg/min) dopamine, a continuous infusion of loop diuretics, intravenous inotropes, or in some cases mechanical fluid removal by means of ultrafiltration, continuous arteriovenous hemofiltration, or dialysis.

Beta-blockers, which have been studied in the treatment of heart failure patients for over twenty years, have recently been accepted as effective therapy for chronic heart failure. In the Metoprolol in Dilated Cardiomyopathy Study, metoprolol decreased the pre-defined endpoint of death and the need for heart transplantation (p=0.058), improved symptoms, and decreased the overall number of admissions to the hospital or emergency department for CHF.[13] Carvedilol, which has vasodilatory and antioxidant properties as well as being a non-specific beta-blocker, has been studied more recently. This drug has been shown to reduce hospitalizations and mortality[14] and a preliminary economic analysis shows that carvedilol is cost effective in the treatment of congestive heart failure.[15] However, beta-blocker therapy should be initiated when patients are in a compensated state on a stable oral regimen of ACE inhibitors, digoxin and diuretics (if needed). It is also important to follow patients closely and inform patients that they may notice an increase in symptoms as beta-blocker therapy is initiated.

Intravenous inotropic agents have long been used in treating hospitalized patients (usually in an intensive care unit) with decompensated congestive heart failure. Indeed, the use of intravenous inotropes and/or vasodilators, particularly when used in conjunction with hemodynamic monitoring with a Swan-Ganz catheter, allows optimization of oral therapy to an extent that patients may notice sustained hemodynamic and clinical improvement for several months.[16,17] Chronic intermittent, and even continuous, therapy with dobutamine, milrinone or amrinone has been used on an outpatient basis in an effort to reduce hospitalization in patients refractory to therapy with standard oral agents. Although the mortality risk/benefit ratio for this type of therapy has not been clearly defined, it has been shown that inotropic infusions improve functional class and decrease the cost of care in patients with advanced (NYHA class IV) heart failure.[18-20] Intermittent intravenous inotropes are often administered in specially designated outpatient clinics with electrocardiographic monitoring capability, where specially trained nurses place intravenous lines, attend patients during infusions (usually lasting four to six hours), and report to the supervising physician any concerns about patient condition which can be addressed (i.e., excessive interval weight gain or the development of edema or pulmonary rales which can be treated with intravenous diuretics or dosage adjustment of oral medications).

It is also important to educate patients with heart failure, and particularly family members who influence the patients' dietary intake, on the importance of sodium and fluid restriction. It must be understood that thirst does not necessarily mean that the patient needs to drink more fluid, and indeed in situations when thirst is most prominent (i.e., situations of highest vasopressin stimulation), the patient is often already volume overloaded. Having a nurse who is well versed in the management of heart failure participate in the education of patients and their families is extremely important. This education should also include the recommendation that the patient be weighed daily. If a weight increase of greater than two pounds occurs in a single day, the medical caregivers should be contacted such that treatment can be provided prior to extreme volume overload, thereby decreasing the need for inpatient therapy. Indeed, every time a patient presents with evidence of decompensated heart failure, attempting to define precipitating causes of the decompensation is important, for only through defining the precipitating causes can such factors be prevented from leading to recurrent cardiac decompensation. Precipitating factors to consider include myocardial ischemia, uncontrolled hypertension, atrial or ventricular arrhythmias, excessive physical activity, noncompliance with the medical regimen, and dietary and/or fluid indiscretion.

EFFECTS OF TREATMENT MODALITIES ON GOALS OF HEART FAILURE THERAPY

Table 2 indicates the ability of each of the therapeutic modalities used in the treatment of heart failure to control symptoms, improve exercise tolerance, improve survival and decrease the number of hospitalizations, a surrogate for the cost of heart failure therapy. It can be seen that the "report card" is the best for the ACE inhibitors, which are beneficial in all these aspects, and for the beta-blockers and beta/alpha blockers, which clearly decrease symptoms and hospitalizations, and, in the case of carvedilol, and perhaps other beta-blockers, improve survival. It is also important to notice in Figure 1 that ACE inhibitors and beta-blockers most specifically block the mechanisms producing progressive cell death and altered gene expression in the heart failure syndrome, and thereby block progression of the heart failure state at a cellular level. It is unlikely that these effects and the proven benefits of ACE inhibitors and beta-blockers in the treatment of CHF are fortuitous.

Table 2. Effects Of Treatment Modalities On Goals Of Heart Failure Therapy

Drug Class	Symptoms	Exercise Tolerance	Survival	Hospitaliz-ations
Diuretics	⇩	⇧	?	?
Digitalis	⇩	?	=	⇩
Vasodilators				
Direct (combo)	⇩	⇧	⇧	?
ACE inhibitors	⇩	⇧	⇧	⇩
Angiotensin II antagonists	⇩	⇧	?	?
Beta-blockers	⇩	?	?	⇩
Beta/alpha blockers	⇩	?	⇧	⇩

THE ROLE OF SPECIALIZED HEART FAILURE TREATMENT PROGRAMS

The initial evaluation and management of patients with congestive heart failure is admittedly the province of the primary care physician. However, it is important that complete patient evaluation and aggressive optimization of therapy (as outlined here and shown to be beneficial in trials) are performed, even if symptoms improve or resolve before these goals are reached. Indeed it is of concern that primary care physicians are less likely to conform with published guidelines for CHF evaluation and management than cardiologists,[21] as less than optimum CHF care can produce a major impact on patient outcome and health care costs. For patients who don't respond readily to medical therapy, and particularly those who require hospitalization or rehospitalization for decompensated heart failure, referral to a designated heart failure program is clearly of benefit. Not only do the physicians in designated heart failure treatment programs have extensive experience in treating patients with severe left ventricular dysfunction, but they have developed a multidisciplinary approach to the care of CHF patients, involving specialized heart failure nurses, home health nurses, patient and family education, social service consultation, and intensive follow-up. Specialized heart failure programs have been shown to be beneficial in terms of improving the functional status of and decreasing hospitalization and medical costs for patients with congestive heart failure, both in this country and abroad.[22-25] Heart failure is not a static condition, but one which requires careful monitoring by the patient and his family, the home health nurse, the nurses of the heart failure program, and physicians, in order to respond promptly to subtle changes in the patient's condition, particularly the patient's volume status, and thus allow for interventions to be carried out prior to the time that readmission to the hospital is required.

AN ALGORITHM FOR CARE OF THE PATIENT WITH CHF

The approach to the evaluation and management of patients with CHF which has been described, and in most cases justified, in this chapter is shown is Figure 2. In closing, two factors deserve emphasis. The first is that cost-effective management of heart failure, particularly in patients who respond poorly to medical therapy or who have frequent exacerbations of heart failure, should include referral to a specialized heart failure program. In addition, due to the dynamic and ever-changing nature of the heart failure syndrome, close patient follow-up, by specially trained home health or office nurses and the physician, allows modification of therapy prior to severe decompensation and can go a long way toward preventing costly hospital admissions.

Figure 2. An Algorithm for Care of the Patient with CHF

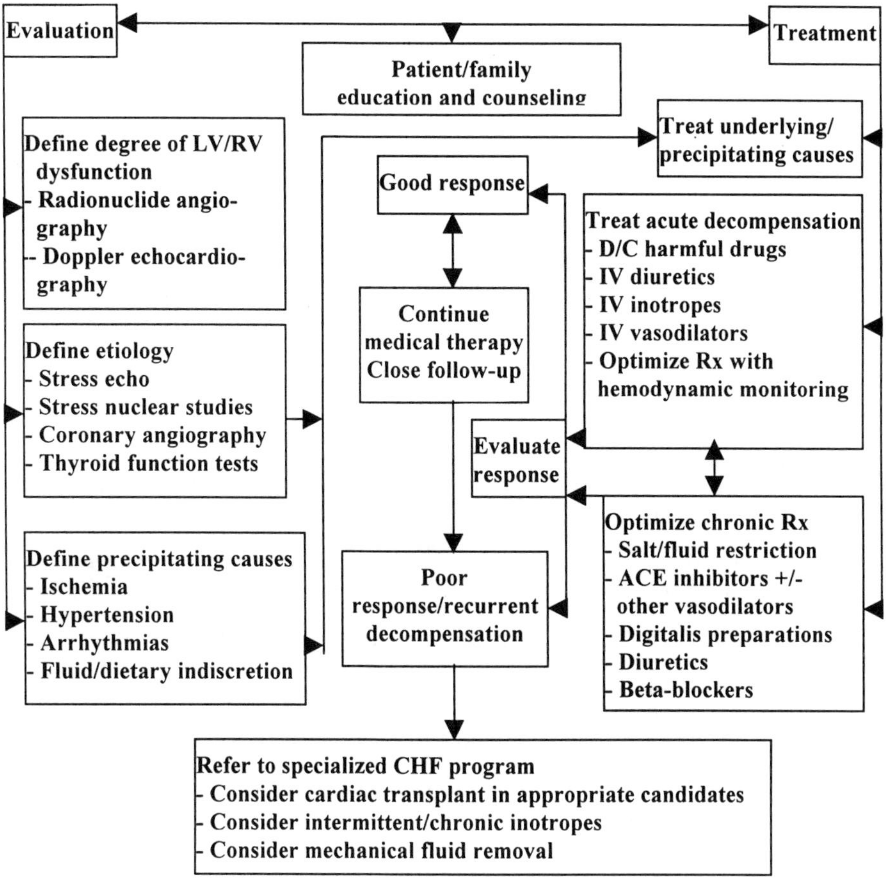

ACE = angiotensin converting enzyme; CHF = congestive heart failure; D/C = discontinue; IV = intravenous; LV = left ventricular; RV = right ventricular; Rx = therapy

REFERENCES

1.   Konstam M, Dracup K, Baker D, et al. Heart failure: evaluation and care of patients with left-ventricular systolic dysfunction. Clinical practice guideline No. 11. AHCPR Publication No. 94-0612. Rockville, MD: Agency for Health Care Policy and Research, Public Health Service, U.S. Department of Health and Human Services. June 1994.

2.   Williams JF Jr., Bristow MR, Fowler MB, et al. Guidelines for the evaluation and management of heart failure. Report of The American College of Cardiology/American Heart Association Task Force on Practice Guidelines (Committee on Evaluation and Management of Heart Failure). J Am Coll Cardiol 1995; 26:1376-98.

3.   The Task Force on Heart Failure of the European Society of Cardiology. Guidelines for the diagnosis of heart failure. European Heart J 1995;16:741-51.

4.   The Task Force of the Working Group on Heart Failure of the European Society of Cardiology. The treatment of heart failure. European Heart J 1997;18:736-53.

5.   The Digitalis Investigation Group. The effect of digoxin on mortality and morbidity in patients with heart failure. N Engl J Med 1997;336:525-33.

6.   Packer M, Gheorghiade M, Young JB, et al. Withdrawal of digoxin from patients with chronic heart failure treated with angiotensin-converting-enzyme inhibitors. N Engl J Med 1993;329:1-7.

7.   Uretsky BF, Young JB, Shahidi FE, et al. Randomized study assessing the effect of digoxin withdrawal in patients with mild to moderate chronic congestive heart failure: results of the PROVED trial. J Am Coll Cardiol 1993;22:955-62.

8.   Ward RE, Gheorghiade M, Young JB, Uretsky B. Economic outcomes of withdrawal of digoxin therapy in adult patients with stable congestive heart failure. J Am Coll Cardiol 1995; 26:93-101.

9.   The CONSENSUS Trial Study Group. Effects of enalapril on mortality in severe congestive heart failure. Results of the Cooperative North Scandinavian Enalapril Survival Study (CONSENSUS). N Engl J Med 1987;316:1429-35.

9.   The SOLVD Investigators. Effect of enalapril on survival in patients with reduced left ventricular ejection fractions and congestive heart failure. N Engl J Med 1991;325:293-302.

11.   The SOLVD Investigators. Effect of enalapril on mortality and the development of heart failure in asymptomatic patients with reduced left ventricular ejection fractions. N Engl J Med 1992;327:685-91.

12.   Glick H, Cook J, Kinosian B, et al. Costs and effects of enalapril therapy in patients with symptomatic heart failure: an economic analysis of the Studies on Left Ventricular Dysfunction (SOLVD) treatment trial. J Cardiac Failure 1995;1:371-80.

13.   Waagstein F, Bristow MR, Swedberg K, et al. Beneficial effects of metoprolol in idiopathic dilated cardiomyopathy. Lancet 1993;342:1441-6.

14.   Packer M, Bristow MR, Cohn JN, et al. The effect of carvedilol on morbidity and mortality in patients with chronic heart failure. N Engl J Med 1996;334:1349-55.

15.   Oster G, Menzin J, Richner RE, et al. Impact of carvedilol therapy for heart failure on costs of cardiovascular-related hospitalization. J Am Coll Cardiol 1997;29:326A (abstract).

16.   Steimle AE, Stevenson LW, Chelimsky-Fallick C, et al. Sustained hemodynamic efficacy of therapy tailored to reduce filling pressures in survivors with advanced heart failure. Circulation 1997; 96:1165-72.

16.   Ruzumna P, Bechtel T, Nee L, et al.. Dramatic improvement in left ventricular ejection fraction following referral to a heart transplant program. J Heart Lung Transplant 1998;17:92 (abstract).

18.   Marius-Nunez AL, Denes P, Silber E, et al. Intermittent inotropic therapy in an outpatient setting: a cost-effective therapeutic modality in patients with refractory heart failure. Am Heart J 1996;132:805-8.

19.   Harjai KJ, Smart FW, Stapleton DD, et al. Home inotropic therapy in advanced heart failure: cost analysis and clinical outcomes. Chest 1997;112:1298-303.

20.   Mehra MR, Smart FW, Zimmerman D, et al. Safety and clinical utility of long-term intravenous milrinone in advanced heart failure. Am J Cardiol 1997;80:61-4.

21.   Edep ME, Shah NB, Tateo IM, Massie BM. Differences between primary care physicians and cardiologists in management of congestive heart failure: relation to practice guidelines. J Am Coll Cardiol 1997;30:518-26.

22.   Rich MW, Beckham V, Wittenberg C, et al. A multidisciplinary intervention to prevent the readmission of elderly patients with congestive heart failure. N Engl J Med 1995;333:1190-5.

22.   Kornowski R, Zeeli D, Averbuch M, et al. Intensive home-care surveillance prevents hospitalization and improves morbidity rates among elderly patients with severe congestive heart failure. Am Heart J 1995;129:762-6.

24.   Fonarow GC, Stevenson LW, Walden JA, et al. Impact of a comprehensive heart failure management program on hospital readmission and functional status of patients with advanced heart failure. J Am Coll Cardiol 1997;30:725-32.

25.   Hanumanthu S, Butler J, Chomsky D, et al. Effect of a heart failure program on hospitalization frequency and exercise tolerance. Circulation 1997;96:2842-8.

12

CORONARY INTERVENTION

Warren K. Laskey, MD
University of Maryland, Baltimore, MD

EXTENT OF RESOURCE UTILIZATION

At the present time over 500,000 catheter-based coronary interventions are performed on an annual basis in the United States alone (1). Although there is tremendous geographic diversity in the number of coronary interventions performed, there are many others factors that may determine the rate and extent to which these procedures are utilized (Table 1).

Table 1. Determinants of Coronary Intervention Utilization Rate

Factor	Reference
geography	(2)
gender	(3)
ethnicity	(4)
insurance status	(5)
care delivery system	(6)
demographics	(7)
physician type	(8)
logistics	(9)
socio-cultural	(10)

An in-depth analysis of the degree to which each of these factors affect utilization rates is beyond the scope of this text. Also, many of these (observational) studies are obtained from non-clinical, e.g., administrative and financial, databases that have failed to encompass the full extent of clinical, physiologic and anatomic information. Furthermore, without a true index of "need", the extent of resource utilization, appropriateness and outcome assessment of coronary inteventions are difficult to put into perspective.

Resources consumed under the rubric of coronary intervention include considerably more than catheter material. Table 2 outlines the additional components of the coronary interventional resource "pie" (data obtained from the University of Maryland Cardiac Catheterization Laboratory, fiscal year 1997-1998). The data in Table 2, however, reflect the use of low osmolarity radiographic contrast media in under 25% of all procedures. Pharmacy costs reflect the use of IIb/IIIa inhibitors in under 20% of all procedures.

Table 2. Resource Components of Coronary Interventional Program

Factor	Relative weight (%)
equipment / inventory	40
radiologic equipment (+ depreciation)	8.5
pharmaceuticals	7
personnel:	
M.D.	20
non- M.D.	20
facility	4
information management	0.5

As the technologic complexity of coronary intervention continues to increase, it is apparent that the logistics and costs of associated personnel, facilities and adjunctive pharmaceuticals will add to the mix. Table 3 summarizes the dramatic changes in the components of a coronary interventional procedure since 1990.

Table 3. "Essential" Tools of the Coronary Interventionalist

pre-1990	post-1990
POBA	stents, stents, stents
DCA	PTCRA
heparin	?laser
aspirin	?IVUS
$\geq$ 8F sheaths	$\leq$ 8F sheaths
	newer anti- thrombotic agents:
	ticlopidine
	GP IIB/IIIA inhibitors
	LMWH

The economic consequences of this hyperplastic change are obvious. Thus, any analysis of coronary interventional resource utilization will be significantly deficient, and misleading, if confined to simple procedural volume. Unfortunately, such ancillary information is difficult to obtain at present except in institutions with sophisticated information systems support enabling the amalgamation of clinical, financial and administrative databases .

What is the appropriate extent of resource utilization in this high profile area? Methodologically speaking, it is the number of procedures and conduct within each of those procedures that results in an optimal level of sustained and improved clinical outcomes in a given population. In contrast to most biologic phenomena, we would prefer if these outcomes were dichtotomized (with the vast majority, i.e., > 95% , of patients having an improved outcome) rather than distributed in a gaussian fashion. The exact "cut-point" for "appropriate" procedural frequency is unknown. Table 4 presents current prevalence data and emphasizes the dependence of this rate on both geography and demographics (Robert A. Vogel, M.D., personal communication).

Table 4. Coronary Intervention Procedure Rates (per 100,000 population)

Insurer	National average	HMO average	HMO average (West Coast)
Commercial	80	45	30
Medicare	480	250	180
age adjusted mean	128	72	48

Not only does the frequency of resource utilization need to be quantified but the characteristics of these procedures must also be scrutinized. Here, too, the nature of coronary intervention is significantly influenced by clinical factors. In Table 5 are summarized data obtained from the University of Maryland Cardiac Network experience over the interval 1995-1997.

Table 5. Resource Utilization and Outcomes Depend on Clinical Presentation

Mode of presentation	Resources	clinical outcome
Chronic stable angina	atherectomy-10% POBA- 40% stent- 50%	98% success
Unstable ischemic syndromes	DCA- 1% POBA- 40% stent- 59% IIB/IIIA inhibitors- 20%	94% success
Acute infarction (primary and "rescue")	POBA- 60% stent- 40% IIB/IIIA inhibitors- 10% additional facility/personnel- ?%	92% success

It is easily appreciated that as the complexity of the presenting illness increases, so too does the likelihood of additional resource consumption. Furthermore, there is significant geographic variation in the frequency of stent utilization as well as the use of adjunctive pharmacotherapy (R. Krone, personal communication). Increased procedural rates as the result of enhanced population screening (11), improved disease detection methods(12) and the changing demographics of the U.S. population will place further pressure on resource allocation.

What are the outcomes we hope to "optimize" with our coronary interventions? Table 6 summarizes "reasonable" endpoints to assess (University of Maryland Cardiac Network, Quality and Outcomes Committee) and the relationship of these endpoints to the clinical well-being of the patient (consensus-derived scale of 1-5: 1 - no relationship, 3 - a modest relationship, 5 -a strong relationship).

Table 6. Endpoints of Coronary Interventional Procedures and Their Clinical Significance

Endpoint	(Relative) Clinical Significance
Decreased medication requirement	2
Life style	2
Anatomic success	3
Procedural success	3
Clinical success:	
short term	4
long term	5

It can be seen, however, that as the endpoints become "softer", i.e., harder to quantify, the substantive benefit from our efforts fails to keep pace with both the effort itself and the attendant risk of that effort. While there have been substantial improvements and impressive growth in the level of technology , commensurate improvements in these "hard" outcomes is difficult to detect (Table 7) (12a).

Table 7. One year adjusted outcomes in NACI and NHLBI II PTCA Registries

outcome	adjusted relative risk (95% CI)
Death	1.0 (0.69, 1.43)
death/MI/repeat revascularization	1.23 (1.10, 1.37)
TLR	1.28 (1.11, 1.49)

Furthermore, the relationship of a "successful" procedure to the long-term diminution of cardiovascular morbidity and mortality, e.g., cardiac death, myocardial infarction, remains to be established (12a). Unfortunately, there is precious little data on the relative efficacy of mechanical intervention compared to medical therapy in either stable or unstable ischemic heart disease on these important outcomes (cf. below). "Open-label", non-comparative observational studies are difficult to interpret given the many potential biases inherent in such appoaches. Only in recent years have properly conducted randomized trials of mechanical vs. surgical intervention been completed. Although signifcant criticism of such trials was not unexpected , the results, to date, fail to support a life-saving role for coronary intervention in the setting of stable coronary heart disease (13). Large scale trials comparing mechanical intervention to intensive medical therapy are conspicuous by their paucity and at this time also fail to identify a life-saving role of coronary intervention (13a). The implications of these data are even more sobering when viewed from the standpoint of aggressive, interventional-minded approaches to the management of unstable ischemic syndromes.

APPROPRIATENESS OF RESOURCE UTILIZATION

Perhaps there is no more controversial area within interventional cardiology than that of the appropriateness of these procedures (14,15). Given the enormous clinical, financial and ethical implications of inappropriate application of coronary intervention, this issue is, indeed, mandatory to discuss. However, no discussion of appropriateness is relevant without reference to a measure of benefit, i.e., without benefit any procedure (irrespective of success) becomes inappropriate . What benefits are to be considered? How should they be weighted, if at all? As discussed above, hard endpoints e.g., cardiac mortality, are relatively infrequent and render rigorous statistical approaches untenable. Conversely, soft endpoints e.g., improvements in life style quality, may be more frequent and lend themselves to highly statistically significant conclusions of questionable clinical relevance.

An extensive literature exists on the appropriateness of diagnostic coronary angiography in a variety of clinical settings(16). However, the literature on the appropriateness of coronary intervention is scant (17). To some degree this may be the result of dynamic changes in the field itself. Incremental benefit from coronary stenting and adjunctive pharmacotherapy have contributed significantly to this "moving target", rendering cross-sectional analysis markedly time-dependent. Nevertheless, most studies of this latter type have limited their analyses to short-term i.e., < one year, follow-up. This limitation effectively eliminates valid comparisons to surgical or pharmacologic trials of disease intervention in which long-term follow-up is available.

The measure of benefit, and therefore, appropriateness, of coronary intervention in patients with stable coronary heart disease is limited to symptom relief and improvements in quality of life as no randomized study has demonstrated a benefit on survival. A recent meta-analysis of trials comparing outcomes of surgical versus catheter-based intervention, in fact, yielded an unfavorable combined end-point relative risk point estimate of 1.1 (95% confidence intervals; 0.89, 1.37) for catheter intervention (13). Intense, although perhaps tendentious, discussion in the wake of publication of the BARI trial has highlighted the difficulties of interpreting outcome data in both surgical and PTCA groups (18). Nevertheless, a reduction in mortality with PTCA was not found. All studies have been remarkably consistent in one important aspect: there is a significant early benefit on symptoms with both modalities although the well-known requirement for repeat procedures in patients undergoing PTCA detracts from its utility in the long term. Unfortunately, there is little comparative data with respect to the incremental benefit of intracoronary stenting in the context of stable coronary heart disease. The reduction in the requirement for repeat revascularization in patients receiving these devices is, at present, limited to the "STRESS" and "BENESTENT" lesion population (19, 20) as reported rates in observational studies of angiographic restenosis rates remain high, i.e., > 30%, in the majority of "real-life" i.e., non- STRESS/BENESTENT, situations (21,22).

The measure of benefit from coronary intervention in patients with unstable ischemic syndromes is more ambiguous. Not only does the underlying disease substrate confer an adverse short- and long term prognosis (23), but the intervention itself has resulted in lower immediate success rates (24   ), higher procedural complication rates (25) and suboptimal long term, i.e. >6 months, morbidity and mortality rates when compared to outcomes in patients with stable coronary heart disease . More disturbing is a trend in large, prospective randomized trials towards worse clinical outcomes with intervention compared to conservative approaches (Table 8).

Table 8. Clinical Outcomes in Comparative Trials of Unstable Ischemic Syndromes

Trial	Death or Non-fatal MI(6 mo,).	Death or Non-fatal MI(1yr.)
TIMI III:		
Invasive arm	9.1%	10.8%
Conservative arm	10.5%	12.2%
		p=NS
VANQWISH:		
Invasive arm	N/A	24%
Conservative arm	N/A	18.5%
		p=0.05

While these recognized sub-optimal outcomes and complication rates in patients undergoing interventional procedures have driven the use of "adjunctive" pharmocotherapies and, in the current era, increased rates of intracoronary stenting, intermediate (30 day) and longer term (> 6 months) clinical outcomes are still characterized by a not insubstantial rate of morbid events and the requirement for repeat intervention(26, 27). Unfortunately, there are no comparative trials in which these modalities are used and in which outcomes are compared to more conservative approaches. The issue of appropriate timing of intervention has also not been adequately studied (28). The immediate success rate of percutaneous intervention varies inversely with the acuity of disease. A highly thrombotic mileau coupled with a mechanically fragile endoluminal surface are recognized risk factors for procedural complications . It may well be that a more "combined" approach of medical stabilization followed by intervention, when indicated, would yield improved clinical outcomes. The emphasis on decreased hospital utilization, increased throughput and earlier intervention precludes any such evaluation of a combined approach . The need for such studies is more acute than ever given the disconcerting long term outcomes noted above.

The rapidly changing nature of coronary intervention as a technical discipline, the emphasis on overall cost reduction, the earlier ascertainment of patients at risk of significant morbidity and mortality and physician-specific issues have added to the inherent difficulty of rating the appropriateness of care. The high rate of performance of coronary angiography in post- myocardial infarction patients has been suitable material for study . However, evaluating the appropriateness of this technology has indicated that there are many more factors impinging on the decision to perform angiography in this setting than consideration of the results of clinical trials with explicit (and hard) end-points (29). The decision to act on the information at hand is equally, if not more so, complex. The increased facility with which coronary intervention can be performed, the remunerative aspect of these procedures and the increasing emphasis (both patient driven and payor driven) on same-sitting intervention have further aggravated the behavior known as the "oculostenotic reflex" (1). Given the misplaced emphasis on visual gratification, it is not surprising that the scientifically verified benefits of coronary intervention in either stable or unstable coronary heart disease are limited to a prompt reduction in symptoms and an enlargement of coronary artery diameter. The benefits to be assessed (and measured) in order that appropriates may be evaluated must include more than immediate outcomes. The clinical, financial and social consequences of procedures that are efficacious in the short term but less so in the long term are disheartening. This is particularly so when viewed from the standpoint of progressive reductions in long term morbid and fatal coronary heart disease events in primary and secondary risk reduction trials (30). The appropriate use of resources in coronary intervention should not be the widespread use of these resources, but the considered amalgam of mechanical and pharmacologic modalities in individual circumstances. Coronary intervention goes far beyond technical expertise. Patient outcomes are not related to structural coronary disease in any simple fashion (except in the instance of left main disease). Therefore, the evaluation of the appropriateness of this treatment modality must include long term outcomes and the link between immediate procedural success (or failure) and these outcomes.

ASSESSING THE EFFECTIVENESS OF RESOURCE UTILIZATION IN CORONARY INTERVENTION

In the same manner that appropriateness is linked to benefit, the effectiveness of resource utilization is linked to overall quality of care. While clinical benefit is the *sine qua non* of overall quality, there is more to the measure of quality than simple outcomes(31). In interventional cardiology it is also important how certain outcomes are arrived at and the mechanism whereby these pathways may be optimized (31a). Although clinical guidelines are one mechanism for accomplishing this end, there are others as well (Table 9).

Table 9. Mechanisms for optimization of quality of care

continuous quality improvement programs
risk adjusted outcome analysis
evidence based decision making
credentialing and clinical competency assessment
patient education
practice guidelines

Ideally, all factors will be invoked, albeit to varying degress, as the process of care develops. Relevant to interventional cardiology is the relationship between quality of care and resource consumption. Given the plethora of technologic and pharmacologic resources, it is intuitive that not all modalities are appropriate or necessary and that the universal application of certain modalities e.g., stenting, requires a critical appraisal of both process and outcomes. While the dynamic nature of this field is defined by the rapid dissemination of new technology, "traditional" means of assessing outcomes and quality indicators have been severely delimited. New methodologies are required that allow for rapidly changing physician behavior and significant alterations in peri- procedural conduct over relatively short intervals of time. If the important clinical end-points don't (and shouldn't) change, then the means whereby they are achieved become essential. Furthermore, in the present environment of substantial cost containment, if not cost reduction, the implications of changes in resource utilization are obvious: there simply will not be sufficient monies to cover true costs if appropriateness of utilization is ignored. Hence, virtually every ongoing major randomized trial in interventional cardiology possesses an economic arm in addition to the clinical objectives.

It is equally germane that every coronary interventional facility possess a program of cost -containment as part of its ongoing quality improvement efforts. While this concept leaves much to interpretation , substantive programs designed to limit (excessive) utilization and reduce expenditures on catheter inventory need to be quite specific. Table 10 outlines several potential means of achieving these ends.

Table 10. Potential Means of Limiting Utilization and Reducing Expenditures

Category	Example
limiting equipment use	revenue sharing on cost savings; physician profiling; reduced (simplified) inventory
reduction of expenditures	"capitation" programs with vendors;" profit sharing programs with facility; bulk purchasing agreements
limiting extent of hospitalization	? ad hoc intervention; 23 hour observational units; improved risk stratification

While each interventional facility must arrive at its own unique solution to these issues, the invariant theme proposed herein is the rational, informed and efficient use of resources to accomplish the irrefutable objective of improvement in clinical outcomes. An algorithm for the reader's consideration is shown below:

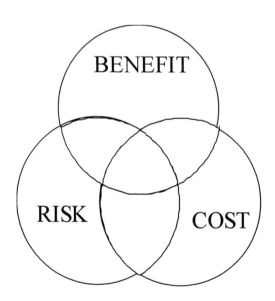

where the function "BENEFIT" is optimized and the co-variables "RISK" and "COST" are minimized. The overall outcome then is expressed as ("BENEFIT") / ("RISK") x ("COST"). In this manner, specific outcomes("hard" or "soft") may be relatively quantified and compared in groups of patients. Clearly, the most desirable benefit of coronary intervention would be a favorable impact on mortality , with secondary benefits being myocardial infarction prevention, diminished need for additional revascularization, symptomatic relief and, finally, entities under the rubric" quality of life", e.g., psychosocial adjustment, employability and general well-being. Having seen that the first two benefits are without scientific basis, the optimization of outcomes with relatively lower order of magnitude of benefit mandates proportional significant reductions in procedural risk and overall costs. While the determinants of procedural risk have been quantified (32, 33) they are far from precise particularly in the instance of the low volume operator (34) and/or low volume institution (35). Quantification of costs is, as well, fraught with difficulty (36, 37) and can only be estimated in very crude form at present. The approach taken herein allows for a "sliding scale" of benefit but necessitates proportional changes in risk and cost in order to maintain a given level of acceptable outcomes. Deviation from this level will require adjustments in all three components of the "process" of coronary intervention.

In summary, the subject of resource utilization in coronary intervention goes considerably beyond catheter inventory. The appropriateness of these interventions must be factored in to properly assess benefit. Cost and risk assessment are integral components of the care process and need to be properly weighted. "Success" is not simply a procedural-outcome but a complex function of benefit, risk and total cost.

References:

1. Topol EJ. Quality of care in interventional cardiolgy in Topol EJ Textbook of Interventional Cardiology (2nd edition). WB Saunders Co. 1994 pp.1354-1366

2. Topol EJ, Ellis SG, Cosgrove DM, Bates ER, Muller DWM, Schork NJ, Schnork MA, Loop FD. Analysis of coronary angioplasty practice in the United States with an insurance-based claims data base. Circulation 1993; 87: 1489-1497

3. Ayanian JZ, Epstein AM Differences in the use of procedures between men and women hospitalized for coronary heart disease. N. Engl. J. Med. 1991; 325: 221-225

4. Wenneker MB, Epstein AM. Racial inequalities in the use of procedures for patients with ischemic heart disease in Massachusetts. JAMA 1989; 261: 253-257

5. Sada MJ, French WJ, Carlisle DM, Chandra NC, Gore JM, Rogers WJ. Influence of payor on use of invasive cardiac procedures and patient outcome after myocardial infarction in the United States. J. Am. Coll.. Cardiol. 1998; 31: 1474-1480

6. Every NR, Fihn SD, Maynard C, Martin JS,Weaver W. Resource utilization in treatment of acute myocardial infarction: staff-model health maintainance organization vs. fee-for-service hospitals. J. Am. Coll. Cardiol. 1995; 26:> 401-406

7. Hadley J, Steinberg E, Feder J. Comparison of uninsured and privately insured hospital patients: condition on admission, resource use and outcomes JAMA 1991; 265: 374-9

8. Borowsky SJ, Kravitz RL, Laouri M, et al Effect of physician specialty on use of necessary coronary angiography J. Am. Coll. Cardiol. 1995; 26: 1484-91

9. Carroll RJ, Horn SD, Soderfeldt B, James BC, Malmberg L. International comparison of waiting times for selected cardiovascular procedures. J. Am Coll. Cardiol. 1995; 25: 557-63

10. Yedidia MJ. The impact of social factors on the content of care: Treatment of ischemic heart disease at a public and voluntary hospital. Arch. Int. Med. 1992; 152: 595-600

11. Wong ND, Defrano RC, Abrahamson D, Tobis JM, Gardin JM. Coronary artery screening by electron beam computed tomography: facts, controversy and future. Circulation 1995; 91:632-36

12. Wilson PWF, D'Agostino RB, Levy D, Belanger AM, Silbershatz H, Kannel WB. Prediction of coronary heart disease using risk factor categories. Circulation 1998; 97: 1837-1847

13. King SB, Yeh W, Holubkov R et al. Balloon angioplasty versus new device intervention: clinical outcomes. A comparison of the NHLBI PTCA and NACI Registries. J. Am. Coll. Cardiol. 1998; 31: 558-566

14. Pocock S, HendersonR, Rickards A, Hampton J, King S, Hamm C, Puel J, Hueb W, Goy J, Rodriguez A. Meta-analysis of randomized trials comparing coronary angioplasty with by-pass surgery. Lancet 1995; 346: 1184-1189

15. RITA-2 Trial Participants. Coronary angioplasty versus medical therapy for angina: the second Randomized Intervention Treatment of Angina (RITA-2) trial. Lancet 1997; 350: 461-468

16. Hilbourne LH, Leape LL, Kahan JP, Park RE, Kamberg CJ, Brook RH. Percutaneous transluminal coronary angioplasty. A literature review and appropriateness ratings and necessity RAND 1991 Santa Monica

17. Ayanian JZ, Landrum MB, Normand S-L T, Guadaguoli E, McNeil BJ. Rating the appropriateness of coronary angiography- Do practicing physicians agree with an expert panel and with each other? N. Engl. J Med. 1998; 338: 1896-904

18. Chassin MR, Kosecoff J, Solomon DH, Brook RH. How coronary angiography is used: clinical determinants of appropriateness. JAMA 1987; 258: 2543-47

19. Hirshfeld JW Jr, Ellis SG, Faxon DP et al. Recommendations for the assessment and maintainance of proficiency in coronary interventional procedures. J. Am. Coll. Cardiol. 1998; 31: 722-43

20. Favoloro RG Critical analysis of coronary artery bypass graft surgery: A 30 year journey. J. Am. Coll. Cardiol. 1998l; 31(suppl B): 1B-63B

21. Fischman DL, Leon MB, Baim DS et al A randomized comparison of coronary stent placement and balloon angioplasty in the treatment of coronary artery disease. N. Engl. J. Med. 1994; 331: 496-510

22. Serruys PW, de Jaegere P, Kiemeneij F on behalf of the BENESTENT Study Group: A comparison of balloon expandable stent implantation with balloon angioplasty in patients with coronary artery disease. N. Engl. J. Med. 1994; 331: 489-95

23. Mehran R, Hong MK, Lansky AJ et al Vessel size and lesion length influence late clinical outcomes after native coronary stent placement (abstr) Circulation 1977; 96(suppl I): I-274

24. Mehran R, Abizaid A, Hoffman R et al Clinical and angiographic predictors of target lesion revascularization after stent placement in native coronary arteries (abstr) Circulation 1997; 96(suppl I): I-472

25. Mulcahy R, Al Awadhi AH, de Buitleer M, Tobin G, Johnson H, Contoy R. Natural history and prognosis of unstable angina Am. Heart J. 1985; 109: 753-58

26. Myler RK, Shaw RE, Stertzer SH et al. Unstable angina and coronary angioplasty. Circulation 1990; 82(suppl II) : II88-95

27. Hong MK, Popma JJ, Baim DS, Yeh W, Detre KM, Leon MB. Frequency and prediction of major in-hospital ischemic complications after planned and unplanned new device angioplasty from the New Approaches to Coronary Intervention (NACI) Registry. Am. J. Cardiol. 1997; 80:40K-49K

28. Topol EJ, Califf RM, Weisman HE et al. Randomized trial of coronary intervention with antibody against IIb/IIIa integrin for reduction of clinical restenosis: results at six months. Lancet 1994; 343: 881-886

29. The RESTORE Investigators. Effects of platelet glycoprotein IIb/IIIa blockade with tirofiban on adverse cardiac events in patients with unstable angina or acute myocardial infarction undergoing coronary angioplasty. Circulation 1997; 96: 1445-1453

30. Kimmel SE, Berlin JA, Hennessy S, Strom BL, Krone RJ, Laskey WK. Risk of major complications from coronary angioplasty performed immediately after diagnostic coronary angiography. J. Am. Coll. Cardiol. 1997l 30: 193-200

31. Phelps CE. The methodologic foundations of studies of the appropriateness of medical care N. Engl. J. Med. 1993; 329: 1241-45

32. The Scandinavian Simvistatin Investigators. Randomized trial of cholesterol lowering in 4444 patients with coronary heart disease: The Scandinavian Simvistatin Survival Study (4S) Lancet 1994; 344: 1383-89

33. 28th Bethesda Conference. Practice Guidelines and the Quality of Care. J. Am. Coll. Cardiol. 1997; 29: 1125-79

34. Heupler FA, Al-Hani AJ, Dear WE et al Guidelines for continuous quality improvement in the cardiac catheterization laboratory. Cathet. Cardiovasc. Diag. 1993; 30: 191-200

35. Ellis SG, Vandormael MG, Cowley MG et al Coronary morphologic and clinical determinants of procedural outcome with angioplasty for multi-vessel coronary disease: implications for patient selection Circulation 1990; 82: 1193-98

36. Kimmel SE, Berlin JA, Strom BL, Laskey WK Development and validation of simplified predictive index for major complications in contemporary PTCA practice. J.Am. Coll.Cardiol 1995; 26: 931-38

37. Ellis SG, Omoigui N, Bittl JA et al Analysis and comparison of operator specific outcomes in interventional cardiology from a multicenter database of 4860 quality-controlled procedures. Circulation 1996; 93: 431-9

38. Kimmel SE, Berlin JA, Laskey WK. The relationship between coronary angioplasty procedure volume and major complications JAMA 1995; 274: 1137-42

39. Dick RJ, Popma JJ, Muller DWM, Burek KA, Topol EJ In-hospital costs associated with new percutaneous coronary devices. Am J. Cardiol. 1991; 68: 879-85

40. Ellis SG, Miller DP, Brown KJ, Omoigui N, Howell GL, Kufner M, Topol EJ. In-hospital cost of percutaneous coronary revascularization. Circulation 1995; 92: 741-747

13

CARDIOGENIC SHOCK

Eric R. Bates, MD
Mauro Moscucci, MD
University of Michigan, Ann Arbor, MI

INTRODUCTION

The organization of coronary care units in the 1960's to treat lethal arrhythmias and the development of thrombolytic therapy in the 1980's to reduce infarct size are the two major therapeutic advances which have reduced mortality due to acute myocardial infarction (MI). Nevertheless, mortality rates associated with cardiogenic shock, the most common cause of death in patients hospitalized with acute MI, remain high and relatively unchanged by modern cardiac intensive care unit interventions including vasopressor and inotropic drug infusions, hemodynamic monitoring, and intraaortic balloon counterpulsation[1]. Preliminary evidence, however, suggests that there may be a survival advantage for selected patients who achieve sustained infarct artery patency and myocardial reperfusion. The economic cost of aggressive and prolonged intensive care, cardiac catheterization, and coronary revascularization in a subgroup of patients with 65-80% hospital mortality rates has obvious medical resource utilization implications. It is the purpose of this chapter to review the acute cardiogenic shock syndrome and current treatment options. A risk stratification scheme will be suggested to assist in selecting those patients who might benefit from the more expensive interventions.

Definition

Circulatory shock is characterized by the inability of tissue blood flow and oxygen delivery to meet metabolic demands. Cardiogenic shock is a type of circulatory shock resulting from severe impairment of ventricular pump function rather than from abnormalities of the vascular system producing vasodilation (septic shock, anaphylactic shock) or from hypovolemia (dehydration, hemorrhage). Diagnosis of cardiogenic shock should include: 1) at least 30 minutes of systolic blood pressure less than 80 mm Hg without inotropic or vasopressor support, or less than 90 mm Hg with inotropic or vasopressor support; 2) low cardiac output (less than 2.0

litres/min^2) not related to hypovolemia (i.e., pulmonary artery wedge pressure less than 12 mm Hg), arrhythmia, hypoxemia, acidosis, or atrio-ventricular block; and 3) tissue hypoperfusion manifested by oliguria (less than 30 ml/hr), peripheral vasoconstriction, or altered mental status. It is important to separate the shock state, in which tissue perfusion is inadequate, from hypotension, in which tissue metabolic demands may be met by increasing cardiac output or decreasing systemic vascular resistance. Ideally, the diagnosis should be confirmed by pulmonary artery catheterization documenting adequate intravascular volume, low cardiac output, and high systemic vascular resistance. Importantly, there is usually a preshock state characterized clinically by severe vasoconstriction and hemodynamically by very high systemic vascular resistance where systemic arterial pressure is preserved. Early recognition by the astute clinician and aggressive treatment interventions may interrupt the hemodynamic and metabolic decline which leads to deteriorating left ventricular function.

Etiology

The most common etiology of cardiogenic shock is an extensive myocardial infarction, although a smaller infarction in a patient with borderline ventricular function may precipitate a low cardiac output state. Large areas of ischemic, nonfunctioning, but viable myocardium occasionally lead to shock. The delayed onset of shock may result from reocclusion of the patent infarct artery, infarct extension, or metabolic decompensation of noninfarct zone regional wall motion. Occasionally, cardiogenic shock is due to right ventricular infarction or mechanical complications including acute mitral regurgitation or rupture of the interventricular septum or free wall. Cardiogenic shock complicates acute MI in 5-10% of patients. Other cardiac causes of cardiogenic shock not emphasized in this discussion include dilated cardiomyopathy, hypertrophic cardiomyopathy, myocardial contusion, myocarditis, valvular heart disease, pericardial disease, and post-cardiopulmonary bypass.

Pathogenesis

Acute thrombosis of the coronary artery supplying a large myocardial distribution without collateral flow recruitment is the most common event. Frequently, this is the left anterior descending artery, although shock may result from coronary thrombosis in other sites if previous myocardial infarction has occurred. Multivessel disease is present in two-thirds of patients. Infarct size exceeds 40% of the myocardium in autopsy studies.

A sequence of events leads to progressive hemodynamic deterioration, initiated by a critical amount of ischemic or necrotic myocardium decreasing contractile mass and cardiac output. When cardiac output is low enough that arterial blood pressure falls, coronary perfusion pressure decreases in the setting of an elevated left ventricular end-diastolic pressure. This decreases the coronary perfusion gradient from epicardium to endocardium, exacerbates myocardial ischemia, further decreases left ventricular function and cardiac output, and perpetuates a vicious downward cycle to hemodynamic collapse. The speed with which this process develops is modified by the infarct zone, noninfarct zone myocardial function, neurohumoral responses, and metabolic abnormalities.

The infarct zone can be stabilized by recruitment of collateral blood flow or by restoration of antegrade coronary flow. Conversely, it can be enlarged by side branch occlusion due to propagation of thrombus, reocclusion of a patent infarct artery, or thrombosis of a second stenosis stimulated by low coronary blood flow and hypercoagulability. Infarct expansion or aneurysm formation can further decrease left ventricular function by reducing mechanical efficiency.

Noninfarct zone hyperkinesis is a compensatory ventricular response in the setting of a large myocardial infarction. This mechanism may be lost when multivessel disease produces ischemia in these segments or when focal areas of necrosis develop due to poor coronary perfusion.

A series of neurohumoral responses is activated in an attempt to restore cardiac output and vital organ perfusion. Catecholamine stimulation increases heart rate, myocardial contractility, venous tone, and arterial vasoconstriction. Angiotensin production stimulates peripheral vasoconstriction and aldosterone synthesis. Aldosterone and antidiuretic hormone increase sodium and water retention.

When compensatory neurohumoral responses are overwhelmed, anaerobic metabolism, lactic acidosis, and depleted ATP stores further depress ventricular function. Arrhythmias may additionally reduce cardiac output and increase myocardial ischemia. Loss of vascular endothelial integrity from ischemia culminates in multiorgan failure. Pulmonary edema impairs gas exchange. Renal and hepatic dysfunction cause fluid, electrolyte, and metabolic disturbances. Gastrointestinal ischemia can lead to hemorrhage or entry of bacteria into the blood stream, causing sepsis. Microvascular thrombosis due to capillary fibrin deposition and platelet aggregation further impairs organ function.

Diagnosis, Risk Stratification, and Management

Diagnosis

The diagnosis of acute MI must first be confirmed by history, electrocardiography, echocardiography, and troponin or creatine kinase measurements. Other cardiac and noncardiac causes of shock need to be ruled out. The average time from chest pain onset to cardiogenic shock is 8-10 hours, so the noninvasive diagnostic evaluation is more likely to occur in the intensive care unit than in the emergency department. The results of the noninvasive evaluation and the response to initial medical interventions should determine which patients will proceed to cardiac catheterization (Table 1) (Figure 1).

Table 1   Early Mortality Risk

	Expected (>80%)	Very High (60-80%)	High (<60%)
	Any of the following features	No features in left column, but any of the following	No features in left or middle columns
Age (yrs)	>80	60-80	<60
Symptom duration (h)	>12	6-12	<6
CPR	Prolonged	Short, successful	Not required
Neurologic status	Unconscious	Arousable	Conscious
Motor tone	Flaccid	Spontaneous movements	Purposeful movements
BP after pressors or IABP (mm)	<60	60-80	>80
Myocardial salvage potential by ECG	Poor	Fair	Good
CAD	Diffuse 3 VD	Focal 2 VD	1 VD

BP = blood pressure; CAD = coronary artery disease; CPR = cardiopulmonary rescucitation; ECG = electrocardiogram; VD = vessel disease

Figure 1   Critical Pathway for Triaging Patients With Cardiogenic Shock

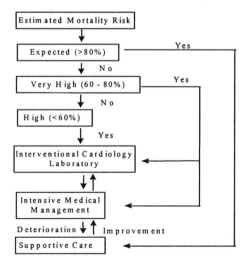

Noninvasive Diagnostic Evaluation

The most important predictor of outcome is age. In the large thrombolytic trials, mortality was 5% for patients less than 70 years and 20% for older patients. The adverse prognosis of older patients is even more dramatic with cardiogenic shock; rarely do elderly patients survive and some have questioned whether any revascularization attempt should be undertaken in this subgroup.

Time to treatment is critical in salvaging ischemic myocardium. Since the only possible way of changing mortality rates in cardiogenic shock is to reperfuse ischemic myocardium and preserve left ventricular function, early intervention is desirable. Reperfusion of nonviable myocardium offers no acute benefits.

Cardiac arrest is another ominous prognostic factor, particularly when resuscitative efforts involve more than one early defibrillation or neurologic status does not return to normal immediately. Cardiac arrest for several minutes results in myocardial dysfunction in the noninfarct zones and global left ventricular dysfunction.

The electrocardiogram offers important information for risk stratification. The potential infarct size is proportional to the number of leads with ST segment deviation. Extensive ST segment elevation suggests a large ischemic zone with good potential for myocardial salvage. New left bundle branch block usually signifies a large anteroseptal infarction. Less ST segment elevation suggests either a smaller infarct zone or more advanced progression to necrosis. Stratifying patients with only ST segment depression is more difficult. Their mortality risk is at least as high as patients with ST segment elevation because they tend to be older, have more comorbid disease, and have a higher incidence of prior MI. Diffuse ST segment depression is also a marker for left main occlusion or severe multivessel disease. However, no study of reperfusion therapy has ever demonstrated a survival advantage in this group of patients. Therefore, whereas patients with extensive ST segment elevation and new left bundle branch block are good candidates for reperfusion therapy, it is unclear whether patients with ST segment depression will benefit. Similarly, evidence for prior Q-wave MI on the electrocardiogram also suggests preexisting left ventricular dysfunction and a worse prognosis. In contrast, patients with inferior MI and right precordial (V4R) ST segment elevation usually have acute thrombosis of the proximal right coronary artery and are excellent candidates for reperfusion because right ventricular function recovers more quickly than left ventricular function and left ventricular function is usually preserved because the low cardiac output state is due to right ventricular dysfunction.

Echocardiography offers valuable information on left and right ventricular function, mechanical complications, and the pericardial space. A dilated, hypokinetic left ventricle suggests left ventricular shock, but a dilated right ventricle suggests right ventricular involvement. Hyperkinesis of noninfarct zones supports single vessel disease, whereas global dysfunction is seen more commonly in multivessel disease. Normal ventricular function, low cardiac output, and mitral regurgitation are consistent with acute severe mitral regurgitation. The Doppler evaluation can easily confirm the presence of significant mitral regurgitation or ventricular septal rupture. Surgical mortality associated with mitral valve repair or ventricular septal repair rises dramatically with left ventricular dysfunction and particularly with right ventricular dysfunction. Pericardial tamponade from hemorrhagic effusion or free wall rupture can easily be detected.

Clinical Stabilization

A number of supportive measures need to quickly be instituted (Table 2). If there is no clinical evidence for pulmonary edema, a fluid bolus should be given to exclude hypovolemia as a cause of hypotension. Patients with a history of inadequate fluid intake, diaphoresis, diarrhea, vomiting, or diuretic use may not have pump failure and will improve dramatically with fluid administration. Because preload is critical in patients with right ventricular shock, fluid support and avoidance of nitrates and morphine are indicated.

Table 2 Conventional Therapy for Cardiogenic Shock

1. Maximize volume (RAP 10-14 mm Hg, PAWP 18-20 mm Hg)
2. Control rhythm (e.g., pacemaker, cardioversion)
3. Maximize oxygenation (e.g., ventilator)
4. Correct electrolyte and acid-base imbalances
5. Sympathomimetic amines (e.g., dobutamine, dopamine, norepi-nephrine).
6. Phosphodiesterase inhibitors (e.g., amrinone, milrinone)
7. Vasodilators (e.g., nitroglycerin, nitroprusside)
8. Intra-aortic balloon counterpulsation.

PAWP = pulmonary artery wedge pressure; RAP = right atrial pressure.

Oxygenation and airway protection are critical. Intubation and mechanical ventilation is usually required, followed by sedation and muscular paralysis. These interventions also improve the safety of electrocardioversion or cardiac catheterization.

Electrolyte abnormalities should be corrected. Hypokalemia and hypomagnesemia predispose patients to ventricular arrhythmias. Because metabolic acidosis decreases contractile function, hyperventilation and sodium bicarbonate administration should be considered.

Arrhythmias and atrio-ventricular heart block have a major influence on cardiac output. Tachyarrhythmias should be electrically cardioverted promptly rather than treated with pharmacologic agents. Severe bradycardia due to excess vagotonia can be corrected with atropine. Temporary pacing should be initiated for high degree heart block, preferably with a dual chamber system. This is especially important in patients with right ventricular infarction who depend on the right atrial contribution to preload.

Table 3.   Pharmacologic Treatment for Cardiogenic Shock

Drug	Dose
Dobutamine	5-15 µg/kg/min IV
Dopamine	2-20 µg/kg/min IV
Norepinephrine	2-16 µg/min IV
Nitroglycerin	10 µg/min, increased by 10 µg every 10 min
Nitroprusside	10 µg/min IV, increased by 5 µg every 10 min
Amrinone	0.75 mg/kg over 2 min IV, then 5-10 µg/kg/min
Milrinone	50 µg/kg over 10 min IV, then 0.375-0.75 µg/kg/min
Furosemide	20-160 mg/IV
Bumetanide	1-3 mg IV

Aspirin and monitored heparin should be administered to decrease the likelihood of reinfarction, ventricular mural thrombus formation, or deep venous thrombosis in the setting of low flow and hypercoagulability. Morphine sulfate, by reducing pain and anxiety, can reduce excessive sympathetic activity and decrease preload and afterload.

Central hemodynamic monitoring is critical for confirming the diagnosis and guiding pharmacologic therapy. Urine output needs to be monitored hourly through catheter drainage. A pulmonary artery catheter should be inserted as soon as feasible to measure intracardiac pressures, cardiac output, systemic vascular resistance, and mixed venous oxygen saturation. An arterial catheter allows constant monitoring of the blood pressure.

Vasopressor and inotropic drug therapy are the major initial interventions for reversing hypotension and improving vital organ perfusion (Table 3). Failure to improve blood pressure with these agents is an ominous prognostic sign. Continued hypotension results in progressive myocardial ischemia and deterioration of ventricular function. Improvement in blood pressure suggests that viable myocardium is present and is a good indication to proceed with cardiac catheterization with a goal toward infarct artery reperfusion. Dobutamine is the agent of choice for patients with systolic pressures >80 mm Hg. Dopamine is required when the systolic pressure is <80 mm Hg. Norepinepherine is used when the systolic pressure is <70 mm Hg. Catecholamine infusions should be carefully titrated. A delicate balance must be obtained between increasing coronary perfusion pressure and increasing oxygen demand so that myocardial ischemia is not exacerbated. Moreover, excessive peripheral vasoconstriction decreases tissue perfusion, increased afterload increases filling pressures, and excessive tachycardia or arrhythmias can be stimulated. Digitalis has no significant inotropic effect, but may be employed for superventricular tachycardias to control heart rate. Nitroprusside and nitroglycerin are vasodilators that can be used if adequate blood pressure and coronary artery perfusion pressure can be restored. Afterload reduction is especially important when mitral regurgitation or ventricular septal rupture is present. Diuretics decrease filling pressures and should be used to control volume. Antiarrhythmic agents are negative inotropes and should be avoided if possible.

When pharmacologic therapy provides insufficient hemodynamic support, mechanical circulatory assistance can be instituted, especially when revascularization or surgical repair of mechanical complications is planned[2]. Intraaortic balloon counterpulsation reduces systolic afterload and augments diastolic perfusion pressure. The usual result is a decrease in filling pressures, systolic blood pressure, heart rate, mitral regurgitation, and left to right shunting across a ventricular septal rupture, along with an increase in diastolic blood pressure, stroke volume, cardiac output, and urine output. Subendocardial blood flow is improved, and in contrast to vasopressor support, oxygen demand is decreased. Unfortunately, there is no improvement in ischemic zone blood flow distal to significant coronary stenoses nor in noninfarct zone wall motion. The failure to improve ischemic zone myocardial blood flow probably explains why, despite temporary hemodynamic and clinical improvement in 75% of patients, no obvious difference in enzyme infarct size or mortality rate has been noted in randomized trials[3,4].

Invasive Diagnostic Evaluation

Coronary angiography should only be considered in salvageable patients whose clinical profile and response to cinitial therapy suggest that ischemic, viable, but nonfunctioning myocardium can be revascularized. Neither intraaortic balloon counterpulsation nor cardiac catheterization and revascularization are likely to alter the outcome in patients with extensively scarred ventricles or persistent hemodynamic deterioration. The procedure is most safely performed with the patient ventilated and paralyzed. Gas exchange is maximized, risk of aspiration minimized, cardioversion can easily be performed, and patient movements do not interfere with the procedure. Patients should have an intraaortic balloon pump and a pulmonary artery catheter in place and access should be available to insert a temporary pacemaker, if needed. Using nonionic contrast medium, two orthogonal views of the left coronary artery and the left anterior oblique view of the right coronary artery can be obtained with less than 20 cc's of contrast medium. Patients with discrete proximal lesions in one or two arteries are good candidates for PTCA; patients with multivessel disease or multiple lesions or diffuse plaque formation are much less attractive candidates. The presence of either a patent infarct artery with slow flow (TIMI-II flow) or retrograde collateral flow increases the probability that viable myocardium exists in the infarct zone, making PTCA more attractive.

Reperfusion Therapy

Several multicenter randomized megatrials have demonstrated that thrombolytic therapy reduces mortality from acute MI. Moreover, the greatest survival benefit has been confirmed for patients with the most jeopardized myocardium (e.g., anterior infarction, new left bundle branch block). It is paradoxical and disappointing that no obvious survival benefit has been realized for the subset of patients with cardiogenic shock[5]. The failure of thrombolytic therapy to affect mortality due to cardiogenic shock may reflect the low cardiac output state which decreases reperfusion rates or increases reocclusion rates. Preliminary preclinical and clinical studies suggest that increasing diastolic perfusion pressure with vasopressors or intraaortic balloon counterpulsation can improve reperfusion rates with thrombolytic therapy and may provide a survival advantage not seen when the therapies are given independently[6,7]. Therefore, thrombolytic therapy should be administered in the absence of contraindications, if angioplasty or surgical revascularization is not available, in combination with vasopressor agents and intraaortic balloon counterpulsation.

Bypass graft surgery potentially offers superior revascularization to patients in whom angioplasty cannot usually be performed safely or who have chronically occluded arteries that cannot be completely revascularized percutaneously. The high degree of surgical expertise required, the inherent time delays, the increasing hesitancy of surgeons to operate on patients with high operative mortality risk because of "score card" medicine, and the generally favorable results with PTCA make bypass graft surgery an increasingly rare intervention.

More than 20 reports have consistently shown a survival benefit for patients in whom reperfusion was successfully obtained with PTCA compared with patients in whom reperfusion was unsuccessful or with historical controls[1]. Unfortunately, none of these reports represented randomized, controlled studies of angioplasty. Although a selection bias undoubtedly influenced the results[8], several studies and clinical experience clearly demonstrate the favorable impact a patent infarct artery can have on reversing the shock state. PTCA should be performed as quickly and efficiently as possible with limited contrast injections. Although PTCA for acute MI is usually limited to the infarct artery, patients in cardiogenic shock with multivessel disease may have the best survival chance with PTCA of all proximal discrete lesions. Early resolution of arrhythmias, conduction blocks, or hypotension suggests an important therapeutic benefit. Conversely, prolonged procedures or failure to improve within the first 24 hours usually predicts mortality.

Recent Advances

Two major advances have occurred in the field of interventional cardiology in the past few years. First, endoluminal stent implantation has dramatically reduced the complication of acute closure of the artery after balloon injury and halved restenosis rates. Second, the development of more potent antiplatelet therapy with a series of drugs that block the glycoprotein (GP) IIb/IIIa platelet receptor and prevent platelet aggregation has decreased thrombotic complications. Both of these interventions should increase PTCA success rates in cardiogenic shock by increasing patency rates in the setting of low cardiac output.

Likewise, two major advances in mechanical support devices now permit patients to be kept alive until a donor heart can be procured for cardiac transplantation. First, extracorporeal membrane oxygenation (ECMO) teams at large medical centers can now quickly place patients on a cardiopulmonary bypass machine that delivers 3-5 liters per minute of nonpulsatile flow and maintains a mean aortic pressure of 50-70 mm Hg despite cardiac standstill. Support can be continued for as long as two weeks, extending the 6-8 hour time limit associated with the percutaneous cardiopulmonary bypass technique. Second, the HeartMate left ventricular assist device has reduced the embolic complication rate from 40% with earlier devices to 2% and is relatively portable such that patients can be discharged home from the hospital.

Resource Utilization

Cardiogenic shock mortality rates are high and treatment options can consume extensive medical resources. Hospital charges in these patients for intensive care exceed $2,000 per day, for cardiac catheterization and angioplasty exceed $10,000, and for cardiac transplantation exceed $100,000. Patients who die within hours of presentation consume the fewest resources. The mortality rate, length of stay, and hospital charges for the last 69 patients selected for cardiac catheterization at our institution are summarized in Table 4. The average charges for survivors was $64,431 compared with $37,212 in non-survivors. Similar data for patients not treated in the cardiac catheterization laboratory are not available.

Table 4. Mortality Rates and Resource Utilization by Age Group (University of Michigan)

Age	<60	60-70	70-80	>80
Number of patients	17	23	18	11
Mortality rate (%)	30	47	39	81
Length of stay (days)	11.5±11.2	9.5±10.7	8.75±11.8	6±4.9
Total charges ($)	55,437	55,263	50,840	34,613

CONCLUSION

Treatment decisions must balance the goal of preventing mortality versus unnecessarily prolonging inevitable death with expensive technology. Resources spent on preserving life are easily justifiable and the majority of hospital survivors have a reasonable short-term prognosis.

The challenge is determining which patients are destined to die and appropriately conserving resources in their care. Although no critical pathway has been prospectively evaluated, the items summarized in Table 4 should help select patients for cardiac catheterization and PTCA.

References:

1. Bates ER, Moscucci M. "Post-myocardial infarction cardiogenic shock", in: Brown DL (ed), Cardiac Intensive Care, WB Saunders Co., Philadelphia 1998, pp215-217.

2. Bates ER, Stomel RJ, Hochman JS, Ohman EM. The use of intraaortic balloon counterpulsation as an adjunct to reperfusion therapy in cardiogenic shock. Int J Cardiol (in press)

3. Flaherty JT, Becker LC, Weiss JL, et al. Results of a randomized prospective trial of intraaortic balloon counterpulsation and intravenous nitroglycerin in patients with acute myocardial infarction. J Am Coll Cardiol 1985;6:434-46.

4. O'Rourke MF, Norris RM, Campbell TJ, Chang VP, Sammel NL. Randomized controlled trial of intra-aortic balloon counterpulsation in early myocardial infarction with acute heart failure. Am J Cardiol 1981;47:815-20.

5. Bates ER, Topol EJ. Limitations of thrombolytic therapy for acute myocardial infarction complicated by congestive heart failure and cardiogenic shock. J Am Coll Cardiol 1991;18:1077-84.

6. Prewitt RM, Gu S, Schick U, Ducas J. Intraaortic balloon counterpulsation enhances coronary thrombolysis induced by intravenous administration of a thrombolytic agent. J Am Coll Cardiol 1994;23:794-8.

7. Kovack P, Rasak MA, Bates ER, Ohman EM, Stomel RJ. Thrombolysis plus aortic counterpulsation: improved survival in patients who present to community hospitals with cardiogenic shock. J Am Coll Cardiol 1997;29:1454-8.

8. Hochman J, Boland J, Sleeper LA, et al. Current spectrum of cardiogenic shock and effects of early revascularization on mortality: results of an international registry. Circulation 1995;91:873-81.

14

THE USE OF CLINICAL PRACTICE GUIDELINES IN CARDIOLOGY

James E. Calvin, MD
Lloyd W. Klein, MD
Rush-Presbyterian-St. Luke's Medical Center, Chicago, IL

Over the past decade, increasing emphasis has been placed on the development of clinical practice guidelines.1-3   The motivations behind this interest are the competitive pressures to reduce costs and the desire by all stakeholders to improve the quality of care by reducing variation in the type of care that patients receive. Clinical practice guidelines should improve care by facilitating access to proven therapy and reducing the use of unproven or harmful therapy.   However, health care providers have embraced clinical practice guidelines as an instrument to reduce cost largely by the use of critical paths. The purpose of this chapter will be to differentiate between clinical practice guidelines and critical pathways, to define what constitutes a good clinical practice guideline, to discuss how to implement clinical practice guidelines, to review their efficacy, and to outline their value in quality improvement efforts.

WHAT IS A CLINICAL PRACTICE GUIDELINE?

A clinical practice guideline is a coherently sequenced set of recommendations that tightly links specific information sources with specific information uses as it relates to health care delivery[4] (Table1).   In general, a guideline provides in a single monograph a convenient summary of the existing medical literature on a particular subject. Clinical practice guidelines are usually authored by experts, the medical evidence reviewed and strength of the evidence graded. The content of practice guidelines requires 3 interrelated descriptors of content: care process, disease severity and timeliness. In particular, the goal of describing the process of care could be paraphrased as doing the right thing at the right time.[5]

While often thought by some to be synonymous with clinical practice guidelines, care maps and critical pathways are different. As shown in Table 2, a care plan is a guideline that details the usual sequence of decisions and the nature

Table 1

Information Needs	↔	Clinical Practice Guideline	↔	Information Sources
-Patient care -Patient education -Care documentation -Care refinement -Care process assessment -Outcomes -Guideline assessment		Recommendations linking specific medical information sources and needs		-Clinical studies -Practice experience -General knowledge -Clinical databases -Results of prior guideline use

JACC 1997; 29: 1125-79

and duration of services for a defined episode of care, a critical pathway is a core set of decisions and services described in an appropriate sequence and schedule most likely to effect an efficient, coordinated program of treatment (Table 2). Both care plans and critical pathways are directed towards improving efficiency and decreasing costs.

Table 2

Definitions

Guideline
   A related set of generalizations derived from past experience arranged in coherant structure facilitate appropriate responses to specific situations
Care Plan
   A clinical practice guideline detailing the usual sequence of decisions and nature and duration of services for a defined episode of care
Critical Pathway
   The core set of decisions and services described in an appropriate sequence and schedule most likely to effect an efficient, coordinated program of treatment.

JACC 1997; 29: 1125-79

STEPS IN CLINICAL PRACTICE GUIDELINE DEVELOPMENT

Several authors have addressed the various ways of developing clinical practice guidelines.[5]   These are summarized in Table 3. Each step is important if the guideline is to be effective. As in most enterprises, having clear goals at the outset is a strong determinant of what the effect of the guideline will have. Goals need to be prioritized, often with the help of experts. An extensive review of the literature is always necessary. This stage is often overlooked in guidelines sponsored by managed care groups. However, the aim should be to develop evidence based guidelines that work for the best interest of the patient. Failure to find an evidence based review in a clinical practice guideline should be treated with a great deal of skepticism. Next, a consensus process should be established and described. There are three common methods of consensus development:[6] nominal group technique, the Delphi process and finally the Rand modification of the Delphi. Finally, guidelines need to be tested and revised.

Table 3. Guides for guidelines

Guidelines programs	Guidelines projects
• Define goals • Set priorities • allocate resources • Monitor impact	• Plan • Develop • Validate • Report • disseminate • Implement • Maintain

Can Med Assoc J 1993; 148 (4): 507-512

GUIDELINE IMPLEMENTATION

While guideline development appears arduous, guideline implementation has proven to be the most perplexing. Little research exists on the best way to implement a guideline and under what circumstances. Various methodologies have been identified each with varying degrees of success. The major categories of interventional strategies are education and direct physician interaction.[7]

I. *Educational Strategies*
  a.) Physician mailing
  Mass mailing of clinical practice guidelines has been used but the published experience has demonstrated limited success.
  b.) Face to face consultation
  This strategy (sometimes referred to as "academic detailing") is a rather involved and expensive intervention that involves several steps. First, surveys are conducted to determine physician knowledge, motivation for change and barriers to implementation of practice guidelines. Efforts are then targeted to categories of physicians whose practice patterns are at most variance with the guideline in question. The intervention is best performed by a respected physician-leader. The guideline should be presented in an authoritative but balanced way. Controversial issues should discussed candidly. Two way discussion should be encouraged. Very little evidence exists on the effectiveness of this method. However, one study suggested that this approach could increase the rate of trials of labor by 46%.[8]
  c.) Opinion Leaders
  While cheaper than an academic counter detailing program, the identification of influential opinion leaders had yet to be rigorously tested and proven to be an effective interventional tool.

II. *Directed Physician Interaction*
  a.) Retrospective Feedback
  Individual physician feedback is usually achieved by medical record audit. Published reviews have suggested that results are best if these reviews are performed by physician leaders, if there is an action plan that can be utilized by the physician and if small group discussion occurs.
  b.) Practice Profiling
  The best example in cardiology of practice profiling has been the publication by the New York State Department of Health of mortality rates from coronary artery surgery.[9,10] Published since 1989, mortality rates have decreased. The reasons for reduction in adjusted mortality rates are not altogether clear. It has been suggested that increased coding of comorbid conditions and referral of high risk patients out of state may, in part be responsible, but there is evidence that low volume operators are performing less surgery. One great limitation of patient profiling is that individual physician numbers of procedures may be too few to generate narrow confidence limits making this approach more applicable to systems than individual physician practices.
  c.) Real time strategies
  These strategies have proven to be the most useful means of implementing clinical practice guidelines. There are two methodologies that are commonly used, guideline reminders and critical pathways. Guideline reminder systems[11-13] provide convenient summaries of clinical practice guidelines made available to the practicing physician at the time of diagnosis, or after a critical physician order or after a critical test result. The reminders can be administered by utilization management, nursing coordinators or by electronic hospital information systems.

THE EFFECT OF CLINICAL PRACTICE GUIDELINES ON CLINICAL PRACTICE AND PATIENT OUTCOME

There have been a number of papers that have looked at the effectiveness of clinical practice guidelines. Some of these have looked at resource limitation, often reflected by length of stay, while others have looked at physician compliance with guidelines. Relatively few have looked at patient outcome. Two studies have demonstrated that clinical pathways have reduced length of stay in cardiovascular disease. One study [14] demonstrated that clinical pathways reduced length of stay by over 3 days and reduced costs by 14 % after coronary bypass grafting. A second study[15] demonstrated reduced length of stay after surgery for congenital heart disease.

Davis et al[16] reported a systematic review of the effectiveness of clinical practice guidelines. They looked at the influence of Continuing Medical Education activities, academic detailing, patient mediated strategies, audit with feedback and reminder systems. Ninety-nine trials testing 160 interventions were identified. Two-thirds of these studies demonstrated improvement in at least 1 major outcome. Seventy percent demonstrated changes in physician performance. Of all the strategies studied, guideline reminders were most effective producing improvements in 22 of 26 studies. Patient mediated strategies, outreach visits and academic detailing were also effective. The least effective were audit with feedback (10 studies +, 14 -), distributing educational materials (only 4/11 +) and CME conferences were the least effective. This review also demonstrated that multiple interventions were even more effective. Sixty-four studies using 2 interventions were effective and 79 % using 3 interventions were effective. Another review performed by Grimshaw[17] also demonstrated that 9 of 11 studies (Table 4) that looked at patient outcome showed improvement and 55 of 59 showed improvement in the process of patient care.

HOW DO YOU JUDGE THE VALIDITY OF CLINICAL PRACTICE GUIDELINES ?

Whether you are a physician, a quality assurance coordinator or a health care administrator, clinical practice guidelines are taking on increasing importance in day to day work life. The quality of clinical practice guidelines varies greatly. Some guidelines developed by health care consultants having little foundation in evidence based medicine. The best of those developed by either federal agencies or peer group organizations are heavily on the medical evidence, externally reviewed by independent experts and tested in real-life situations.

There are some useful tips to keep in mind when assessing how guidelines might affect the care of the average patient.[2, 29] The first tip is to determine whether the recommendations are evidence based. based. It is very useful if the strength of the medical evidence has been objectively graded. Several grading systems have

Table 4. Studies of effect of guidelines on patient outcome

Author (s) (years)*	Effects on outcome of care
Sanzaro and Worth[18]	No significant change
Hopkins et al[19]	Patient requiring ventilation reduced by 19% (33% to 14%)
Linn[20]	Early complications in patients admitted to study hospital reduced by 15% (45% to 30%) and patient non-compliance after 2 wks in study hospitals reduced by 5% (10% to 5%)
Barnett et al[21]	After 2 yrs patients with diastolic BP < 100 mm Hg or on treatment increased by 18% (52% to 70%)
Thomas et al[22]	No significant change
McDonald et al[23]	Patients eligible for pneumococcal or influenza vacinnation suffered fewer winter hospitalizations and emergency room visits during years with influenza epidemics
McAlister et al[24]	In newly detected hypertensives number of days per year with diastolic BP < 90 mmHg increased by 19% (from 255 to 323)
Wilson et al[25]	Patients who reported not smoking after one year increased by 4.4% (4.4 to 8.8%)
Cohen SJ et al[26]	Patients not smoking after 1 yr increased by 8.4% (2.7% to 11.1%)
Cummings et al[27]	Patients not smoking after 9 mo increased by 1.1% (1.5% to 2.6%) (not significant); motivated patients not smoking after 9 mo increased by 2.2% (1.7% to 3.9%)
North of England Study[28]	Developing (but not receiving) internal guidelines improved patient outcomes for only one of the five study conditions (recurrent wheezy chest) including: patient compliance increased by 14% (79% to 91%) and patient breathlessness decreased by 40% (4.2 to 1.7 days/mo)

Lancet 1993; 342:1320

been promulgated for this purpose. Essentially, the highest grade is based on high quality randomized controlled clinical trials with sufficient power (in the case of a single trial) or with homogeneity (in the case of multiple trials) of results. Weaker evidence is based on heterogeneous trials and prospective trials. One should also ask whether the primary objectives of the guideline the same as your objectives. For instance, a guideline developed by insurers may draw different conclusions about the medical evidence or a different views about its importance than the practitioner. Finally, one should ask whether the guidelines are applicable to the individual patient.

As discussed below, improving a health care process as suggested by clinical guidelines is based first on understanding the process, defining, measuring and analyzing process indicators, and implementing changes in the process for subsequent measurement of improvement. Intertwined with this idea of process improvement is an understanding of what quality health care and outcomes management are. The concepts can be related. Outcomes measurement is best served when it uses the techniques of statistical control of processes (a central tool of quality assessment and improvement).

Quality Of Care

Any definition of quality of health care involves a description of the efficacy and appropriateness of care.[30] Quality improvement is aimed at improving the general level of standard medical practice. Quality assessment identifies and corrects serious failures in care and creates an environment of attentive care. The most contemporary models of quality improvement, which have been championed for industry by Deming,[31] are based on the premise that inspection is an inadequate method for quality improvement and that problems are deep rooted within the system of health care. Therefore, the system and processes of health care must be studied and understood. Variations of the processes of care must be clarified and classified as resulting from special causes (isolated problems), or common causes intrinsic to the system giving rise to stable variation. Understanding the processes of health care is difficult but critical to these models.

Outcome Management

In order for a hospital or a unit to analyze its performance, it must be prepared to analyze and evaluate patient outcomes and costs.[32, 33] However, its focus must shift away from centering this analysis around a single or individual episode of patient care towards patient- or disease-specific processes. In this way, institutions can evaluate the factors that are influencing cost, separate the direct and indirect costs by patient acuity and diagnosis, and bring the processes under statistical control.

Implicit in this discussion is a need to eliminate barriers between clinical and administrative computing. Management of services should be developed along a product line which is multidisciplinary rather than departmentally based. These assumptions have significant impact on the hospital information system, discussed below.

MEASURING OUTCOMES

The measurement of outcomes is integral to both cost containment and maintaining or improving cost-effectiveness. It is the major tool of analysis for evaluation, strategic planning, and quality improvement. Table 5 list the widely recognized elements of the data collection.[32] Describing patients in terms of their demographics, risk factors, and disease would appear to be obvious. Assessment of patient acuity can be extremely helpful and scoring systems now exist that have been prospectively evaluated.[34, 35] Both APACHE II[33, 36-39] and III have been advocated.[40] Their value as a predictive instruments depends on the disease process, but disease and acuity should be coupled in a predictive model. Quantifying acuity on the basis of nursing intensity has also been used.[33, 41]

Table 5. Data Elements Required to Measure Outcomes
Patient demographics
Patient risk factors (disease-specific)
Patient acuity (TISS,APACHE II or III)
Procedural data (disease-specific)
Administrative data
Insurance descriptors
DRG or case-mix measures
Admission descriptors (LOS, surgery, etc.)
Outcome Data
Short-term (pre-discharged)
Quality of care (health outcome)
Mortality
Morbidity
Quality of service (patient satisfaction)
Cost of service
Charges vs. Actual costs
Departmental/subaccount charges
Lost work time, lost earnings
Long-term
Survival
Subsequent physiologic events/complications
Subsequent treatment/resource use
Patient functional status
Patient reported sense of well-being
TISS = Therapeutic Intervention Scoring System
APACHE = Acute Physiologic Assessment and Chronic Health Evaluation
DRG = diagnosis-related group
LOS = Length of stay

(From Calvin JE: Balancing cost considerations and quality of care. In Parrillo JE and Bone RC, editor: Critical Care Medicine Principles of diagnosis and management, St. Louis, 1995, Mosby)

Fiscal data including charges, costs, and insurers must be merged with both descriptive data and clinical data. The latter should include outcomes (morbidity, mortality, physiologic derangement, quality of life), patient satisfaction, and resource utilization.

It is important that the institution develop its own strategy to collect this information completely and accurately and use adequate software and hardware to support the necessary analysis. In general, a relational database accessible by standard query language is recommended so that analysis can be directed along disease-specific lines.

A general model for auditing a critical care unit was proposed by Byrick and Caskennette[33] (Figure 1). Although implementation costs were significant, the operating cost was under $10,000 per year.

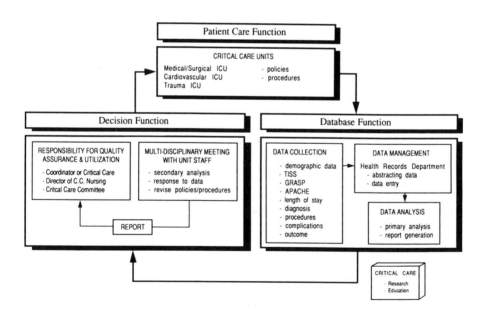

Figure 1. A schematic representing the functions of the "audit cycle," which involves administrative responsibility, data collection, management, and theanalysis procedure. Critical care research and education are also supported and enhanced by this "audit cycle." *(From Byrick RJ, Caskennette GM: Audit of cirical care: aims, uses, costs and limitations of a Canadian system, Can J Anaesth 39:260, 1992; with permission.)*

ASSESSING QUALITY

W. Edwards Deming has been called the Father of the New Industrial Age and the Founder of the New Economics Era. His visits to Japan in 1950 had tremendous influence in their emphasis on quality and the application of statistical principles to assess it.[31]   Although this approach has been most widely applied to manufacturing in post-war Japan, it has been more commonly practiced in North America in the last decade.   Although the principles Deming[31] espoused were developed in particular for manufacturing, they can be easily applied to health care

Deming's approach focused less upon managing and rewarding by results and more upon improving quality of the product and the manufacturing processes.   In health care, the product really is a process leading to a favorable outcome; therefore the quality and cost effectiveness of patient care can be analyzed using statistical techniques that Deming espouses.

The basic principle of the statistical approach to quality assessment and management is to assess variation in outcome measurements that are felt to be meaningful.   Variation can result from: *common* causes and *special* causes. Common cause variation reflects the overall sum of small variations inherent to the process and determines the limits and capabilities of current operation. As an example, measurement of length of stay can be summarized for a given diagnosis each quarter. This summary provides an average number of days that are inherent for treating a specific condition and its standard deviation (SD). If the length of stay in general is too long, independent of time period, common causes of variation must be sought out and analyzed so that it can be reduced. Large variability, suggested by a large SD, is readily identified as a problem requiring analysis.

In contrast, a large difference in complication rates between time periods may indicate special cause variations which are not part of the process all the time. A large increase in the incidence of hemorrhage, for instance, may indicate problems with prescribing practices or variation in pharmaceutic preparation. These types of problems can be resolved by addressing their special causes rather than the overall process of care delivery itself.

In Figure 2 we have summarized how one can determine, hypothetically, common and special cause variations in mortality from myocardial infarction. The average mortality rate is $7.2 \pm 1.5\%$ (mean ± SD) for a hypothetical hospital.   Two observations can be made using such analysis. First, the overall mortality rate can be compared to currently published mortality rates for myocardial infarction. If the hospital's overall mortality is consistent with or better than currently reported mortalities, the level of care is probably acceptable. This is called benchmarking.

If not, common causes of variation should be analyzed, such as the variation in the frequency of use of thrombolytic therapy or other adjunctive therapy (which can be

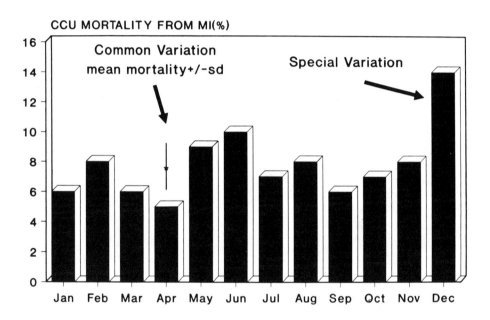

Figure 2. Demonstration of the common and special variation in myocardial infarction mortality in a hypothetical coronary care unit. (*From Calvin JE: Balancing cost considerations and quality of care. In Parrillo JE and Bone RC, editor: Critical Care Medicine: principles of diagnosis and management, St. Louis, 1995, Mosby*)

compared to recently published benchmarks), use of older technologies in monitoring, or the lack or delay in access to cardiac catheterization or cardiac surgical facilities necessary for complicated cases. Each potential issue can be each analyzed in a systematic fashion. On the other hand, if the variation in mortality is large, and particularly if an unusually high rate occurs in one time period, a special cause of variation should be sought out, identified, and corrected. Special causes of variation could be related to higher patient acuity or comorbidity, higher complication rates, or changes or breaches in existing policy or procedure, all of which should be sought out and corrected.

Measuring Quality Indicators

Health care quality can be assessed by using structural, process or outcome indicators (Table 6). Structural indicators include standards for physical plant and administrative structures.

Physical plant guidelines are frequently established by government (federal or state) or peer review organizations such as the Society of Critical Care Medicine. These guidelines cover the size of the unit, environmental controls, lighting, power, security, and preventive maintenance.

Table 6. Necessary Indicators for Quality Review and Management

Structural indicators:
   Physical plant guidelines
      Size of unit (federal guidelines exist)
      Environmental control
      Lighting
      Power source/supply
      Security
      Planned preventive maintenance
Administrative
   Departmental philosophy/mission
   Job descriptions
   Credentialing
   Role of ancillary services
   Activity levels (occupancy rates)
   Case mix
   Turnovers rates
   Absenteeism indicators
Process indicators:
   Rules/regulations
   Professional guidelines (i.e., nursing, respiratory therapy, medical staff, etc.)
   Admission/discharge criteria
   Case management guidelines (treatment, assessment, evaluation, etc.)
   Transfer guidelines (to and from critical care units)
   Investigation guidelines (i.e., routine order formats)
   Acuity scoring systems/workload management
Outcome indicators:
   Mortality/morbidity
   Timeliness of diagnosis and treatment
   Quality of life (levels improved, maintained, deteriorated)

(From Calvin JE: Balancing cost considerations and quality of care. In Parrillo JE and Bone RC, editor: Critical Care Medicine Principles of diagnosis and management, St. Louis, 1995, Mosby)

Administrative structures include the presence of a mission statement, job descriptions, credentialing, definition of roles and responsibilities, staffing requirements, ancillary services, occupancy rates, case mix, and staff turnover rates.

The quality of the process of health care which is the central theme of this discussion can be assessed by comparing specific processes of health care to clearly defined criteria or by implicitly auditing departures from a desired standard of practice based on judgments of the individual reviewer.[30] The former mechanism has many advantages. It is fair and credible. It can be applied by trained staff without a major time commitment from experts. It can judge the appropriateness of proposed interventions. Commonly, compliance with policies and procedures, rules and regulations, admission and discharge criteria, and professional guidelines is used as indicator of process. Other indicators of efficiency can include length of stay and waiting times for major investigations or interventions, which can contribute to overall cost and may either reflect or be in part responsible for complications.

Outcome indicators of quality usually include mortality; physiologic, functional, and health status outcomes; and major morbidities. Obviously the cost of care, especially when analyzed by disease-specific criteria, is a powerful means of measuring effectiveness and efficiency.

Outcome Management: The Feedback-Evaluation Loop

Once causes of variation in process indicators or outcome indicators have been ascertained and analyzed, improvement should be initiated. This requires certain organizational structures, policies and procedures. In the case of medical outcomes, it is generally part of the medical director's job description to measure the outcomes and analyze the processes involved.

Once analysis has been completed, some recommendations should follow. The use of a so-called CRAE (Conclusions, Recommendations, Action and Evaluation) report provides a structure and the necessary documentation for this process. Completion of all four sections provides a powerful tool for both quality assessment, management and improvement.

The next issue that needs to be addressed in order to make important changes in patient care is the reporting structure within the hospital. As an example, a model reporting structure is depicted in Figure 3.

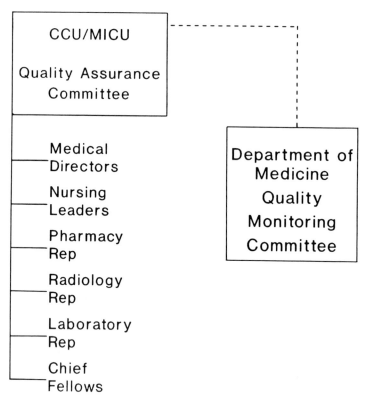

Figure 3. A model organizational structure for both quality assurance and improvement. (*From Calvin JE: Balancing cost considerations and quality of care. In Parrillo JE and Bone RC, editor: Critical Care Medicine: principles of diagnosis and management, St. Louis, 1995, Mosby*)

In this example, the directors of critical care units report to a Critical Care Quality Assurance Committee (CCQAC), which is multidisciplinary and involves the leadership of critical care. Most quality assurance issues can be resolved at this level. The CCQAC also reports to a departmental Quality Monitoring Committee to ensure adequate documentation and follow-up. These reporting structures provide the communication necessary for improvement by formalizing linkages to general medical staff, the responsible hospital departments and to other stakeholders. Without this type of communication, it would be impossible to implement change when necessary. This acknowledges that the unit is not isolated, but part of a larger entity and it is that understanding and awareness that facilitates improvement.

Improving cost-effectiveness involves more than measuring quality. Evaluating length of stay, waiting times for essential tests and procedures provide a means to analyze a hospital's efficiency. However, the need to improve efficiency is a multidisciplinary and multidepartmental task. For instance, length of stay for chest pain could be lengthened by a cardiac catheterization laboratory or exercise testing facility with an excessive waiting time. Thus, solving the problem may involve services that are external to the intensive-care unit. Therefore, the institution and its departmental directors must be committed to a process of evaluation and management that is multidisciplinary. The critical care medical director may be in a position to identify and to evaluate a problem, but solving it often will require the help, commitment and support of other services and departments.

The recent development of critical paths for patient diagnoses and treatment plans may be helpful in improving efficiency and reducing unnecessary delay especially when a case manager is part of the team.[42] This is an area of continuing interest in general. The impact of critical care treatment paths on cost of care is not yet well studied.

SUMMARY

In this chapter, general cost-containment strategies both at a macro (system) and micro (unit) level have been reviewed. These have been focused primarily on the utilization and restraint of resources, only one component of a health-care system. This chapter has also focused on the analysis of processes of care and measurement of both outcome and quality indicators as the primary means to maintain and improve outcome while containing cost in critical care.

References:

1.   Woolf, S. and H. Steven Practice Guidelines: A New Reality in Medicine. Archives of Internal Medicine 1993; 153:2646-2655.

2.   Girotti, M. and S. Brown Reducing the costs of ICU admission in Canada without diagnosis-related or case-mix groupings. Canadian Anaesthesia Society Journal 1986; 33:765-772.

3.   Gottlieb, L., C. Margolis and S. Schoenbaum Clinical Practice Guidelines at an HMO: Develpment and implementation ina quality improvement model. QRB 1990; February:80-100.

4.   Ritchie, J., J. Forrester and R. Jones 28th Bethesda Conference: Introduction. JACC 1997; 29(6):1130-1132.

5.   Jones, R., J. Ritchie and B. Fleming Task Force 1: Clinical Practice Guideline Development, Dissemination and Computerization. JACC 1997; 29(6):1133-1140.

6.   Fink, A., K. J, C. M, et al. Consensus Methods: Characteristics and Guidelines for Use. American Jounral of Public Health 1984; 74 (9):979-983.

7.   Eagle, K., T. Lee, T. Brennan, et al. 28th Bethesda Conference: Practice Guidelines and Quality of Care. JACC 1997; 29(6):1141-1147.

8.   Lomas, J., M. Enkin, G. Anderson, et al. Opinion leaders vs audit and feedback to imlement practice guidelines. Delivery after previous cesarean section. JAMA 1991; 265(17):2202-7.

9.   Hannan, E., H. Kilburn, M. Racz, et al. Improving the outcomes of coronary artery bypass surgery in New York State. JAMA 1994; 271(10):761-6.

10.   Hannan, E., A. Siu, D. Kumar, et al. The decline in coronary artery bypass graft surgery mortality in New York State. The role of surgeon volume. JAMA 1995; 273(3):209-13.

11.   McDonald, C., S. Hui, D. Smith, et al. Reminders to physicians from an introspective computer medical record: a two-year randomized trial. Annals of Internal Medicine 1984; 100:130-138.

12.   Tierney, W., S. Hui and C. McDonald Delayed feedback of physician performance versus immediate reminders to perform preventive care: effects on physician compliance. Medical Care 1986; 24:659-666.

13.   Tierney, W., J. Overhage and C. McDonald Toward electronic medical records that improve care. Annals Internal Medicine 1995; 122:725-726.

14.   Velasco, F., W. Ko, C. Roge, et al. Cost containment in cardiac surgery: results with a critical pathway for coronary bypass surgery at the New York Hospital-Cornell Medical Center. Best Practices and Benchmarking 1996; 1:21-8.

15.   Turley, K., M. Tyndall, C. Roge, et al. Critical pathway methodology: effectiveness in congential heart surgery. Ann Thorac Surg 1994; 58(1):57-63; discussion 63-5.

16.   Davis, D., M. Thomson and A. Oxman Changing Physician Performance: A systematic review of the effect of continuing medical education strategies. JAMA 1995; 274(9):700-705.

17. Grimshaw, J. and I. Russell Effect of clinical guidelines on medical practice: a systematic review of rigorous evaluations. Lancet 1993; 342:1317-22.

18. Sanzaro, P. and R. Worth Concurrent quality assurance in hospital care. N Engl J Med 1978; 298:1171-77.

19. Hopkins, J., W. Shoemaker, S. Greenfield, et al. Treatment of surgical emergencies with and without an algorithm. Arch Surg 1980; 115:745-50.

20. Linn, B. Continuing medical education: Impact on emergency room burn care. JAMA 1980; 244:565-70.

21. Barnett, G., R. Winickoff, M. Morgan, et al. A computer-based monitoring system for follow-up of elevated blood pressure. Med Care 1983; 21:400-09.

22. Thomas, J., A. Moore and P. Qualls The effect on cost of medical care for patients treated with an automated audit system. J Med Syst 1983; 7:307-13.

23. McDonald, C., S. Hui, D. Smith, et al. Reminders to physician rom an introspective computer medical record: A two year randomized trial. Ann Intern Med 1984; 1984(100):130-38.

24. McAlister, N., H. Covvey, C. Tong, et al. Randomised controlled trial of computer assisted management of hypertension in primary care. BMJ 1986; 293:670-4.

25. Wilson, D., D. Taylor, R. Gilbert, et al. A randomized trial of family physician intervention for smoking cessation. JAMA 1988; 260:1570-74.

26. Cohen, S., M. Weinberger, S. Hui, et al. The impact of reading on physicians non adherence to recommended standards of medical care. Soc. Sci Med 1985; 21:909-14.

27. Cummings, S., T. Coates, R. Richard, et al. Training physicians in counsellilng about smoking cessation: a randomized trial of the "Quit for Life" program. Ann Intern Med 1989; 110:640-47.

28. North, o. England, S.o. Standards, et al. Medical audit in general practice: Effects on doctors' clinical behaviour and the health of patients with common childhood conditions. BMJ 1992; 304:1480-88.

29. Daly, B., E. Rudy, K. Thompson, et al. Development of a special care unit for chronically critically ill patients. Heart & Lung 1991; 20 (1):45-51.

30. Group, H.S.R. Quality of care: 1. What is quality and how can it be measured? Canadian Medical Association Journal 1992; 146:2153-2158.

31. Deming, W., Out of the Crisis. 1986, Cambridge, Mass: MIT, Center for Advanced Engineering Study.

32. Lansky, D., Hospital-based outcomes management: enhancing quality of care with coorindated data systems., in Proceedings: Symposium on Computer Applications in Medical Care, Nov.5-8 1989., L. Kingsland, Editor. 1989, Institute of Electrical and Electronic Engineers: New York. p. 732-736.

33. Byrick, R. and G. Caskennette Audit of critical care: aims, uses, costs and limitations of a Canadian system. Canadian Journal of Anaesthesia 1992; 39:260-269.

34.   Lemeshow, S., D. Teres, J. Avrunin, et al. Refining intensive care unit outcome prediction by using changing probabilities of mortality. Critical Care Medicine 1988; 16:470-477.

35.   Lemeshow, S., D. Teres, J. Avrunin, et al. A comparison of methods to predict mortality of intensive care unit patients. Critical Care Medicine 1987; 15:715-722.

36.   Knaus, W., E. Draper, D. Wagner, et al. APACHE II: A severity of disease classification system. Critical Care Medicine 1985; 13:818-829.

37.   Chang, R.W., S. Jacobs and B. Lee Predicting outcome among intensive care unit patients using computerized trend analysis of daily APACHE II scores corrected for organ system failure. Intensive Care Medicine 1988; 14:558-566.

38.   Kruse, J.A., M.C. Thill-Baharozian and R.W. Carlson Comparison of clinical assessment with APACHE II for predicting mortality risk in patients admitted to a medical intensive care unit. Journal of American Medical Association 1988; 260:1739-1742.

39.   Jacobs, S., R.W. Chang and B. Lee Audit of intensive care: A 30 month experience using the APACHE II severity of disease classification system. Intensive Care Medicine 1988; 14:558-566.

40.   Knaus, W.A., D.P. Wagner, E.A. Draper, et al. The APACHE III prognostic system: Risk prediction of hospital mortality for critically ill hospitalized adults. Chest 1991; 100:1619-1636.

41.   Cullen, D. Results and costs of intensive care. Anesthesiology 1977; 47:203-216.

42.   Moher, D., A. Weinberg, R. Hanlon, et al. Effects of a medical team coordinator on length of hospital stay. Canadian Medical Association Journal 1992; 146:511-515.

15

INFORMATION SYSTEM REQUIREMENTS

William S. Weintraub, MD
Emory University, Atlanta, GA

INTRODUCTION

Clinical databases have been used in cardiovascular medicine at leading institutions such as Duke University for over 25 years (1). In recent years clinical databases have become much more popular for a variety of reasons. The first issue to consider when deciding on whether to develop a clinical database in an institution or cooperatively between institutions is the reason for having the database in the first place. Failure to articulate the reason for the database may result in the development of a database that will not meet the needs of the institution or cooperative group. Another critical point when considering databases is to identify the primary unit for analysis. Generally in clinical databases this is a patient. Remarkably, large databases have been developed in which a patient cannot be recognized. Databases require careful design and adequate resources. A sloppy design and inadequate resources generally will result in a database that cannot be maintained. Finally, dedication to accurate and complete data collection is essential. Each of these issues, as well as several others, will be considered in detail.

The Purpose of a Clinical Database

Databases are often created without adequate consideration of what the database might be used for. Generally there are several aims, some of which might act in synchrony and some in conflict. A clinical database may be used to create daily reporting such as admission notes, catheterization and angioplasty reports, discharge summaries and letters to referring physicians. These are worthwhile goals, and help ensure local participation. By themselves these goals are probably inadequate to justify the database as computerized notes have not been shown to be either less expensive or better than dictation. In addition, the data collection needed to create clinical reporting is probably more extensive than is needed for outcome reporting. If the database is used for other purposes, the additional expense and extra data points needed may be warranted if this helps data collection. A related operational use of a clinical database is to provide on-line availability of data. In this regard the database forms part of an electronic medical record that may be made widely available. This may be of great value, and the datasets needed should be quite congruent with those needed for daily reporting. Additional, user-friendly, software will be necessary to make the data available to clinicians with varying degrees of computer sophistication. Using a clinical database for daily reporting and to provide ready access to patient data in a clinical setting requires that data capture be kept up-to-date.

Essentially all other uses of data involve some form of outcome reporting concerning grouped data. Types of outcome reporting include internal quality assurance and/or continuous quality improvement, understanding and control of local finances, local research efforts, and participation in various local, regional or national registries. While the data sets needed for these efforts will be less than are needed for clinical reports, various organizations requesting data may have different requirements, making it difficult to respond to all needs. There is an ongoing activity of the American College of Cardiology Database Committee to try to standardize this type of activity. Data collected for outcome reporting must be complete, within some pre-defined bounds. In this regard more extensive data collection for daily reporting may result in less complete data collection and thus interfere with outcome reporting.

Institutional Culture and Organizational Structure

Perhaps the biggest obstacle to the creation of a clinical database is to overcome cultural barriers within an institution. Medical institutions are all complex, and institutions vary. When deciding to develop a clinical database in a catheterization laboratory, it is necessary to decide who will run the database. It may be run by the hospital information services department, the catheterization laboratory administrative staff, the interventional cardiologists or other cardiologists on the staff. In any case, it will be necessary to assure wide by-in by a broad group of people including the hospital personnel and cardiology staff. In addition, the clinical leadership and hospital leadership must be behind the effort or it will falter. The risks are both that there will not be adequate financial support as well lack of cooperation in data collection if a broad by-in is not achieved. The clinical database will have to be coordinated with other clinical computing activities and should not duplicate what is already being done. In addition the database will need to be placed on a sound financial footing. It is necessary to recognize that the database will always be a cost center and cannot be expected to be a source of revenue. The economic justification for most databases is substantiated in the ways they are able to provide information that allows the physicians and hospitals to obtain, sustain and enhance programs that generate revenue for the organization. A detailed business plan for the data center should, at least in principle, be in place prior to its creation.

As the institutional barriers are being overcome, it will also be necessary to develop a sound internal administrative structure. The database will need both clinical and administrative champions as well a dedicated and probably full time leadership. The size of the staff that will be needed will depend on the goals of the database, size of the institution and ability to build the database into the clinical care process.

Personnel Requirements

Once the institutional and cultural hurdles are overcome, leadership and staff are required to make the effort successful. The clinical leadership is essential and it must be recognized that this is a process which will require a considerable and sustained time commitment, although this can be less than full time. The leader of the effort should be a clinician who is able to garner the respect of colleagues as well as the support of the overall clinical leadership. The leader of this effort cannot be an individual acting alone as in such a situation the constant support and cooperation that is needed will not be forthcoming. The other skill sets which are required are management, computer science, biostatistics and office support staff. Generally the clinical leader of a database effort will be a physician with neither the training nor inclination to act as manager. The manager may be a full time position in a larger institution or part time in a smaller one.

Computer science support is essential. If the database is going to be built entirely with commercial software, then some part time local support from the hospital information system department may prove satisfactory. If, at the other extreme, a deeper informatics solution is required in which the computerized reporting and data availability is built into the day to day structure of practice, then a considerable dedicated programming staff may be required.

Data outcome reporting may be limited to stored programs provided by a software vendor or comprehensive, detailed reporting with considerable ad hoq. In the former case, there may be no need for biostatistical staff. In the latter case a biostatistical staff led by a doctorally prepared biostatistician with one or more masters level people may be appropriate.

If data collection is built into care, then there may be no need for dedicated data collection personnel. In other situations data center staff may be required for data collection. Similarly, if data entry into the computer is built into the process of care, then special personnel may not be needed. However, if the data center will have data input responsibilities, then dedicated data entry personnel may be necessary.

Most sites with databases ignore followup. This can be a mistake after considerable resources have already been expended. A small, dedicated followup staff can turn an in-hospital database into a longitudinal database of much greater value and interest.

Database Scope and Depth

Clinical databases in cardiovascular medicine have most often focused around cardio-thoracic surgery, catheterization and catheter based coronary intervention (2,3,4). Other procedural areas such as electrophysiology, nuclear cardiology and echocardiography are suitable for databases. Process of care areas such as acute myocardial infarction (5,6), heart failure and medical management may also be of interest. Many institutions see the goal as trying to ultimately establish a comprehensive database at least for cardiovascular medicine in which patient care as a whole can be covered. To date there is probably no cardiovascular clinical database which has accomplished this broad goal. In any case, it is generally better to succeed first in a narrowly defined area, such as the catheterization laboratory plus cardiac surgery and then to slowly and deliberately branch into other areas rather than to try to cover all of cardiovascular medicine at once. Proper design will allow a database developed in one area to be expanded into additional areas.

The amount of data which is required for outcome reporting is much less than for day to day reporting. This is because the amount of information required to offer an accurate clinical picture of a single individual, whether undergoing coronary surgery, angioplasty or other care, is much greater than the fields necessary to understand outcomes. If an outcomes database is the sole requirement, then a simple database solution from a commercial vendor may be satisfactory. If, on the other hand, detailed daily clinical reports are required, then a much more extensive database will be needed. Detailed clinical reports offer the clinician computerized reports, and decrease dictation and transcription. However, detailed clinical reporting can greatly increase the burden of data collection. An understanding of the local institutional culture and data needs is necessary to may the decision on depth of clinical data collection.

Similarly, financial data can be collected in a simple fashion or in great depth. The simplist is length of hospital stay, which in almost all studies correlates will with hospital cost. All reasonable database efforts should be able to collect this simple variable. Beyond this, it is possible to collect hospital bills and determine overall costs (see below). It is also possible to collect detailed resource utilization, such as time in the catheterization laboratory and equipment utilization. Staff time can also be measured. Once again, a decision on depth of data collection must reflect informational needs and ability to collect the information. A particularly difficult area is professional resource utilization. This is generally not included in the hospital bill, and thus many studies ignore professional costs. Effort to account for professional costs and to integrate these costs fully with hospital costs remain experimental. A major effort to use the Resource Based Relative Value Scale to account for all professional costs for episodes of care is underway at Emory University (7).

Coordinating a Clinical Database With Hospital Information Systems

Although historically hospitals have had very weak information systems, this is beginning to change. While the medical industry still lags behind many others, a clinical database will no longer be developed in an institution where there are no other clinical computer systems. Some institutions will have systems that will relate to a cardiovascular database quite directly. This may create both opportunities as well as problems. There may be order entry systems, computerized care maps, laboratory systems, ATD (admission, transfer, discharge), dictation systems, laboratory systems, global registrations systems and clinical repositories. A clinical repository is a relatively poorly defined term generally meaning a database with information of varying sorts not having the controlled definitions and fields of a clinical database. Clinical repositories often contain a lot of information in the form of text, such as admission notes and discharge summaries. A clinical repository may have some conflicting goals with a clinical database. An important point that is often overlooked in the zeal to collect data is that parallel data collection efforts in which multiple groups collect overlapping data is a waste of precious resources and generally leads to poor quality data compared to a more cooperative integrated effort.

Care maps offer different challenges and opportunities. Care maps are often developed by multidisciplinary teams with the goal of streamlining services and controlling costs. A related goal is the computerization of guidelines. Guidelines generally are concerned with larger, often more scholarly considerations about the appropriateness of care than care maps. Efforts to combine clinical databases with care maps and guidelines are just beginning at a number of institutions and by several software companies. The goals of clinical databases, care maps and guidelines may differ sufficiently that close coordination may be difficult.

Hospitals have long kept financial records on computers. The simplest data set is ATD (admissions, transfers, discharges). Interaction with the ATD computer (or global registration system if there is one) can obviate the need for separate registration. This assumes that the primary unit of consideration, the patient, can be identified. Hospitals also create bills that may be of interest to people running the clinical database. Most non-federal hospitals in the United States create a form of the hospital bill called the UB-92. The charges on the bill may be reduced to cost, using either whole institution or departmental cost to charge ratios, permitting assessment of the relationship of clinical activities to cost if these financial data are incorporated into the clinical database (8).

One of the best services a hospital can provide is access to an intranet in the institution and the internet outside the institution. The intranet will permit multiple computers to access the data in the clinical database, as long as the database computer is on the network and has appropriate software.

Software Considerations

The choice of software depends on what the goals of the database are. If the goals are only to collect data for outcome reporting, then the software can be relatively simple. Software aimed at daily reporting will need to be more sophisticated, but can then readily used to collect data for outcome reporting as well. Software aimed at offering ready access at multiple locations, including remote locations, poses additional software needs. There are multiple commercial firms offering database software. In addition, multiple institutions have developed software locally for their database and reporting needs. The choice of developing software locally or buying commercial software needs to be based on needs assessment and financial considerations. It will generally be less expensive to buy commercial software than to develop it, but commercial software may not be suitable for complex clinical environments. Software development is a time consuming process. The most important consideration is to be quite clear on what is to be collected.

Clinical databases are generally oriented around the patient. This is by its very nature what is called in the database world a hierarchical design. However, almost all database software today is relational, which means that there are separate sets of data (called tables) for different categories of activities (such as catheterization and discharge) without a prearranged relationship between the tables. It is necessary to impose a patient oriented hierarchy on top of the relational tables to make the database patient oriented. Thus, all tables should relate to an enrollment or registration table. The data in a clinical database can largely be collected in defined fields (such as is hypertension present, yes or no). Such a database can have a very simple design for its user interface (called character cell). However most contemporary software uses a graphical user interface (GUI) in which most operations can be controlled with a mouse. GUI's are easier to use, to look at and provide a relatively straight forward path to integration of multiple applications (such as database activities, graphical display and word processing), but add considerably to software development. No matter what the goals and choice of vendor or local development, the user interface will almost certainly be a GUI and the back end will almost certainly be a relational database.

The other software concern is the ability to query and report grouped data. Database software has highly variable ability to access data and provide grouped reporting. The standard querying language for relational databases is called SQL. The most limited form of query is to write SQL code in a scripting or programming language. To simplify this process, some database management systems use pointing and clicking with a mouse to develop SQL code. This is relatively simple to do, with a reasonable learning curve. However, such queries are relatively limited. Other databases use more difficult but also more powerful scripting languages, sometimes called 4gl's (for Fourth Generation Language), to manipulate data as it is retrieved from the database with embedded SQL statements. The choice of method to query the database will depend on the skill of those querying the database and the complexity of the queries needed.

To turn data retrieved from the database into useful information it is generally necessary to have a path to reporting. This will generally involve the use of a major statistical package as well as word processing and presentation software. A well constructed environment will permit virtually seamless query, statistical analysis and the development of outcome reporting.

Hardware Considerations

Historically hardware considerations were a major concern because there was an up front fee to buy a computer that might have amounted to several hundred thousand dollars before anything else was purchased. With the decline in computer hardware prices and vast improvements in performance this is much less of a concern. In general it is difficult to overbuy on the power of a computer. Buying a more expensive computer generally has the principle effect of prolonging its useful life and thus paying for itself. It is possible to construct a clinical database on a computer running almost any commercial operating system including Windows or NT, Apple and Unix. Each has its distinct advantages and disadvantages that must be weighed and evaluated in each specific location. Local database needs will be quite important. For instance a very large institution or group of institutions may choose Unix for its power, stability and scalability. A small institution may choose Apple for its simplicity and ease of use. An institution may choose Windows or NT for it ubiquitous availability and familiarity. The hardware chosen should accommodate the software chosen and also fit into the organization and existing computer infrastructure.

Patient Identification, Confidentiality and Security

As has been stated above, clinical databases, by their very nature, are patient oriented. Procedures are performed on patients who have histories, physical exams and who have other things happening to them. Failure to properly identify patients will result in a database that is not useful. Proper software design can readily overcome this problem if the organizational aspects are resolved. Patient identification requires within the database a unique identifier such as the social security number or medical record number. Whatever number is used, great care must be made in collecting and entering this number accurately and consistently.

Correction of errors is also a never ending problem. This may best be accomplished in institutions which use a unique identifier. Such institutions may also be best able to identify patients from the ATD database, avoiding reregistration. However, many institutions do not have a unique identifier and thus the clinical database may have to pick one of several in the institution or develop an independent identifier.

There are basically two types of identifiers: social security number and everything else. Similar numbers to the social security number will exist in most countries. The arguments in favor of the social security number is that it is relatively universal, most patients know their social security number and it may be used in multiple institutions, permitting integration of outside databases such as the National Death Index and Medicare databases (such as MEDPAR). Arguments against the social security number are that not everybody has one and that it is relatively long, leading to key stroke errors. The first argument is readily addressable as patients without a social security number (often small children) can get one, and in the mean time they can be given an assigned number. The error rate is a problem, but may be more apt to become apparent and then be corrected with the social security number than other numbers as patients often know their social security numbers or carry with them identification with the social security number. The key point is that whatever number is used, the process will have to be handled with care to preserve the integrity of the system.

An argument that is made against positive patient identification in general and about the social security number in particular is that patient confidentiality and security may be compromised. Part of the answer to this is that it does not make sense to have a database at all if this is an overriding concern. If confidentiality is a concern that is recognized but not seen to be so important as to preclude the development of the database, then it may be dealt with, although not solved. Within an institution this is less of a problem, as it is appropriate and necessary to be able to identify a patient for patient care. Nonetheless, even within an institution there may be concerns about inappropriate access to patient data. While within an institution access may be controlled, it must be wide enough for the care givers to be able to function and use the database appropriately. Access that is too restrictive may compromise the functioning of the database. Access that is not restrictive enough may risk the loss of patient confidentiality for no gain in information or quality of care.

Outside the boundaries of an institution the problems of confidentiality and security are murkier. Access to data distributed outside an institution may be more limited, as it will not be necessary for day to day care. Nonetheless, there will be concern because an institution sharing patient identifiers with outside databases will not be able to control what is done with the data and there may be a perception of legal vulnerability. Cooperative databases seeking identifiers may offer a contract to participating institutions stating that identifiers will not be shared except as part of a process of discovery in a court of law. This is relatively good protection if the outside database is run by a responsible organization well known to the participating institution. In the end some privacy must be lost to permit the construction of useful cooperative databases. Security can be guaranteed to a much greater extent than confidentiality through the use of encryption. Data may be encrypted by scrambling it such than it cannot be read without the appropriate key. By limiting access to the key to appropriate people, security may be largely, although not absolutely assured.

Data Dictionaries and Data Standards

Data in databases can only be useful if the data elements are carefully defined. For instance, there may be somewhat variable definitions of unstable angina. If there is not one definition used in the collection of the data, it is not possible to consistently establish, for example, the prevalence of stable versus unstable angina in patients undergoing angioplasty. For this reason it is an intrinsic part of database design to define all variables in a data dictionary. The dictionary then must be made widely available to users of the database, especially those collecting the data. Most data elements in clinical databases will not be new and have been defined before. Data dictionaries are available from many clinical trial databases as well as multiple institutional and cooperative databases (see below).

Beyond data dictionaries, there is a growing recognition of the importance of developing standards for communication. This involves definitions, but also the identification of data elements that may be useful for specific tasks. An example of this is the effort to develop core elements to predict mortality after coronary surgery (9). Standard definitions and data elements should facilitate communications across different databases and permit easier interpretation of data and comparison of outcomes. In this regard the American College of Cardiology has developed a core dataset for the catheterization laboratory, which will be described in detail below.

Data Quality

It is a truism that a database is only as good as the quality of data in the database. Thus, if there is to be a database, the idea of collecting complete data on all appropriate patients must be widely accepted in the institution. Completeness is, in principle, a simple idea, but may be hard to achieve unless the database is built carefully into the structure of clinical medicine. Thus, if the database is used for daily reporting and there is no other path, this will help data collection. On the other hand, it is much easier to collect a small dataset than a large one (the term that is often used is a parsimonious set of data), and as noted above the dataset for daily reporting is often relatively large. One way of dealing with this issue is to have the software demand complete data for the key (or core) data elements and allow missing data in other areas. Even for daily reporting limiting the dataset to those areas of real interest is the correct thing to do.

Assuring the accuracy of collected data is more complicated. This may in principle require auditing. Certainly range checks and acceptable values may be build into the software, although is must be recognized that this will produce acceptable values, not necessarily correct ones. A logical problem presents itself if there is no independent data to audit against. If the database is used to produce medical record material including admission notes, catheterization notes, angioplasty notes and discharge summaries, then audit against the database will essentially mean using the database to audit itself. Individual institutions will have to decide for themselves what is a suitable level of audit as there is at present not standard for local databases. Audit issues for cooperative databases will be discussed below.

Outcome Reporting

Clinical databases may be used for quality assurance and continuous quality improvement on the one hand and for clinical research on the other. By using a clinical database for both types of purposes, it is possible to improve data collection and to have the two processes work synergistically. Furthermore, the information needed is much the same. That being said, clinical research is probably easier to do (albeit requiring more creativity) than routine reporting. This is because when doing clinical research it is possible to pick and choose data of interest and then to fill in gaps in the data by retrospective review. For routine reporting this may not be the case. Thus routine reporting may require greater effort to maintain complete data. Choice of software to accomplish good quality outcome reporting is essential. Properly done, much of the process can be automated and routine reports can be produced quite rapidly and reliably. However, software to accomplish such tasks may result in a steep learning curve for users.

Even more important than software is to have staff that are capable of querying the database and analyzing the data. In non-academic centers where there is not ready access to biostatisticians, this can be a major limitation. It is also necessary to be realistic about the budgetary implications of having adequate staff to analyze and interpret data. Attempts to have programming staff, who do not have a medical or analytic background, double as data analysts is dangerous, and may result in incorrect information being put before clinicians who do not understand how the data were produced. Thus, there must in the end be a responsible individual or group who can stand behind the correctness of summary data.

Once a database is in place there may be an attempt to embed randomized clinical trials (RCTs) within the database. This is possible, but it is difficult and the experience with this has been less than satisfactory. The goals of RCTs and clinical databases are different. In general when running RCTs there has to be absolute dedication to the RCT, and if the RCT is used to push a secondary agenda, there may be considerable difficulty. This is probably one area in which parallel data collection is usually the prudent choice.

Cooperative Databases

There are multiple multi-institutional databases in the United States and additional cooperative databases in other countries as well. These databases are of several types. The best know are claims databases such as those in insurance companies or the Health Care Financing Agency (the MEDPAR database). Claims databases have limited clinical data, and thus there has been interest in developing cooperative clinical databases.

There are state clinical databases for cardiovascular medicine, such as the one in New York State (10). Many states have established or are considering the establishment of a state database. These databases have the advantage that data collection can be mandated by law. They have the disadvantage of leaving physicians disenfranchised without input into the database design or reporting. Developing the infrastructure for a database may be an unrealistic burden for many states as well. There is a commercial cooperative database for the National Cardiovascular Network (NCN), where the database is used to support NCN contracting. There is the highly regarded Northern New England regional database (11), which is used for clinical outcome reporting including both clinical research and quality improvement. There are subspecialty databases such as the Society of Cardiac Angiography and Intervention (12) and the Society of Thoracic Surgeons (13) databases. These subspecialty databases are by now well known and established. Some databases were developed and the effort was abandoned when the effort was seen to be unrealistic, such as the Academic Medical Center Consortium. The last is a case in point of a database for which the data collection activities were perceived to be unrealistically complicated. All of the cooperative databases within any area, such as coronary surgery, collect similar datasets, but the datasets are not exactly the same and the definitions used vary. This can create a difficult situation for institutions seeking to participate in multiple databases.

Data quality in cooperative databases is recognized to be a major problem. In the absence of an audit, data quality in a cooperative database cannot be assured. Software that catches out of range or in valid values may be helpful, but is probably not sufficient. Thus, audit by an external review must be at least considered. Several databases, such the one from New York State, have an ongoing audit procedure. There are no agreed upon standards for audits of data in databases, and no established mechanisms for addressing infrequent events where statistically meaningful audits may be unrealistic or for situations where there is no gold standard to audit against. What is certainly possible is to audit the process of data collection and reporting from participating institutions in a cooperative database. A process audit would examine activities such as how data collection is performed, whether staffing adequate, if there is adequate documentation and if data quality is stressed. In contrast, a content audit would exam the data directly and compare it to a gold standard (usually the somewhat tarnished gold standard of the medical record).

The cardiovascular database with the broadest perspective, which may reduce some of the uncertainty and anarchy in data collection activities is the American College of Cardiology National Database Registry (14). This database has focused to date largely on cardiac catheterization and catheter based coronary intervention. However, it is within the purview of this organization and this database to look broadly across cardiovascular medicine. The American College of Cardiology will seek to encourage software development and availability which will allow participation in multiple cooperative databases. The American College of Cardiology has completed a two year process of developing a 141 element core data set with detailed coding and definitions to define the most important points concerning description of the patients, procedures and outcome of catheterization and catheter based coronary intervention. This process involved examining multiple databases, cooperating specifically with the Society of Thoracic Surgeons and the Society of Cardiac Angiography and Intervention, considering variables shown to predict outcome after angioplasty, field testing of the elements and review by a wide ranging group of cardiologists. The core elements will be updated on an annual basis, with an attempt to maintain compatibility with past data collection. The use of these core elements by multiple cooperative database may decrease the burden of responding and improve the quality of collection. This process may also facilitate communication between multiple organizations with outcome oriented databases. The American College of Cardiology Database Committee may be expected to develop, with the aid of sister societies, clear standards, core data elements and registries in broad areas of cardiovascular medicine.

CONCLUSIONS

There has now been over 25 years of experience with clinical databases in the United States. These databases have been important in understanding the clinical course, outcome and impact of therapy on cardiovascular diseases, especially coronary artery disease. The human as well as technical problems in the development of clinical databases are well understood and acknowledged. Nonetheless, cardiovascular medicine is becoming increasingly data driven and this trend may be expected to continue. Cardiovascular practitioners could shrink from the demands for data and let others evaluate outcome of care or they could become increasingly engaged in the process. Good quality databases, and where the problems are dealt with as well as they can be, where there is broad and deep clinical input and support, should be seen as vehicles for increasing our understanding and for improving cardiovascular patient care.

References:

1   Rosati RA, McNeer JF, Starmer CF, Mittler BS, Morris JJ, Wallace AG. A new information system for medical practice. Arch Intern Med 1975;135:1017.

2   Harris PJ, Harrell FE, Lee KL, Behar VS, Rosati RA. Survival in medically treated coronary artery disease. Circulation 1979;60:1259-1269.

3   Vigilante GJ, Weintraub WS, Klein LW, Schneider RM, Seelaus PA, Parr GVS, Lemole G, Agarwal JB, Helfant RH. Medical and surgical survival in coronary artery disease in the 1980's. Am J Cardiol 1986;58:926-931.

4   Talley JD, Hurst JW, King SB, Douglas JS, Roubin GS, Gruentzig AR, Anderson HV, Weintraub WS. Clinical outcome 5 years after attempted percutaneous coronary angioplasty in 427 patients. Circulation 1988;77:820-829.

5   Davis HT, DeCamilla J, Bayer LW, Moss AJ. Survivorship patterns in the posthospital phase of myocardial infarction. Circulation 1979;60:1252-1258.

6   Behar S, Gottlieb S, Hod H, Benari B, Narinsky R, Pauzner H, Rechavia E, Faibel HE, Katz A, Roth A, Goldhammer E, Freedberg NA, Rougin N, Kracoff O, Shapira C, Jafari J, Lotan C, Daka F, Weiss T, Kanetti M, Klutstein M, Rudnik L, Barasch E, Mahul N, Blondheim D, et al. The outcome of patients with acute myocardial infarction ineligible for thrombolytic therapy. Israeli Thrombolytic Survey Group. American Journal of Medicine. 1996;101:184-191.

7   Weintraub WS, Connolly S, Canup D, Deaton C, Culler S, Becker E. Total Hospital Costs for Coronary Revascularization: Hospital (UB92) and Professional (RBRVS) Components (abstr). In Press, J Am Coll Cardiol.

8   Mauldin PD, Weintraub WS, Becker E. Predicting hospital charges and costs for coronary surgery from pre-operative and post-operative variables. Am J Cardiol 1994;74:772-775.

9   Jones RH, Hannan EL, Hammermeister KE, DeLong ER, O'Connor GT, Luepker RV, Parsonnet V, Pryor DB for the Working Group Panel on the Cooperative CABG Database Project. J Am Coll Cardiol 1996;28:1478-1487.

10   Hannan EL, Sui AL, Kumar D, Kilburn HJ, Chassin MR. The decline in coronary artery bypass graft surgery mortality in New York State. The role of surgeon volume. JAMA 1995;273:209-213.

11   Malenka DJ. Indications, practice, and procedural outcomes of percutaneous transluminal coronary angioplasty in northern New England in the early 1990s. The Northern New England Cardiovascular Disease Study Group. American Journal of Cardiology. 1996;78:260-265.

12   Krone RJ, Johnson L, Noto T and the registry committee of the Society for Cardiac Angiography and Interventions. Five Year trends in Cardiac Catheterization: A report from the Registry of the Society for Cardiac Angiography and Interventions. Cathet and Cardiovasc Diagn 1996;39:31-35.

13   Edwards FH, Clark RE, Schwartz M. Coronary artery bypass grafting: the Society of Thoracic Surgeons National Database Experience. Ann Thorac Surg 1994;57:12-19.

14   Weintraub WS, McKay CR, Riner RN, Ellis SG, Frommer PL, Carmichael DB, Hammermeister K, Effros MN, Bost JE, Bodycombe DP. The American College of Cardiology National Database: Progress and Challenges. In Press, J Am Coll Cardiol.

16

MANAGEMENT OF PATIENTS WITH LIFE-THREATENING VENTRICULAR TACHYARRHYTHMIAS: FOCUS ON THE PREEMINENT ROLE OF THE IMPLANTABLE CARDIOVERTER-DEFIBRILLATOR

Sergio L. Pinski, MD
Richard G. Trohman, MD
Rush-Presbyterian-St. Luke's Medical Center, Chicago, IL

INTRODUCTION

Survivors of life-threatening ventricular tachyarrhythmias (hemodynamically unstable ventricular tachycardia or ventricular fibrillation) represent an important therapeutic target because of their high risk of arrhythmia recurrence and sudden death. The widespread availability of the implantable cardioverter-defibrillator (ICD) has revolutionized the management of these patients.[1] However, the expense and special expertise required for implantation and follow-up of this sophisticated device make the design of efficient clinical pathways for treatment of these patients crucial. In the next few years, the number of survivors of near-fatal ventricular tachyarrhythmias will increase significantly as a result of the broader utilization of automatic external defibrillators and public access defibrillation.[2] Evaluation and management of these patients (including the identification of those needing an ICD) will constitute an important public health issue that will consume significant health care resources.

RESULTS OF RANDOMIZED STUDIES

Several randomized trials have shed light on the role of different treatment strategies in patients with life-threatening ventricular tachyarrhythmias. Despite lack of strong evidence, pharmacological treatment guided by serial electrophysiological studies (EPS) (complemented by map-guided surgical ablation in selected patients) was the preferred treatment modality until the late 1980s.[3] A series of controlled studies questioned such approach. Steinbeck et al. randomized 115 patients with spontaneous sustained ventricular tachyarrhythmias inducible at EPS to therapy with antiarrhythmic drugs (guided by EPS) or empiric metoprolol and found similar outcomes in both groups.[4] The Cardiac Arrest in Seattle: Conventional versus Amiodarone Drug Evaluation (CASCADE) trial randomized 288 survivors of out-of-hospital ventricular fibrillation not associated with a Q-wave myocardial infarction to empiric treatment with amiodarone or treatment with class I antiarrhythmic drugs guided by EPS, Holter monitoring, or both. After a follow-up of 6 years, survival free of cardiac death, resuscitated ventricular fibrillation, or syncopal defibrillator shock was significantly better in the group assigned to empiric amiodarone (2 year actuarial survival: 82% versus 69%; 6 year actuarial survival: 53% versus 40%; p=0.007).[5] The Electrophysiologic Study Versus Electrocardiographic Monitoring (ESVEM) Trial randomized 486 patients with ventricular tachycardia or ventricular fibrillation to treatment with antiarrhythmic drugs guided by EPS or Holter monitoring. During long-term follow-up of the 296 patients discharged on a drug predicted to be effective, there were no differences in overall survival or arrhythmia recurrence in patients on the EPS or Holter limb.[6] In a separate analysis from the same study, arrhythmia recurrence after predicted drug efficacy by either strategy was significantly lower for patients treated with sotalol than for patients treated with the 6 class I drugs evaluated (risk ratio, 0.43; 95 percent confidence interval, 0.29 to 0.62; P < 0.001). Sotalol was associated with lower risks of death from any cause (risk ratio, 0.50; 95 percent confidence interval, 0.30 to 0.80; P = 0.004), death from cardiac causes, (0.50; P = 0.02), and death from arrhythmia (0.50; P = 0.04).[7]

These studies, together with the CAST trials (which demonstrated detrimental effects of class I agents in patients with prior myocardial infarction and ventricular ectopy),[8] led to the conclusion that the outcome of pharmacological treatment of ventricular arrhythmias depended more on the drugs administered than on the methods used to assess their efficacy. Beta-blockers, sotalol, and amiodarone emerged then as the preferred options. At approximately the same time, improvements in ICD technology (especially the advent of nonthoracotomy systems) set the stage for large multicenter randomized trials comparing pharmacologic and device therapy in patients with life-threatening ventricular tachyarrhythmias.

The final results of three such trials have become recently available. In the Antiarrhythmics Versus Implantable Defibrillators (AVID) Trial, 1,016 patients with ventricular fibrillation, documented syncopal ventricular tachycardia, or sustained ventricular tachycardia (with severe symptoms and left ventricular ejection fraction < 0.40) not due to reversible causes were randomized to receive an ICD or antiarrhythmic drugs (empiric amiodarone or guided sotalol).[9] ICD patients had better survival throughout the course of the study (unadjusted survival at 1 year: 89% versus 82%; at 3 years: 75% versus 61%; p <0.02). The corresponding reduction in death rates were 39% and 31%, respectively. The benefits of ICD therapy were consistent among prespecified subgroups categorized according to age, degree of left ventricular dysfunction, presence of coronary artery disease, or presenting rhythm.

The Cardiac Arrest Study-Hamburg (CASH) trial randomized cardiac arrest survivors to ICD implantation or treatment with propafenone, metoprolol or amiodarone. The propafenone limb was prematurely concluded when interim analyses suggested higher mortality than the ICD limb. The trial continued comparing ICDs, metoprolol and amiodarone in 288 patients. Nearly half of the ICDs were implanted by thoracotomy. Two-year mortality rate was 12.1% for the ICD arm and 19.6% for the combined arms of amiodarone and metoprolol (37% mortality reduction; one-sided p value 0.047). The sudden cardiac death rate was significantly lower in the ICD arm (2% versus 11%; p <0.001). There were no statistically significant differences in global or sudden death rates between patients randomized to amiodarone or metoprolol.[10]

The Canadian Implantable Defibrillator Study (CIDS) randomized 659 patients with resuscitated cardiac arrest, syncopal ventricular tachycardia, ventricular tachycardia (with presyncope or angina and left ventricular ejection fraction <0.36 or ventricular tachycardia rate > 150 beats per minute), and unmonitored syncope (with subsequently monitored or inducible ventricular tachycardia) to ICD implantation or treatment with empiric amiodarone. Three-year mortality rate was 25% in the ICD arm and 30% in the amiodarone arm (19.6% mortality reduction; one-sided p value 0.072).[11]

There is a remarkable concordance in the degree of benefit conferred by the ICD among these 3 studies. Although formal metanalyses have not been published, it appears safe to conclude that early use of the ICD in patients with life-threatening ventricular tachyarrhythmias results in a 20 to 30% reduction in total mortality at 2 to 3 years. The AVID trial is particularly valuable because it maintained a comprehensive registry of patients with qualifying arrhythmias seen at the participating centers. The fact that there were no significant baseline clinical differences between randomized and nonrandomized patients, and that their outcome was similar allows for the extrapolation of the main trial results to the broad population of patients with ventricular tachyarrhythmias.[12]

INDICATIONS

On the basis of the previously discussed studies, ICDs should be considered first-line therapy in patients who have survived episodes of cardiac arrest or hemodynamically significant sustained ventricular tachycardia not due to reversible causes.[13] Patients with syncope of undetermined origin in whom sustained ventricular tachycardia is induced during an EPS have a high incidence of appropriate ICD discharge,[14] and also appear to benefit from implantation.

ICDs should not be implanted in response to ventricular arrhythmias that have been triggered by acute myocardial infarction, correctable toxic or metabolic factors, or rapid atrial fibrillation complicating the Wolff-Parkinson-White syndrome. Ruling out reversible or correctable causes is an important component of the initial evaluation of patients with life-threatening ventricular tachyarrhythmias. Patients with very frequent ventricular tachycardia or fibrillation unresponsive to drugs, ablation, or antitachycardia pacing should not receive ICDs, as frequent painful shocks would be delivered. Although the low morbidity associated with current ICD implant techniques has made surgical or medical contraindications less relevant than in the past, patients with a life expectancy of less than a year are not appropriate candidates for ICD therapy. Patients awaiting cardiac transplantation have a high incidence of sudden death,[15] but the merit of the ICD as a "bridge" to transplantation is uncertain.[16]

INITIAL EVALUATION OF THE PATIENT

After their acute stabilization, patients who have suffered a life-threatening ventricular arrhythmia require a thoughtful, systematic approach to evaluate the cause and substrate of their event. They not only need evaluation of myocardial structure and function, but they need an arrhythmia specialist to plan the most appropriate form of therapy. [17]

Role of the EPS

Electrophysiological studies have been used in the diagnosis and treatment of patients with sustained ventricular tachyarrhythmias for the past two decades. Initially, EPS was used to induce ventricular arrhythmias and test the ability to reinduce them after the administration of antiarrhythmic agents. Multiple (generally unfruitful) procedures were the rule. Because the accumulated evidence suggests that the EPS has limited value to stratify the risk of recurrence in patients with sustained ventricular tachyarrhythmias[18] and ICDs provide superior outcomes than antiarrhythmic drugs, the role of routine baseline EPS in these patients needs to be carefully reevaluated. Although current ACC/AHA guidelines recommend performing a baseline electrophysiological evaluation in all survivors of cardiac arrest without evidence of acute Q wave myocardial infarction,[19] a consensus is emerging that the decision should be individualized on the basis of expected benefits, risks, and costs.

Differential Diagnosis of Wide Complex Tachycardia

A regular wide QRS complex tachycardia may represent ventricular tachycardia, supraventricular tachyarrhythmia conducted with bundle branch block or preexcited supraventricular tachyarrhythmia. Some clinical features like older age, previous history of myocardial infarction, or left ventricular dysfunction favor the diagnosis of ventricular tachycardia. Younger age and ventricular preexcitation during sinus rhythm favor supraventricular tachycardia. Several algorithms for the electrocardiographic differential diagnosis of wide complex tachycardia with good sensitivity and specificity have been proposed,[20] but their use is limited when only single-lead strips from a bedside monitor (instead of a 12-lead ECG) are available. Intravenous administration of adenosine during tachycardia may also aid in the diagnosis.[21] However, the clinical diagnosis of wide complex tachycardia is imperfect, and supraventricular tachycardia with aberrancy or preexcited supraventricular tachycardias may be mistaken for ventricular tachycardia. The EPS remains the gold standard for the differential diagnosis of regular wide QRS tachycardia, and should be used liberally whenever the clinical diagnosis is uncertain.[22]

Identification of Reversible or Correctable Causes

The EPS is also useful in the characterization of substrates and mechanisms of ventricular tachyarrhythmias that are amenable to specific therapy (including radiofrequency catheter ablation) and in which implantation of an ICD should not be considered first-line therapy (Figure 1).

Idiopathic ventricular tachycardias originating in the right or left ventricle occur in the absence of structural heart disease and have typical, easily recognized electrocardiographic patterns. Clinical recognition of these patients is important since more than 90% can be cured via catheter ablation.[23]

The optimal management of patients with structural heart disease (most often coronary artery disease with prior myocardial infarction) and hemodynamically stable sustained monomorphic ventricular tachycardia is controversial. Their risk of sudden death during antiarrhythmic drug treatment is lower than for patients with less tolerated tachyarrhythmias,[24] and depends on the underlying left ventricular function.[25] These tachycardias may also be amenable to radiofrequency catheter ablation, with success rates close to 80% in experienced hands.[26] Advances in 3 dimensional mapping techniques may improve results. Non-contact mapping catheters allow computer generation of a tachycardia map from a few beats and may facilitate ablation of some hemodynamically unstable ventricular tachycardias. However, most patients have more than one morphology of inducible tachycardia, a concomitant hemodynamically unstable tachyarrhythmia, or both. Because ischemic heart disease is an evolving substrate, most electrophysiologists prefer the comprehensive treatment and protection afforded by the ICD. Some studies have shown a relatively high incidence of shocks for rapid, potentially life-threatening ventricular arrhythmias in patients with stable ventricular tachycardia receiving ICDs.[27] Ablation is in general regarded as palliative, and reserved to reduce shock frequency in patients with drug-refractory hemodynamic stable tachycardias.[28]

Bundle branch reentry is responsible for approximately 6% of all monomorphic ventricular tachycardia. This percentage may increase to 40-50% in patients with nonischemic (dilated or valvular) cardiomyopathies. The arrhythmia should be suspected in patients with significant left ventricular dysfunction (especially of nonischemic etiology), intraventricular conduction defects, and a wide complex tachycardia with a left bundle branch block pattern (the tachycardia typically uses the right bundle branch for antegrade conduction and the left bundle branch for the retrograde limb of the reentrant circuit).[29] Definitive diagnosis and treatment can be provided during a single invasive electrophysiology session. The right bundle branch potential is easily recorded and ablated during sinus rhythm This allows for cure of the tachycardia without the need for detailed mapping during the often hemodynamically unstable tachycardia.

Interfascicular reentry is an uncommon cause of ventricular tachycardia due to reentry within the two fascicles of the left bundle branch. It may coexist with bundle branch reentry or be present as an isolated entity. Ablation of either the anterior or posterior fascicle, or the common left bundle branch can be curative, but clinical experience is very limited.[30] The risk of creating complete heat block (due to the close proximity of the ablation targets to the penetrating His bundle) or worsening the hemodynamic status (by inducing asynergic left ventricular contraction) with these procedures is not negligible. Ablative approaches to these arrhythmias should only be undertaken by experienced interventional electrophysiologists.

Because most patients with bundle branch reentry have severe left ventricular dysfunction, they are susceptible to other forms of ventricular arrhythmia. Approximately 25% of patients will have another inducible ventricular tachycardia. A comprehensive electrophysiologic evaluation aimed at ruling out concomitant "myocardial" ventricular tachycardia is necessary. Prognosis is favorable in patients with isolated bundle branch reentry tachycardia who undergo right bundle branch ablation, but patients with residual inducible or spontaneous ventricular tachycardia should be offered further therapy. Those with residual significant His-Purkinje system conduction delay (i.e., HV interval >90 ms) should be considered for permanent pacing. Most other sustained ventricular tachyarrhythmias that occur in nonischemic cardiomyopathies are difficult to induce at EPS. Hemodynamically unstable sustained ventricular arrhythmias should be managed with ICDs. Many electrophysiologists also believe that unexplained syncope (negative EPS) in these patients should also be managed with an ICD. Symptomatic nonsustained arrhythmias may be managed with amiodarone without fear of increasing mortality via proarrhythmia.

In occasional patients, true ventricular tachycardia or fibrillation is initiated by a supraventricular arrhythmia. Ventricular fibrillation resulting from the degeneration of atrial fibrillation in patients with the Wolff-Parkinson-White syndrome constitutes the classic example, but a similar circumstance can occur secondary to accelerated AV nodal conduction.[31] In most instances, the diagnosis can be documented from electrocardiographic recordings during the event or is strongly suspected (i.e., ventricular preexcitation in the ECG). Demonstration of rapid conduction via the AV node during EPS in patients with documented ventricular fibrillation and structural heart disease is of uncertain relevance. Most electrophysiologists would hesitate in limiting therapy to this target.

Supraventricular tachycardia may coexist with ventricular tachycardia and result in spurious ICD interventions. If a concomitant supraventricular tachycardia has been documented or is strongly suspected, comprehensive EPS should be performed before ICD implantation to identify its mechanism and select specific therapy (catheter ablation or pharmacological suppression). Routine use of EPS to disclose clinically unsuspected supraventricular tachyarrhythmias appears unwarranted. We have seen patients in whom clinically unsuspected AV nodal reentrant tachycardia triggered spurious ICD interventions after a standard EPS before implantation was nonrevealing. Induction of the clinical tachycardia at repeat EPS post-implant required atrial stimulation during isoproterenol infusion.

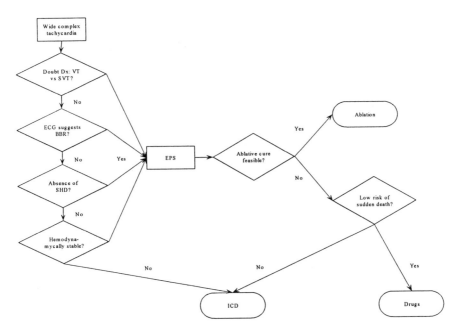

Figure 1. Algorithm for treatment of patients presenting with wide complex tachycardia. BBR: bundle branch reentry; SHD: structural heart disease.

Management of Coronary Disease

It is frequent to find severe coronary disease (with or without clinical evidence of ischemia) during the initial evaluation of patients with life-threatening ventricular arrhythmias. The optimal management of these patients is controversial. There are no prospective, randomized studies comparing the merits of myocardial revascularization, antiarrhythmic strategies (including the ICD), or their combination in this population. A few generalizations can be made on the basis of observational studies. The prognosis is good with revascularization alone in patients with ventricular fibrillation and normal left ventricular function, but patients with ventricular tachycardia, large   fixed perfusion defects, or left ventricular dysfunction remain at high risk without specific treatment. Some groups have found programmed ventricular stimulation after myocardial revascularization of value in the   risk stratification of these patients[32,33] while others reported a relative high incidence of ICD shocks in patients who were noninducible after bypass surgery.[34,35] In the past, it was common to implant an ICD (or at least the epicardial patches and leads) at time of CABG. However, this practice was associated with increased morbidity and mortality, and it is no longer recommended.

Analysis of the AVID Registry suggests that the clinical impression of a transient or correctable cause of ventricular tachycardia or fibrillation may not be accurate. Coronary artery disease was present in 81.5% of 270 patients in the AVID Registry felt to have ventricular tachycardia or fibrillation due to transient or correctable causes. Revascularization was performed in approximately half of the patients, and most of them were discharged without specific antiarrhythmic treatment. Actuarial 3-year survival was only 71% (lower than the 73% observed in patients with ventricular fibrillation not thought to be of correctable cause in the same registry).[12] The decision to perform surgical or percutaneous revascularization in patients with life-threatening ventricular arrhythmias should be based on similar grounds to other clinical settings (e.g., presence of large areas of viable, ischemic myocardium). In most patients, further antiarrhythmic treatment will be necessary. Implantation of a transvenous ICD after patient recovery will be the preferred strategy in most cases.

Management of Patients with Less Common Substrates

For the vast majority of patients with life-threatening ventricular arrhythmias that have coronary artery disease or dilated cardiomyopathy, ICDs represent the therapy of first choice. Identification of less common substrates (with different natural history) may at times allow the selection of more individualized therapy (Figure 2).

Sustained ventricular tachycardia of right ventricular origin frequently occurs (as previously noted) in the absence readily discernible cardiac abnormalities. When significant right ventricular disease is obvious, the diagnosis of arrhythmogenic right ventricular dysplasia (ARVD) can be made. ARVD typically occurs in young patients (80% of patients are diagnosed before the age of 40). Males are predominantly affected. Although ARVD may be familial (an abnormal locus has been mapped to chromosome 14 q 13-24), most cases are sporadic. Ventricular arrhythmias may be catecholamine-dependent, and are exacerbated during exercise tolerance testing in 50% of patients. ARVD is an important cause of sudden death in young patients. However, it should be emphasized that the overall risk of sudden death is low (~ 2% per year).[36] Sotalol[37] and amiodarone seem to be effective in patients with ARVD, whereas catheter ablation has more of a palliative, complementary role. Recurrences at new foci may develop after apparent success. There is limited experience with ICDs in ARVD. Patients resuscitated from cardiac arrest or those poorly responsive (or intolerant of drugs) appear to be good candidates.

The congenital long QT syndrome (LQTS) results from a variety of genetic mutations in ionic channels that prolong ventricular repolarization. The three main features of congenital LQTS are prolongation of the QTc, syncope or cardiac arrest secondary to torsades de pointes ventricular tachycardia and QTc prolongation, syncope, or premature sudden death in family members. Syncope often occurs in association with physical or emotional arousal.[38] Beta-blockers are the mainstay of treatment in patients with LQTS. Permanent pacing is beneficial in patients who fail beta-blockade or develop excessive bradycardia. There is limited experience with left cervicothoracic sympathetic gangliectomy in drug-refractory patients. The ICD can be recommended as a fail-safe device in high-risk patients, including those with recurrent syncope despite beta-blockers, aborted cardiac death or a strong family history of sudden death. Although the short-term effects of gene-specific therapy (e.g., mexiletine in patients with sodium-channel defects, potassium plus spironolactone in patients with potassium-channel defects) on the QT interval are encouraging, there is no information on its long-term efficacy in preventing arrhythmias in patients with congenital LQTS.[39]

Coronary artery spasm with overt or silent myocardial ischemia may result in cardiac arrest due to ventricular fibrillation. Recognition of this uncommon cause of cardiac arrest is critical. Management of spasm-mediated ischemia (primarily with calcium channel blockers) appears to be the treatment of choice. Titration of calcium channel blocker dose to prevent ergonovine-induced spasm resulted in elimination of arrhythmia in one small series.[40]

Idiopathic ventricular fibrillation is a diagnosis of exclusion in patients without apparent structural heart disease.[41] In some of them, a genetically determined molecular substrate can be identified.[42] A subset of patients (including young men of Southeastern Asian origin with nocturnal cardiac arrest[43] and those with so-called Brugada's syndrome[44]) present labile right bundle branch block, J waves and ST segment elevation in precordial leads V1 to V3 in sinus rhythm. Although the natural history of all the variant forms of idiopathic ventricular fibrillation is not well-defined, the risk of recurrences is not negligible.[45] The EPS has limited value in risk-stratification. It appears prudent to recommend ICD implantation in all patients with idiopathic ventricular fibrillation.

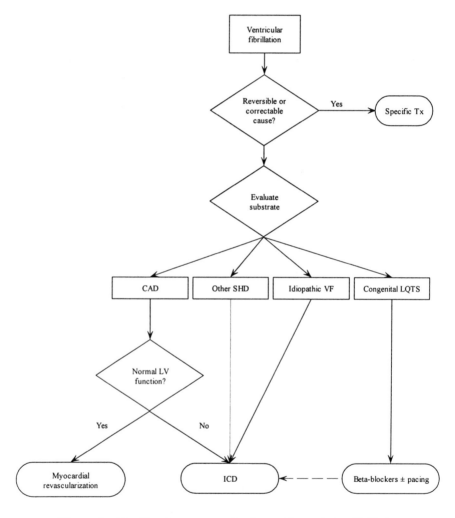

Figure 2. Algorithm for treatment of patients with ventricular fibrillation. CAD: coronary artery disease; SHD: structural heart disease.

RESOURCES FOR IMPLANTATION AND FOLLOW-UP OF THE ICD

Implantation

Current ICDs are <60 ml in size and are implanted transvenously with techniques similar to those used for standard pacemakers. In the US, the cost to the hospital of a modern ICD system ranges between $20,000 and $27,000. Meanwhile, the 1998 estimated Medicare reimbursement at our institution (a large urban teaching hospital) for ICD implantation was $39,320 when a cardiac catheterization or EPS had been performed during the same admission (DRG 104), and $30,250 when the ICD was implanted without cardiac catheterization or EPS (DRG 105). Because the cost of the hardware has remained stable in absolute terms, cost-containment strategies have focused on the design of more efficient clinical pathways for in-hospital management (Table 1).

	Day 1	Day 2	Day 3	Day 4	Day 5
Monitoring	ICU	ICU	Step-down unit	Step-down unit	Telemetry unit
Tests	Chemistries Serial CK Serial ECG Chest X ray	2-D echo	Cardiac cath (Stress test if CAD unlikely) ± EPS		Bedside ICD check (pacing & sensing thresholds) Chest X ray
Therapy	± CHF drugs ± AADs	Consider β-blockers		ICD implant	
Patient and family education	ICU routine	SCD mechanism and risk of recurrence Rx options	ICD function Driving restrictions ICD implant		Wound care ICD follow-up schedule

Table 1. Critical pathway for a patient with ventricular fibrillation or unstable ventricular tachycardia without reversible or correctable cause. AAD: antiarrhythmic drugs; CAD: coronary artery disease; CHF: congestive heart failure; ICU: intensive care unit; Rx: treatment; SCD: sudden cardiac death.

Initially, implantation of the ICD required a cardiothoracic surgeon, a cardiac electrophysiologist and an anesthesiologist. However, miniaturization of the generators and more efficacious lead electrode systems have greatly reduced the surgical skills needed for implantation. Thorough knowledge of the subtleties of defibrillation threshold testing and the value and limitations of different shocking pathways and waveforms remain essential. Therefore, the cardiac electrophysiologist has emerged as the most efficient provider for ICD implantation. The safety of ICD implantation by trained clinical electrophysiologists is well described .[46,47] Similar high rates of success and acceptable complication rates can be achieved whether the implant is performed in the electrophysiology laboratory or in the operating room.[48] In most institutions, cost considerations favor the use of the electrophysiology laboratory. The shortened procedural times and reduced tissue dissection have essentially eliminated the need for general endotracheal anesthesia. Implantation can be safely performed under local anesthesia supplemented with intravenous sedation administered by non-anesthesiologists.[49,50] Guidelines for the administration of intravenous sedation by non-anesthesia personnel during ICD implantation have been published,[51] and need to be interpreted in light of local institutional (along with state board) rules and regulations.

Competence should be determined by the proper training and sufficient ongoing experience of the implanting physician. Training guidelines for ICD implantation from the American College of Cardiology require 20 procedures as primary operator.[52] Maintenance of established competence is also critical. For pacemaker implantation, inexperience (e.g., <12 implants per year) is the main determinant of surgical complications,[53] and a similar association can be expected for ICDs. Interestingly, the most recent survey of pacing practices in the US showed that the majority of implanters would qualify as low volume.[54] Thus, the concentration of procedures in high-volume centers represents a rational strategy for the achievement of superior results. The availability of ancillary services at the implanting institution may impact on the surgical results. Specifically, anesthesiology and thoracic surgery expertise may be necessary to manage patients with obstructive airway disease, high defibrillation thresholds, or occasional catastrophic complications, and should be available on an urgent basis during every procedure.

Current ICDs can deliver not only high-energy defibrillation shocks, but also low-energy shocks and antitachycardia pacing for ventricular tachycardia and back-up ventricular pacing for bradyarrhythmias. The use of "shock-only" ICDs is not recommended because they are only marginally cheaper and most patients benefit from one or more of the refinements in detection and treatment afforded by the tiered-therapy devices. ICDs that incorporate an atrial pacing lead provide more physiological pacing and better discrimination between ventricular and supraventricular arrhythmias by augmenting the detection algorithms with information originating in the atrium. Their universal use cannot be recommended at the present time because they are significantly more expensive and implantation of the extra lead can increase morbidity. However, up to 40% of patients undergoing ICD implantation appear to benefit from their use. They should be strongly considered in patients with more than infrequent bradycardia, when the need for drugs with negative chronotropic effects is anticipated, and in those with atrial tachyarrhythmias that could trigger spurious shocks with conventional systems. Implantable devices capable of electrical therapy for both ventricular and atrial tachyarrhythmias are undergoing clinical evaluation. It is too early to predict their ultimate role in the therapeutic armamentarium.

Postoperative management has also evolved. Admission to an intensive care unit is not necessary after uncomplicated implants. Most patients can be discharged home in less than 24 hours. The role of predischarge testing of defibrillator function via arrhythmia induction using noninvasive stimulation[55] has been the subject of controversy. Potential advantages include confirmation of a safety margin for defibrillation and programming predictably successful antitachycardia pacing schemes for ventricular tachycardia.[56] On the other hand, these tests consume valuable hospital and staff resources, can delay hospital discharge and are inconvenient for the patient. When appropriate sensing and defibrillation are confirmed during implantation, the yield of routine predischarge arrhythmia induction testing is very low, and should be reserved for selected patients. Furthermore, most clinically relevant problems (e.g., early lead dislodgment) can be identified via chest radiography and bedside assessment of pacing thresholds, intracardiac electrograms and lead impedance.[57,58] Predischarge ICD testing is not indispensable for programming of antitachycardia pacing for ventricular tachycardia. Limited data suggest that success rate and incidence of tachycardia acceleration are similar for standardized protocols programmed empirically and for those programmed on the basis of predischarge testing.[59]

Follow-Up

Follow-up of ICD patients is best delivered in a focused "device clinic" staffed by cardiac electrophysiologists and dedicated nurses or technicians. The increasing versatility of these devices has made programming and troubleshooting complex and time-consuming. The untrained physician who is a "casual" follower of ICDs may rely excessively upon the expertise of manufacturer representatives to determine appropriate device function. This practice is questionable on both medical and ethical grounds.[60] Routine follow-up should include a careful history regarding cardioactive drugs, interim symptoms of tachyarrhythmias and ICD discharges, device interrogation (including real-time telemetry of battery status and retrieval of diagnostic data from the memory), and determination of pacing and sensing thresholds and measurement of lead impedances. Periodic routine radiological examination is probably not necessary. It demonstrates lead displacement or migration, but is less useful for the identification of lead fracture. The ability of current devices to automatically reform the capacitors after periods without charging has reduced the frequency of required clinic visits to 2 or 3 a year. Patients should be seen sooner when symptoms change or more than sporadic shocks occur.

Routine clinic evaluations should become more frequent once the battery status approaches the elective replacement indicator (ERI). The longevity of ICD generators depends on the model, the frequency of shocks (delivered or aborted), the proportion of time that the device paces, and the pacing output settings. It is anticipated that current generators should last more than 7 years in average. However, it should be noted that manufacturers' longevity prediction for previous models were generally too optimistic. Replacement of an ICD generator (including those older systems implanted in an abdominal pocket) can also be performed safely by cardiac electrophysiologists in the electrophysiology laboratory.[61]

Multiple defibrillator discharges in a relative short period of time (e.g., ≥ 3 discharges in ≤ 24 hours) constitute a serious situation which requires prompt attention.[62] Implanting institutions should provide 24-hour patient response systems with available personnel experienced in the management of defibrillator patients.[63] A discussion of the evaluation and management of the many causes of multiple defibrillator shocks is beyond the scope of this chapter. It is important to evaluate these patients in a setting in which electrocardiographic monitoring and advanced cardiac resuscitation are possible and to interrogate the device as soon as possible.

COST-EFFECTIVENESS OF THE ICD

Continuous technological advances and streamlining of practice patterns make ICD therapy a "mobile target". Therefore, published analyses of the cost-effectiveness of ICDs tend to become obsolete rapidly.[64]. There is no doubt that ICD therapy is expensive. So far, competition among ICD manufacturers has not resulted in the substantial decreases in price that would be expected in an economically efficient market. In comparison to the $23,000 cost of a standard ICD system, the retail cost of a one year supply of 400 mg of amiodarone daily is $2,200. The fact that ICD patients continue to accrue expenses during follow-up due to severe underlying cardiac disease with recurrent arrhythmic and nonarrhythmic morbidity[65] should also be taken into account in long term analyses..

The cost-effectiveness of the ICD has been estimated in mathematical models and from empiric data collected during the conduct of randomized studies. Both approaches have limitations. The conclusions of cost-effectiveness models differ greatly according to many assumptions introduced. Cost-effectiveness should be most favorable in patients at high-risk for sudden death but at low risk of dying from competing causes. In a detailed analysis, Owens et al. estimated that to become economically "attractive" (i.e., cost less than $50,000 per quality-adjusted life year gained), the ICD would have to reduce total mortality by at least 30% relative to amiodarone (a plausible benefit according to the results of randomized studies)[66]. For example, assuming a reduction in total mortality rate of 40%, the cost of one quality-adjusted life year afforded by treatment with the ICD was $37,300. Sensitivity analysis showed that reductions in perioperative death and implantation costs, and prolongation of battery longevity (already realized in current practice), would significantly improve the cost-effectiveness of the ICD (Figure 3).

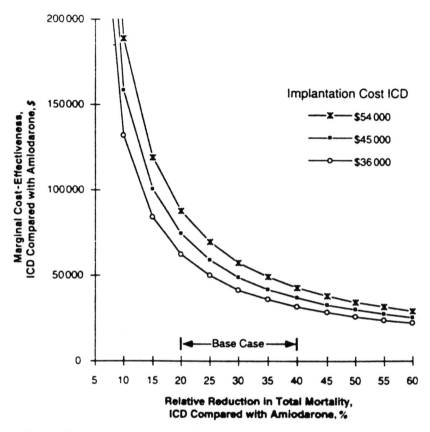

Figure 3.   Effect of cost of implantation of ICD on cost-effectiveness. The middle line
shows the base-cost estimate for ICD implantation; the top and bottom lines show how
cost-effectiveness varies if implantation costs are increased or decreased by 20%.
From Owens DK, et al,[66] with permission from the American College of Physicians.

Measurement of costs (or charges) has been an integral part of randomized studies
comparing the ICD and pharmacological therapy of ventricular tachyarrhythmias.
These analyses depend critically on the representativeness of the control maneuver
and the treatment effect observed in the study. Furthermore, changes in ICD
technology and practice patterns tend to make results less relevant by the time they
become available. An early, small study by Wever et al in survivors of cardiac arrest
with prior myocardial infarction compared early ICD implantation to the (then more
conventional) strategy of serial electropharmacological testing, followed by direct
arrhythmia surgery or ICD implantation in case of drug failure. The study was
terminated prematurely after the enrollment of 60 patients because of a nonsignificant
survival advantage in the ICD limb. After a follow-up of 24 months, 13% of patients
died in the early ICD group versus 35% in the conventional strategy group (p=0.07).

The costs per patient per day alive were $63 and $94 for the early ICD and electrophysiology-guided strategies, respectively. This amounted to a net cost-effectiveness of $11,315 life year saved by early ICD implantation. The early ICD group also underwent fewer invasive procedures and spent fewer days in the hospital.[67] Although in this small study early ICD implantation was dominant (i.e., more effective and cheaper), the results are difficult to extrapolate because the control group did not reflect current optimal management.

The Multicenter Automatic Defibrillator Implantation Trial (MADIT) examined the efficacy of a "prophylactic" ICD versus conventional therapy in 196 patients with prior myocardial infarction, left ventricular ejection fraction $\leq$ 0.35, spontaneous nonsustained ventricular tachycardia and inducible ventricular tachycardia not rendered suppressible with intravenous procainamide at electrophysiological study. A significant 54% reduction in death from all causes was observed in the patients randomized to ICD therapy compared to those treated conventionally (mostly with amiodarone).[68] Although the population studied in MADIT does not constitute the topic of this chapter (i.e., the patients did not have clinical episodes of ventricular fibrillation or sustained ventricular tachycardia), its cost-effectiveness study is the most exhaustive currently available. In MADIT, the cost per life year gained with defibrillator treatment was $27,000.[69] Sensitivity analyses highlighted the impact of technological advances and hardware prices in the cost-effectiveness of ICD therapy. Exclusive use of transvenous systems (which in MADIT were only used in half of the patients) would decrease the cost per life year gained to $22,800; a 25% drop in device cost would decrease the cost per life year gained to $13,100. The very favorable cost-effectiveness ratio in MADIT was partially driven by the impressive survival benefit conferred by the ICD. As discussed earlier, a survival benefit of around 30% is more plausible in unselected patients with life-threatening tachyarrhythmias. Final reports of the cost-effectiveness analyses in AVID, CASH and CIDS are eagerly awaited.

THE FUTURE

The development of safe and widely effective pharmacological or ablative therapies for ventricular arrhythmias does not appear likely in the foreseeable future. Therefore, the ICD will become the key clinical tool in the fight against sudden death. Results from ongoing and planned controlled trials may expand the role of ICD therapy in patients at high risk for life-threatening ventricular arrhythmias. In view of the potential allocation of scarce resources to diverse therapies and populations, society will have to decide the extent of ICD use. In the next few years, controversy will focus on the cost-effectiveness as well as the optimal providers and settings for this sophisticated therapeutic modality. Prospective data collected in randomized trials will help identify the optimal threshold above which implantation of an ICD becomes cost-effective when compared to other accepted therapies like treatment of mild hypertension, cardiac transplantation or hemodialysis.

The currently available results of ICD therapy have been reported from high-volume institutions and dedicated investigators. Diffusion of ICD therapy will result in the proliferation of lower-volume, less-focused providers, and there is no data on the outcomes of ICD therapy provided in those settings. ICD therapy will become the target of close scrutiny, and its continuing development will require the implementation of mechanisms for quality assurance. Components of a quality improvement strategy should include timely publication of evidence-based practice guidelines, credentialing of physicians and institutions based on objective criteria, training of sufficient number of subspecialists to cope with the growing demand for ICD-related services,[70] and tracking of outcomes by (or for) each implanting center. Ideally, those outcomes should be continuously compared with the nationwide experience to assure that minimum standards are maintained. Efforts from professional organizations to develop confidential national registries and risk-adjustment models for ICD therapy will eventually provide the tools for such assessment. Finally, the potential for overuse of ICDs is present, and future allegations of inappropriate use of ICD therapy (as has happened with pacemakers[71]) will not be unexpected. As a "big ticket" item, ICD implantation may become a target for preprocedural review (and even rationing) by HMOs and other medical insurers, thus creating further tension among consumers, providers and payers of medical care. Hopefully, streamlining of clinical practices, combined with reductions in device price, will result in improved cost-efficiency and will make ICD therapy more accessible to the populations likely to benefit from it.

References:

[1] Pinski SL, Chen PS. Implantable cardioverter-defibrillators. In: Topol EJ, ed. Textbook of Cardiovascular Medicine. Lippincott-Raven Publishers, Philadelphia, 1997, 1913-1931.

[2] Nichol G, Hallstrom AP, Kerber R, et al. American Heart Association report on the Second Public Access Defibrillation Conference, April 17-19, 1997. Circulation 1998;97:1309-1314.

[3] Swerdlow CD, Winkle RA, Mason JW. Determinants of survival in patients with ventricular tachyarrhythmias. N Engl J Med 1983;308:1436-1442.

[4] Steinbeck G, Andresen D, Bach P, et al. A comparison of electrophysiologically guided antiarrhythmic drug therapy with beta-blocker therapy in patients with symptomatic, sustained ventricular tachyarrhythmias. N Engl J Med 1992 ;327:987-992.

[5] The CASCADE Investigators. Cardiac Arrest in Seattle: Conventional versus Amiodarone Drug Evaluation (The CASCADE Study). Am J Cardiol 1991;67:578-584.

[6] Mason JW, for the ESVEM Investigators. A comparison of electrophysiologic testing with Holter monitoring to predict antiarrhythmic-drug efficacy for ventricular tachyarrhythmias. N Engl J Med 1993;329:445-451.

[7] Mason JW, for the ESVEM Investigators. A comparison of seven antiarrhythmic drugs in patients with ventricular tachyarrhythmias. N Engl J Med 1993;329:452-458.

[8] The Cardiac Arrhythmia Suppression Trial (CAST) Investigators. Preliminary report: effect of encainide and flecainide on mortality in a randomized trial of arrhythmia suppression after myocardial infarction. N Engl J Med 1989; 321: 406-412.

[9] The Antiarrhythmics versus Implantable Defibrillators (AVID) Investigators. A comparison of antiarrhythmic-drug therapy with implantable defibrillators in patients resuscitated from near-fatal ventricular arrhythmias. N Engl J Med 1997;337:1576-1583.

[10] Kuck KH. Presented at the 47th Annual Scientific Session of the American College of Cardiology, Atlanta, Georgia, March 30, 1998.

[11] Connolly S. Presented at the 47th Annual Scientific Session of the American College of Cardiology, Atlanta, Georgia, March 30, 1998.

[12] Anderson JL, Hallstrom AP, Epstein AE, et al. Design and results of the Antiarrhythmics Versus Implantable Defibrillators (AVID) Registry. (in press).

[13] Gregoratos G, Cheitlin MD, Conill A, et al. ACC/AHA guidelines for implantation of cardiac pacemakers and antiarrhythmia devices: a report of the American College of Cardiology/American Heart Association Task Force on Practice Guidelines (Committee on Pacemaker Implantation). J Am Coll Cardiol 1998;31:1175-1209.

[14] Link MS, Costeas XF, Griffith JL, et al. High incidence of appropriate implantable cardioverter-defibrillator therapy in patients with syncope of unknown etiology and inducible ventricular arrhythmias. J Am Coll Cardiol 1997;29:370-375.

[15] DEFIBRILAT Study Group. Actuarial risk of sudden death while awaiting cardiac transplantation in patients with atherosclerotic heart disease. Am J Cardiol 1991;68:545-546.

[16] Sweeney MO, Ruskin JN, Garan H, et al. Influence of the implantable cardioverter-defibrillator on sudden death and total mortality in patients evaluated for cardiac transplantation. Circulation 1995;92:3273-3281.

[17] Josephson ME. ICD implantation: cost conscious or patient conscious. J Cardiovasc Electrophysiol 1996;7:203-205.

[18] Poole JE, Mathisen TL, Kudenchuk PJ, et al. Long-term outcome in patients who survive out of hospital ventricular fibrillation and undergo electrophysiologic studies: evaluation by electrophysiologic subgroups. J Am Coll Cardiol 1990;16:657-665.

[19] Zipes DP, DiMarco JP, Gillette PC, et a.l. ACC/AHA Task Force Report. Guidelines for clinical intracardiac electrophysiological and cathter ablation procedures. A report of the American College of Cardiology/American Heart Association task force on practice guidelines. J Am Coll Cardiol 1995;26:555-573.

[20] Wellens HJJ, Brugada P. Diagnosis of ventricular tachycardia from the 12 lead electrocardiogram. Cardiol Clin 1987;5:511-526.

[21] Pinski SL, Maloney JD. Adenosine: a new drug for termination of ventricular tachycardia. Clev Clin J Med 1990;57:383-388.

[22] Pinski SL, Maloney JD. Indications for electrophysiologic study in patients with ventricular arrhythmias. Clev Clin J Med 1992;59:175-185.

[23] Varma N, Josephson ME. Therapy of "idiopathic" ventricular tachycardia. J Cardiovasc Electrophysiol 1997;8:104-116.

[24] Sarter BH, Finkle JK, Gerszten RE, Buxton AE. What is the risk of sudden cardiac death in patients presenting with hemodynamically stable sustained ventricular tachycardia after myocardial infarction? J Am Coll Cardiol 1996; 28:122-129.

[25] Caruso AC, Marcus FI, Hahn EA, et al. Predictors of arrhythmic death and cardiac arrest in the ESVEM trial. Circulation 1997;96:1888-1892.

[26] Rothman SA, Hsia HH, Cossu SF, et al. Radiofrequency catheter ablation of postinfarction ventricular tachycardia: long-term success and the significance of inducible nonclinical arrhythmias. Circulation 1997;96:3499-3508.

[27] Böcker D, Block M, Isbruch F, et al. Benefits of treatment with implantable cardioverter-defibrillators in patients with stable ventricular tachycardia. Br Heart J 1995;73:158-163.

[28] Strickberger SA, Man KC, Daoud EG, et al. A prospective evaluation of catheter ablation of ventricular tachycardia as adjuvant therapy in patients with coronary artery disease and an implantable cardioverter-defibrillator. Circulation 1997;96:1525-1531.

[29] Tchou P, Mehdirad AA. Bundle branch reentry ventricular tachycardia. Pacing Clin Electrophysiol 1995;18:1427-1437.

[30] Helguera ME, Trohman RG, Pinski SL, et al. Radiofrequency ablation of the left bundle branch or its fascicles for treatment of interfascicular reentrant ventricular tachycardias. *Pacing Clin Electrophysiol* 1998; 21:843.

[31] Wang Y, Scheinman MM, Chien WW, et al. Patients with supraventricular tachycardia presenting with aborted sudden death: incidence, mechanism and long-term follow-up. J Am Coll Cardiol 199;18:1711-1719.

[32] Kelly P, Ruskin JN, Vlahakes GJ, et al. Surgical coronary revascularization in survivors of prehospital cardiac arrest: its effect on inducible ventricular arrhythmias and long-term survival. J Am Coll Cardiol 1990;15:267-273.

[33] Pinski SL, Mick MJ, Arnold AZ, et al. Retrospective analysis of patients undergoing one- or two-stage strategies for myocardial revascularization and implantable cardioverter-defibrillator implantation. Pacing Clin Electrophysiol 1991;14:1138-1147.

[34] Natale A, Sra J, Axtell K, et al. Ventricular fibrillation and polymorphic ventricular tachycardia with critical coronary artery stenosis: does bypass surgery suffice? J Cardiovasc Electrophysiol 1994;5:988-994.

[35] Daoud EG, Niebauer M, Kou WH, et al. Incidence of implantable defibrillator discharges after coronary revascularization in survivors of ischemic sudden cardiac death. Am Heart J 1995;130:277-280 .

[36] Marcus FI, Fontaine G. Arrhythmogenic right ventricular dysplasia/ cardiomyopathy: a review. Pacing Clin Electrophysiol 1995;18:1298-1314.

[37] Wichter T, Borggrefe M, Haverkamp W, et al. Efficacy of antiarrhythmic drugs in patients with arrhythmogenic right ventricular disease. Results in patients with inducible and noninducible ventricular tachycardia. Circulation 1992;86:29-37.

[38] Roden DM, Lazzara R, Rosen M, et al. Multiple mechanisms in the long-QT syndrome. Current knowledge, gaps, and future directions. Circulation 1996;94:1996-2012.

[39] Moss AJ. Management of patients with the hereditary long QT syndrome. J Cardiovasc Electrophysiol 1998;9:668-674.

[40] Myerburg RJ, Kessler KM, Mullon SM, et al. Life threatening ventricular arrhythmias in patients with silent myocardial ischemia due to coronary artery spasm. N Engl J Med 1992;326:1451-55.

[41] Joint Steering Committees of the Unexplained Cardiac Arrest Registry of Europe and of the Idiopathic Ventricular Fibrillation Registry of the United States. Survivors of out-of-hospital cardiac arrest with apparently normal heart. Need for definition and standardized clinical evaluation. Circulation 1997;95:265-272.

[42] Chen Q, Kirsch GE, Zhang D, et al. Genetic basis and molecular mechanism for idiopathic ventricular fibrillation. *Nature* 1998;392:293-296.

[43] Nademanee K, Veerakul G, Nimmannit S, et al. Arrhythmogenic marker for the sudden unexplained death syndrome in Thai men. Circulation 1997;96:2595-2600.

[44] Brugada J, Brugada R, Brugada P. Right bundle-branch block and ST-segment elevation in leads V1 through V3: a marker for sudden death in patients without demonstrable structural heart disease. Circulation 1998;97:457-460.

[45] Meissner MD, Lehmann MH, Steinman RT, et al: Ventricular fibrillation in patients without significant structural heart disease: a multicenter experience with implantable cardioverter – defibrillator therapy. J Am Coll Cardiol 1993;21:1406-

[46] Strickberger SA, Hummel JD, Daoud E, et al. Implantation by electrophysiologists of 100 consecutive cardioverter defibrillators with nonthoracotomy lead systems. Circulation 1994;90:868-872.

[47] Kleman JM, Castle LW, Kidwell GA, et al. Nonthoracotomy versus thoracotomy implantable defibrillators: intention-to-treat comparison of clinical outcomes. Circulation 1994; 90:2833-2842.

[48] Strickberger SA, Niebauer M, Man KC, et al. Comparison of implantation of nonthoracotomy defibrillators in the operating room versus the electrophysiology laboratory. Am J Cardiol 1995;75:255-257.

[49] Pinski SL, Sgarbossa EB, Trohman RG, et al. Safe ICD implantation without anesthesiologist support. Circulation 1997;96:4434.

[50] Pacifico A, Cedillo-Salazar FR, Nasir N Jr, et al. Conscious sedation with combined hypnotic agents for implantation of implantable cardioverter-defibrillators. J Am Coll Cardiol 1997;30:769-773

[51] Bubien RS, Fisher JD, Gentzel JA, et al. NASPE expert consensus document: use of IV (conscious) sedation/analgesia by nonanesthesia personnel in patients undergoing arrhythmia specific diagnostic, therapeutic and surgical procedures. Pacing Clin Electrophysiol 1998;21:375-385.

[52] Josephson ME, Maloney JD, Barold SS, et al. Task Force 6: training in specialized electrophysiology, cardiac pacing, and arrhythmia management. J Am Coll Cardiol 1995; 25:23-26.

[53] Parsonnet V, Bernstein AD, Lindsay BD. Pacemaker-implantation complication rates: an analysis of some contributing factors. J Am Coll Cardiol 1989;13:917-921.

[54] Bernstein AD, Parsonnet V. Survey of cardiac pacing and defibrillation in the United States in 1993. Am J Cardiol 1996;78:187-196.

[55] Pinski SL, Shewchik J, Tobin M, Castle LW. Safety and diagnostic yield of noninvasive ventricular stimulation performed via tiered-therapy implantable defibrillators. Pacing Clin Electrophysiol 1994;17:2263-2273.

[56] Pinski SL, Simmons TW, Maloney JD: Troubleshooting antitachycardia pacing in patients with defibrillators. In: Estes NAM, Wang P, Manolis A, Eds. Implantable Cardioverter-Defibrillators: A Comprehensive Textbook. New York: Marcel Dekker, 1994:445-477.

[57] Higgings SL, Rich DH, Haygood JR, et al. ICD restudy: results and potential benefit from routine predischarge and 2-month evaluation. Pacing Clin Electrophysiol 1998;21:410-417.

[58] Weiss DN, Zilo P, Luceri RM, et al. Predischarge arrhythmia induction testing of implantable defibrillators may be unnecessary in selected cases. Am J Cardiol 1997;80:1562-1565.

[59] Schaumann A, von zur Mühlen F, Herse B, et al. Empirical versus antitachycardia pacing in implantable cardioverter-defibrillators: a prospective study including 200 patients. Circulation 1998;97:66-74.

[60] Schoenfeld MH. Quality assurance in cardiac electrophysiology and pacing: a brief synopsis. Pacing Clin Electrophysiol 1994;17:267-269.

[61] Pinski SL, Kleman JM, Morant VA, et al. Defibrillator generator replacement performed by cardiologists. Pacing Clin Electrophysiol 1994; 17:800.

[62] Pinski SL, Trohman RG. Implantable cardioverter-defibrillators: implications for the non-electrophysiologist. Ann Intern Med 1995;122:770-777.

[63] Lehman MH, Saksena S. Implantable cardioverter-defibrillators in cardiovascular practice: report of the policy conference of the North American Society of Pacing and Electrophysiology. Pacing Clin Electrophysiol 1991;14:969-978.

[64] Kupersmith J, Hogan A, Guerrero P, et al. Evaluating and improving the cost-effectiveness of the implantable cardioverter-defibrillator. Am Heart J 1995;130:507-515.

[65] Fahy GJ, Sgarbossa EB, Tchou PJ, Pinski SL. Hospital readmission in patients treated with tiered-therapy implantable defibrillators. Circulation 1996;94:1350-1356.

[66] Owens DK, Sanders GD, Harris RA, et al. Cost-effectiveness of implantable cardioverter-defibrillators relative to amiodarone for prevention of sudden cardiac death. Ann Intern Med 1997;126:1-12.

[67] Wever EF, Hauer RN, Schrijvers G, et al. Cost-effectiveness of implantable defibrillator as first-choice therapy versus electrophysiologically guided tiered strategy in postinfarct sudden death survivors: a randomized study. Circulation 1996;93:489-496.

[68] Moss AJ, Hall WJ, Cannom DS, et al. Improved survival with an implanted defibrillator in patients with coronary disease at high risk for ventricular arrhythmia. N Engl J Med 1996;335:1933-40.

[69] Mushlin AI, Hall WJ, Zwanziger J, et al. The cost-effectiveness of automatic implantable cardiac defibrillators: results from MADIT. Circulation 1998;97:2129-2135.

[70] Saksena S. Manpower needs in pacing and electrophysiology: taking a closer look. Pacing Clin Electrophysiol 1996;19:858-860.

[71] Greenspan AM, Kay HR, Berger BC, et al. Incidence of unwarranted implantation of permanent cardiac pacemakers in a large medical population. N Engl J Med 1988;318:158-163.

INDEX